RWD '02

(3) WS 465
02507   P6T

D1628552

The Supportive Care
of the Child with Cancer

The Supportive Care of the Child with Cancer

Edited by

Anthony Oakhill MB, ChB, DCH, MRCP
Consultant Paediatric Oncologist,
Bristol Royal Hospital for Sick Children

WRIGHT
London Boston Durban Singapore Sydney Toronto Wellington

John Wright
is an imprint of Butterworth Scientific

First published 1988

© **Butterworth & Co. (Publishers) Ltd,** 1988

British Library Cataloguing in Publication Data
The Supportive care of the child with
  cancer.
  1. Tumors in children——Treatment
  I. Oakhill, Anthony
  618.92′99406   RC281.C4

ISBN 0 7236 0745 1

Photoset by BC Typesetting, 39 Marsh Green Road, Exeter EX2 8PN
Printed and bound in England by Page Bros. Ltd, Norwich, Norfolk

Preface

The successful management of the child with cancer requires great co-operation and understanding within and between professional groups. Specialist centres will usually arrive at the diagnosis and decide an appropriate treatment regimen. The supportive care that is necessary for the child and her family, however, will be divided between many different people, from a wide range of backgrounds— for example, nurses, social workers, pharmacists, physicians, nutritionists, psychologists.

It is the intention of this book to provide a basic understanding of supportive care and, where appropriate, to give practical advice.

Bristol, 1988   A.O.

Acknowledgement

Mrs Anne Galton for her patient construction of the manuscript.

Contributors

Dr L. Owen Caul PhD
Bristol Virus Laboratory,
Myrtle Road,
Kingsdown,
Bristol BS2 8EL
Jointly

Dr N. A. G. Coad MB ChB MRCP
Senior Registrar (Renal),
The Children's Hospital,
Ladywood Middleway,
Ladywood,
Birmingham B16 8ET
Jointly

Dr Janice A. Culling MB BS MRCPsych
Consultant Child Psychiatrist,
Southmead Hospital,
Southmead Road,
Bristol BS10 5NB

Dr P. J. Darbyshire MB ChB MRCP MRCPath
Consultant Paediatric Haematologist,
Department of Haematology,
The Children's Hospital,
Ladywood Middleway,
Ladywood,
Birmingham B16 8ET

Mr Donal A. Donnelly-Wood
Malcolm Sargent Social Worker,
Royal Liverpool Children's Hospital,
Eaton Road,
Alder Hey,
Liverpool L12 2AP

Miss Jan Drakeford
Dietitian,
Bristol Royal Hospital for Sick Children,
St Michael's Hill,
Bristol BS2 8BJ

Mr E. M. St Gerard Kiely MB BCh BAO NUI FRCS FRCSI
The Hospital for Sick Children,
Great Ormond Street,
London WC1N 3JH

Mr James W. Kuykendall
Child Life and Adolescent Specialist,
Charing Cross Hospital,
Fulham Palace Road,
London W6 8RF

Dr Jillian R. Mann MB BS FRCP MRCS LRCP DCH
Consultant Paediatric Oncologist,
The Children's Hospital,
Ladywood Middleway,
Ladywood,
Birmingham B16 8ET
Jointly

Dr Anthony Oakhill MB ChB DCH MRCP
Consultant Paediatric Oncologist,
Bristol Royal Hospital for Sick Children,
St Michael's Hill,
Bristol BS2 8BJ

Dr A. P. C. H. Roome MB ChB FRCPath
Consultant Virologist,
Public Health Laboratory,
Myrtle Road,
Kingsdown,
Bristol BS2 8EL
Jointly

Ms S. Siddall
Pharmacist,
Alderhey Children's Hospital,
Eaton Road,
West Derby,
Liverpool L12 2AP

Dr Elaine M. Simpson MB ChB MRCP DCH MRCPath
Consultant Haematologist,
Department of Haematology,
The Royal Hospital for Sick Children,
Yorkhill,
Glasgow G3 8SJ

Dr Paul Ward MB ChB DCH MRCP
Paediatrician,
Addenbrooke's Hospital,
Cambridge CB2 2QQ

Dr David Warnock PhD MRCPath
Top Grade Mycologist,
Bristol Royal Infirmary,
Bristol BS2 8HW

CONTENTS

1 **Bacterial Infection**
  P. J. Darbyshire   1

2 **Viral Infection**
  L. Owen Caul and A. Roome   26

3 **Fungal Infection**
  D. Warnock   43

4 **Haematological Support**
  Elaine M. Simpson   60

5 **Metabolic Problems in Children with Leukaemia
  and Lymphoma**
  N. A. G. Coad and Jillian R. Mann   76

6 **Acute Medical Problems**
  A. Oakhill   90

7 **Chemotherapy: Problems and Precautions**
  S. Siddall   98

8 **Antiemesis**
  P. Ward   121

9 **Nutrition**
  Jan Drakeford   142

10 **Central Venous Catheters**
  E. Kiely   163

11 **Play Therapy**
   J. W. Kuykendall   172

12 **Oncology Social Work**
   D. Donnelly-Wood   180

13 **The Psychological Problems of Families of Children
   with Cancer**
   Janice A. Culling   204

14 **Terminal Care**
   P. Ward and A. Oakhill   238

15 **Late Effects of Treatment**
   A. Oakhill   260

Index   271

1. Bacterial Infection

P. J. Darbyshire

INTRODUCTION

Bacterial infection remains one of the major obstacles to the successful treatment of children with malignant disease. The most common
risk factor for the development of severe bacterial infection is the
degree and duration[1] of neutropaenia. It is the diagnosis and treatment of this complication which will occupy a substantial part of this
chapter. Neutropaenia is, however, but one aspect of the immunodeficiency caused by malignant disease and its treatment. For successful therapy, many other factors may have to be taken into account.

The role of the mucosal barriers in acting as a primary barrier
against pathogens has long been understood.[2] The skin, mucous
membranes and gastrointestinal tract may be breached directly by
tumour invasion; much more commonly, however, it is therapy-
related. The use of cytotoxic agents, such as cytosine arabinoside and
the anthracyclines, produce dose-related mucosal damage[3] and this
damage leads to more ready access to the circulation by the gut
microbial flora. The mucous membranes, particularly of the mouth,
are susceptible to damage in a similar way leading to overgrowth by
organisms, often commensals, again with easy access to the circulation through the eroded mucosa. The skin is readily breached by
the insertion of cannulae and indwelling lines. Whilst scrupulous
aseptic technique will limit the colonization of indwelling catheters,
such infections have emerged as a major drawback to their routine
use. A more detailed account of this problem will be given later.

The role of neutropaenia is central in considering bacterial
infection, but other elements of the immune system are also likely to
be severely compromized. The ability of the other elements to
respond normally will be impaired most severely in a child after bone
marrow transplantation (BMT). Whilst immunoglobulin production
may soon resume, the immune memory may be damaged for several

years[4] and this effect is made worse by graft versus host disease. After BMT, cell numbers return quickly but it is emerging that immune function takes much longer to normalize[5] and 'functional immuno-suppression' will continue for several years.

Splenectomy is now rarely performed in childhood, as staging for Hodgkin's disease is becoming less popular.[6] However, it is still performed in hereditary spherocytosis, thallasaemia major, haemo-lytic anaemia and a few other rare childhood conditions. It causes a specific immunodeficiency, the child being unable to respond adequately to infection with encapsulated organisms, such as *Streptococcus pneumoniae* and *Haemophilus influenzae*. The risk of overwhelming infection is greater, the younger the child.[7,8]

One common factor linking many of these elements is that of nutrition. Quite rightly, great emphasis is placed in modern paediatrics on achieving adequate nutritional intake often under difficult circumstances, either by enteral or parenteral hyper-alimentation. The immune system is but one area which suffers in the face of malnutrition. Depression of neutrophil function, impaired phagocytosis, depressed lymphocyte function are all reported[9,10] In addition, malnutrition will worsen other aspects of the child's response to treatment, particularly the ability of the bone marrow and GI tract mucosa to recover from cytotoxic drug damage.

The treatment of bacterial infection in a child with cancer is there-fore not solely a question of administering the appropriate antibiotic cocktail in the face of fever and neutropaenia. Indeed, a great deal may be done to minimize the risks of acquisition of infection, by assessment of an individual child's particular risk factors and inter-vention to reduce them.

PREVENTION OF INFECTION

The risks of increasing depth and duration of neutropaenia have already been mentioned as the major risk factor in the development of septicaemia. Whilst the neutropaenia may be predictable, using present antimitotic drug combinations, it is not possible to eliminate this factor. Hence, much effort has been expended attempting to reduce the bacterial and fungal colonization of the patient, based upon the fact that 80 per cent of bacterial infections in the neutro-paenic patient are caused by endogenous flora, usually from the gastrointestinal tract.[11] The methods used have varied from simple handwashing to the provision of totally protected environments, many regimens containing drug combinations aimed at reducing the bowel colonization. Some of these techniques do not easily transfer from adult to paediatric practice, the acceptability of prolonged isolation and the palatability of the antibiotics being two particular drawbacks.

Protected environments and gut decontamination

When used in their most complete form, these aim to reduce the patient's endogenous bacterial and fungal flora at all sites (but particularly in the GIT) and also to prevent the acquisition of new infectious agents. The measures to be taken include the provision of sterile food, an oral, usually non-absorbable antibiotic combination, filtered air, ideally by a laminar air flow system and almost inevitably physical isolation. Most units limit the visitors to one or two close relatives.[12] There is no doubt that regimens such as these, when rigidly adhered to, reduce the number of septicaemic episodes[13] despite slight differences in practice. However, septicaemia does still occur and is often with unusual and resistant organisms.[14,15] Precisely which components of this type of regimen confer most benefit is difficult to ascertain due to wide variation in trial methodology.

The use of laminar air flow systems which incorporate some form of particulate filtration will remove over 99 per cent of bacteria and fungi.[16] There is no doubt that it has one great value, the elimination of *Aspergillus*[17] which remains a very difficult organism to treat once infection is established. Its effect alone upon septicaemia is uncertain, some groups claiming great benefit,[14,18] others much less,[19] probably reflecting differences in technique in other areas. Many studies have shown the value of the combination of a protected environment with gut decontamination.[20,21]

The logic behind eliminating potentially pathogenic organisms from the GI tract is incontrovertible, given that the majority of endogenous septicaemias originate from this site.[11] Not surprisingly, the total elimination of such potential pathogens is not always achieved, or may be achieved only to be replaced by a more resistant pathogen. The most widely used oral combination was of gentamicin, vancomycin and nystatin.[22] In general, the use of this combination alone produced little effect, although some studies did show benefit,[23] particularly when combined with the use of a protected environment.[18] This initial regimen also illustrated all the potential difficulties: overgrowth with gentamicin resistant organisms.[24] High cost, a high level of microbiological monitoring and, most significantly, its unpalatability. There have been many attempts to evolve combinations free of some of these problems, FRACON (framycetin, colistin and nystatin), NEOCON (neomycin, colistin and nystatin) and a gentamicin/nystatin combination being three prominent regimens. The consensus view appears to be that such combinations may confer significant benefit in reducing bacterial infection, particularly when used in conjunction with a protected environment. However, if not properly monitored, the emergence of resistant strains can create a far worse problem than that which they were introduced to solve.

The problems of expense, in terms of capital outlay and antibiotics are common to both the adult and paediatric age groups when the combination of a protected environment and oral non-absorbable antibiotics is being instituted. In addition, it requires constant vigilance by staff and microbiology departments to ensure the systems adopted work to the full. The child, however, may tolerate the isolation very poorly and many simply cannot be persuaded to take the antibiotic cocktails orally. One element the literature does agree on is that, unless the regimens are rigidly adhered to, any potential benefit will be lost. There is only a small part for these regimens in the treatment of children, notably in bone marrow transplantation and aplastic anaemia where longer periods of neutropaenia are anticipated. The careful preparation of the child beforehand may go some way to minimize the problems of prolonged isolation, and the provision of constructive play and teaching may relieve the boredom whilst in isolation.

There is little evidence that simple protective isolation confers any advantage[25] when used alone. It produces the social isolation without any benefit. The most important single measure which has been shown to be of benefit (in all areas of infection control) is simple handwashing.[26] If this is not adhered to, the most completely protected environment will fail.

Recently, the concept of selective GI tract decontamination has emerged.[27] This approach aims to kill selectively potentially pathogenic organisms whilst leaving the anaerobic bacteria untouched, allowing their role in preventing colonization by resistant organisms to continue. The drug combination most often used has been trimethoprim-sulphamethoxazole (TMP-SMZ). Other drugs which confer some degree of colonization resistance (i.e. leave the anaerobic gut flora intact) include erythromycin and nalidixic acid. TMP-SMZ has been widely adopted in adult practice in an attempt to reduce septicaemic episodes.[28–32] *Table* 1.1 summarizes 5 large studies which examined the use of this combination. As can be seen, all 5 found some advantage in the combination but other groups have not been able to demonstrate this.[33,34] Overall, the majority of studies and trials do show some significant benefit. The EORTC study, for instance, showed that the infection rate in the TMP-SMZ arm was 26 per cent compared to 44 per cent in the placebo arm.[35] The doubts about this combination have centred, not only on its effectiveness, but also on the potential side-effects. TMP-SMZ does have some antifolate effect and the fear was that this would delay marrow

Table 1.1. Effectiveness of TMP–SMZ prophylaxis

Reference	No.	Effectiveness
Hughes et al.[28]	160	More effective than placebo
Preisler et al.[29]	40	Effective
Watson et al.[30]	88	More effective than oral non-absorbable antibiotics
Pizzo et al.[31]	150	More effective than placebo
Wade et al.[32]	62	More effective than oral non-absorbable antibiotics

reconstitution in a neutropaenic patient. Whilst *in vitro* effects can be demonstrated,[36] when examined *in vivo* at a standard dose, no effect could be seen on the speed of reconstitution.[37] However, at high dose (40mg TMP/200mg SMZ kg^{-1} day^{-1}) a delay was seen. Hence, it seems unlikely that this effect is an important consideration in the majority of patients. Work examining other drugs such as erythromycin also suggests that they may be of benefit.[31] However, the number of trials reported with agents other than TMP-SMZ is small.

The use of selective gut decontamination certainly is much more attractive than the oral non-absorbable alternative. It is inexpensive, palatable and requires less microbiological support. The fact that the use of TMP-SMZ has become so widespread (largely before evidence of its efficacy was available) speaks volumes for its acceptability. However, it must be remembered that the resistance patterns may change and its present position may soon need to be superceded by other agents.

There are several other agents available, some of which have been in widespread use for many years, e.g. prophylactic penicillin in splenectomized patients. The use of prophylactic penicillin usually in conjunction with pneumococcal vaccination has been in use for 15 years. Recently, there have been several fatal pneumococcal septicaemias post BMT,[38] particularly in patients with significant graft versus host disease. This group is certainly immunosuppressed, but may have functional hyposplenism in addition, hence prophylactic penicillin would be logical. This approach has not yet been tested in a clinical trial.

Newer agents which are becoming available include anti-*Pseudomonas* vaccines and antisera to lipopolysaccharide core antigens of gram negative organisms. The latter has been shown to be of benefit in treating gram negative infections, but not yet in prophylaxis.[39,40] The use of immunoglobulin preparations has long been a routine part of therapy in patients with hypogammaglobulinaemia, in preventing and treating bacterial infections.[41] Recently, a variety of more specific intravenous preparations has emerged which is at present being evaluated. It may be possible, in the future, to give combinations of specific immunoglobulins which will protect against the majority of potentially infectious agents. Such developments are awaited with interest.

In general, children with cancer have short-lived periods of neutropaenia, in contrast to adults who may have granulocytopaenia lasting several months. It is doubtful if, in the majority of children, most of the measures above are justified. However, there is a small group of children undergoing BMT or with aplastic anaemia in which some of the experience outlined above, gained mainly in adult practice, could be usefully applied.

THE PROBLEM OF FEBRILE NEUTROPAENIA

The management of patients with febrile neutropaenia is now well-established in all centres treating children with malignant disease. The prompt investigation of a febrile episode, the taking of appropriate cultures and the starting of an empiric antibiotic combination are all now taken for granted. It is worth noting that this practice has only emerged in the last 15–20 years. Early trials of antibiotic therapy had poor success[42] as they waited for culture results—more than half of the patients dying in some series. The realization that the neutropaenic patient could not await results was, at the time, a spur to a variety of empiric antibiotic regimens being introduced.

The criteria used in the definition of neutropaenia vary from centre to centre, some centres taking $1000 \times 10^6/1$ neutrophils as a criteria, others $500 \times 10^6/1$. There is not surprisingly an increasing risk of bacteraemia the lower the neutrophil numbers, until by $20 \times 10^6/1$, bacteraemia within a few days can be expected in the majority.[1] The duration of neutropaenia and the rate of fall of the neutrophil count are both further factors. It is worth emphasizing that a child with malignant disease can develop significant bacterial infection even with adequate neutrophil numbers. The use of protocols setting out treatment plans should not overshadow the clinical examination. If the child is febrile and ill, empiric antibiotic therapy may well be justified, whatever the neutrophil count.

The perfect antimicrobial drug or combination for broad spectrum empiric cover of febrile neutropaenia does not yet exist, nor is it likely to in the immediate future. Ideally, the drug or combination should be non-toxic: it must cover all the potential pathogens seen or likely to be regularly seen at a particular hospital: it should, if used in combination, be synergystic and, lastly, it should be cheap! Hardly a group of characteristics that are easily fulfilled. It is obvious that local

Table 1.2. Organism isolated between 1981–3, Bristol Children's Hospital, Paediatric Oncology Unit

Organism	No.	
Staph. aureus	3	
Strep. pneumoniae	2	
Strep. faecalis	1	55% Gram-positive organisms
Strep. sanguis	1	
B. Haemophilus Streptococcus	1	
Staph. epidermidis	3	
E. coli	5	
Pseudomonas aeruginosa	1	45% Gram-negative
Enterobacter cloacae	1	
Lactobacillus jensenii	1	

organisms and their resistance patterns must be of paramount importance when electing to use a particular set of drugs, hence what is ideal for one institute may not cover all the needs of another. There is no substitute for this careful local evaluation. *Table* 1.2 shows the organisms isolated over a 2-year period at Bristol HSC between 1981–3.[43,44] It can be seen that gram positive organisms, particularly *Staphylococcus aureus* and *Staphylococcus epidermidis*, accounted for 55 per cent. Historically, this figure is usually smaller, *Escherichia coli, Klebsiella, Pseudomonas aeruginosa* and *S. aureus* accounting for 85 per cent of organisms seen. However, if one examines the organisms seen after BMT, then a different picture will emerge.[45] The decline in recent years of pseudomonal sepsis has been noted in several centres[46] and can be seen in our Bristol figures (*Table* 1.2) as can the increase in gram positive infection. This has been, in part, attributed to the more widespread use of indwelling i.v. lines.[47]

THE CHOICE OF ANTIBIOTICS FOR EMPIRIC THERAPY

The EORTC trials are a good forum in which to trace the evolution of empiric antibiotic combinations. Whilst these large multicentre studies have undoubted advantages in terms of the number of patients accrued, the disadvantage may be the different resistance patterns seen between hospitals and countries.

The first trial compared three drug combinations of gentamicin and carbenicillin, gentamicin and cephalothin, and carbenicillin and cephalothin. It found the first combination the best in terms of cure (69 per cent) but also the least nephrotoxic.[48] Results using a very similar combination involving all 3 of the above agents[49] give very similar results in single centre studies. The major drawbacks of these initial combinations were the nephrotoxicity with gentamicin and cephalothin (15 per cent) and the solute load associated with carbenicillin use.

Two major groups of drugs have emerged and are now in routine use. They are the semisynthetic penicillins, e.g. azlocillin or ticarcillin which have a much broader antimicrobial range and the third generation cephalosporins, ceftazidime and moxolactam being two recent examples. The third EORTC trial[50] compared an aminoglycoside with the addition of either ticarcillin, azlocillin or cefotaxime. Cefotaxime has little anti-pseudomonal activity and came out least well in a provisional analysis of this trial.

The third generation cephalosporin, ceftazidime, has been the source of much interest. It does possess a very broad antimicrobial range, having extremely good activity against pseudomonas, but also activity against many other organisms. It possesses relatively poor activity against *S. aureus* and this was confirmed in an initial assessment of this drug used as a single agent in Bristol.[43] This experience has been confirmed by others;[51,52] some groups have found this agent satisfactory when used alone.[53,54] Certainly ceftazidime is the nearest we have yet come to providing adequate broad spectrum cover by a single agent.

There is now a wide range of studies using particularly cefotaxime, moxolactam, ceftazidime, piperacillin and azlocillin, usually in combination with an established aminoglycoside. Of these studies, the ones using a double beta-lactam combination[55] are amongst the most interesting. On initial assessment, the combination of moxolactam and piperacillin proved more effective than moxolactam plus amikacin in proven infections. The same combination has been tested by another group who have found less ototoxicity when the aminoglycoside was omitted.[56]

In summary, the best choice of antibiotics would appear to be a combination of an aminoglycoside with an extended range penicillin or third generation cephalosporin. These can be expected to produce response figures in patients with documented infection of 70–80 per cent.[57] This compares very favourably with the best of the older three drug combinations.[58] The combination of two beta-lactams is, at present, being investigated and may have some advantage in lowering toxicity. It seems that local factors such as the resistance pattern of 'in house' organisms and cost may, in the future, play more of a role, given the overall excellence of many of these combinations. It should be remembered that, whilst these combinations are excellent today, the need for constant review will remain; the organisms seen may soon develop resistance.

MANAGEMENT

Many of the most difficult questions in infection management are no longer so much concerned with which drugs to employ, but are of how long to use them for, and what to do if they are failing.

The situation in the 25–30 per cent of patients (often less in paediatric series) with proven bacterial infection is relatively straightforward. The patient will usually be changed to the most specific and safe agent. There is some evidence that, if a single antibiotic is continued for longer than 7 days, then a new septicaemia is possible, whereas this does not happen if 2 active agents are used.[59] Conversely, the incidence of fungal overgrowth is likely to be increased by such a policy. Most units give 10–14 days of antibiotics for proven sepsis. There is no evidence, even in *S. aureus* infection, that a longer course is of any benefit.[60]

The more major management problem is of fever without documented infection and persisting granulocytopaenia, despite antibiotics. This is not very common in paediatric practice, most neutropaenias resolving within a week. However, with increasingly intensive protocols and after BMT, it will be encountered more frequently. The group of Pizzo et al. have confronted this problem and are developing and testing therapeutic strategies.[61] They have found that, in the patient who has become afebrile but remains neutropaenic, if antibiotics are stopped, 40 per cent of patients will have a new septicaemia. If antibiotics are stopped after 7 days in the group of patients who remain febrile and neutropaenic, then over 60 per cent will have further septicaemia. However, if antibiotics alone are continued in these circumstances, then 30 per cent of patients were found to develop invasive fungal disease.[62] Most paediatric units give a standard empiric course of antibiotics of 5 or 7 days and, if the patient is afebrile and well, then stop. This approach is justified in view of the high incidence of fungal overgrowth associated with prolonged use.

Conversely, it seems that the patient who remains febrile and granulolcytopaenic is still at very high risk of further sepsis if antibiotics are stopped, and fungal disease if they are continued. This is, essentially, the argument that has led to empiric antifungal therapy.

There is no doubting the risks of invasive fungal disease associated primarily with prolonged neutropaenia; this is attested to by many post mortem studies.[63,64] There are other risk factors which predispose to fungal disease; these include the previous use of steroids, broad spectrum antibiotics and evidence of fungal colonization at other sites. Most febrile neutropaenias in children are short-lived; this, combined with the toxicity of amphotericin B may explain the reluctance of many paediatricians to consider empiric antifungal therapy (*see* p. 58).

GRANULOCYTE TRANSFUSION

Like many other areas of infection prophylaxis and treatment, an assessment of the value of granulocyte transfusion is hampered by the wide variation in methodology in such areas as methods of collection, cell numbers transfused and whether or not HLA matching is performed, leaving aside criteria for entry into such a study.

The use of granulocyte transfusion is considered on p. 68.

PULMONARY COMPLICATIONS

The constellation of fever, dyspnoea and pulmonary infiltration is a frequent problem in paediatric oncology. It is noteworthy that the lung is the single site most commonly infected;[65] it may be with a wide variety of organisms which occur with increased frequency in particular settings (e.g. CMV pneumonitis post-BMT). However, bacteria, fungi, viruses and protozoae may all give this picture on occasion.

Even in the neutropaenic patient, the adage that common conditions are common still holds. Faced with a febrile patient with patchy pulmonary infiltrates, it is far more likely to be due to *S. pneumoniae* or *H. influenzae* than due to exotic fungal or protozoal causes. Respiratory viruses are also common in all children; adenovirus, respiratory syncytial virus, and parainfluenzae will be seen, as in the general population. Hence the basics of microbiological investigation must not be forgotten. The sputum with gram stain will still yield results. Other techniques, such as tracheal aspiration and the early detection of pneumococcal and other antigens, may both be useful. A variety of gram negative organisms causes pneumonias more commonly in the immunosuppressed; *Klebsiella, Legionella* and *P. aeruginosa* must be considered.[66] The initial investigation and treatment of such problems, therefore, usually follows conventional lines. Only rarely will an organism be isolated initially; more commonly a broad spectrum of cover will be embarked upon before more specific therapy is given later.

The situation of the child with fever and diffuse pulmonary infiltration is rather different. Here the diagnosis may vary considerably depending upon the clinical setting. It is again worth remembering, however, that conventional organisms should not be dismissed. It is widespread paediatric practice to use high-dose TMP-SMZ when faced with fever, neutropaenia and pulmonary infiltrates, on the assumption that *Pneumocystis carinii* is the aetiologic agent. This is very likely in the setting of a patient with acute lymphoblastic leukaemia on maintenance therapy. Gram negative bacteria and fungi can, on occasion, produce at least initially, very similar radiographic appearances. The incidence of *Pneumocystis carinii* pneumonia (PCP) has diminished markedly since the introduction of TMP-SMZ prophylaxis.[67] However, the drug does cause bone marrow suppression in a substantial number of patients, when given in combination with methotrexate, requiring it to be stopped. It is this group that remain at high risk of PCP. The incidence in the UK ALL trials before the introduction of TMP-SMZ prophylaxis was nearly 20 per cent,[68] the major risk factors being the time from diagnosis (6–12 weeks) and the degree of lymphopaenia. The diagnosis may rarely be made by demonstration in sputum or aspirates of pneumocysts by methionine silver staining but all too commonly such efforts produce no results. The use of an immunofluorescent dye test to confirm the diagnosis is valuable,[69] particularly if a substrate of human lung heavily infected with pneumocysts is used. The titre, on occasion, may rise early confirming the diagnosis on the first sample; more commonly only a convalescent sera will confirm the diagnosis.[68]

Another particular clinical setting which gives rise to a specific infection is the susceptibility of the child after BMT to cytomegalovirus pneumonitis. This virus may account for 30 per cent of early post-transplant deaths.[70] The clinical picture is again of fever, dry cough, tachypnoea and a radiograph showing pulmonary infiltrates. Characteristically, this infection occurs rather later in the BMT course, often when the neutrophil count has recovered. In adult patients, drug-induced lung damage due to bleomycin or cyclophosphamide may enter the differential diagnosis, but these are less of a consideration in children.[71] At present, CMV pneumonitis is still widely feared, mortality being < 90 per cent. Two therapies are showing promise, the first using a high titre specific immunoglobulin[72] and the second the new agent foscarnet.[73] The early results show that, if diagnosed early, the pneumonitis is reversible with therapy. It may be that a rapid immunofluorescence test[74] for CMV, looking for the virus in lung washings and other tissues, will be a valuable aid in early diagnosis.

The occurrence of pulmonary infiltrates whilst a patient is on broad spectrum antibiotics is a not uncommon problem and one that has been studied in detail.[75] It is here that empiric antifungal therapy is again of value. Most clinicians would give a trial of antifungal therapy before considering a more invasive diagnostic procedure. The question of when to perform an invasive procedure is a difficult one and still hotly debated. Essentially, it is balancing the risk between the empiric therapy being envisaged, against the risks of the procedure. Hence, most clinicians would give a trial of high-dose TMP-SMZ if PCP was suspected but yet many would embark upon an invasive procedure if amphotericin B, as empiric therapy, was being considered. At present, open lung biopsy remains, in most centres, the best technique for obtaining a diagnosis[76,77] usually in 80–90 per cent of cases depending upon pre-biopsy treatment. In addition, properly performed, its complications may be more manageable than those caused by bronchoscopic biopsy. In one study[78] patients, before open lung biopsy, had bronchial aspirates and transbronchial biopsy performed. These yielded a diagnosis in 30 per cent and 50 per cent of patients respectively compared to 94 per cent by open lung biopsy.[74] One not uncommon reason for failing to make a diagnosis at open lung biopsy is failure to alert all the relevant specialties; virologists, microbiologists, mycologists and pathologists should all be involved to get the maximum information. There is still a need for a clinical trial comparing early open lung biopsy with management by empiric therapy.

In summary, what general guidelines can be given when dealing with pulmonary infections in immunosuppressed children? Firstly, common bacteria and viruses, when the correct methods are employed to detect them, will be the most common infecting agents. Secondly, there are several specific areas where a specific agent may be very strongly suspected in the clinical setting, e.g. fungal disease with new pulmonary infiltration or PCP early in ALL therapy. Lastly, the risks of lung biopsy in any given situation must be carefully weighed against the toxicity of proposed empiric therapy. At present, the lack of comparative data makes this decision a very difficult one.

INFECTION RELATED TO CATHETERS AND OTHER IMPLANTED DEVICES

The importance of the skin as a natural barrier to infection has been mentioned earlier. Increasingly, paediatric oncologists are breaching this in several different ways, the two most common being the use of implanted indwelling central venous catheters of 'Broviac' or 'Hickman' type[79] and the use of Ommaya reservoirs for the prophylaxis and treatment of meningeal disease.[80]

The impact of the first of these developments has been very considerable. They are surgically implanted via a subcutaneous tunnel and can remain in situ for many months or even years. They have revolutionized the care of small children undergoing intensive therapy, not however, without a great increase in catheter-related bacteraemia. The second development, the Ommaya reservoir, has not found the general acceptance in the UK that the device seems to have in the USA, despite some evidence of increased efficacy of intraventricular therapy compared to intralumbar when treating CNS leukaemia. Again, their use is associated with infection by very similar organisms to that seen in catheter-related bacteraemia.

It has long been the practice that once any implanted device becomes infected, it should be removed. We recently analysed our experience in Bristol[81] of the first 3 years' use of such indwelling catheters, looking particularly at our success in eradicating infection without removing the central line. We found a high incidence of infection (we were looking solely at bacteraemia, not exit site or tunnel infection) of 0·68 episodes of bacteraemia per 100 days' catheter use. *Table* 1.3 shows the organisms isolated. The high proportion of *S. epidermidis* is obvious. This probably accounts in part for the increasing preponderance of gram positive organisms seen in many series over the last 5 years.[47] This incidence of infection is broadly in keeping with other units. Shapiro et al.,[82] in a paediatric population, reported 14 episodes in 174 patient months' of use (0·27 episodes per 100 days' catheter use), with only 3 episodes involving coagulase negative *Staphylococci*. Reed et al.[83] give a figure of 0·46 episodes per 100 days' use and Sanz et al.[84] found half of their 23 episodes (in 34 patients) were due to coagulase negative *Staphylococci*. Only the last group were regularly placing their lines before intensive induction chemotherapy as we were in Bristol. We found that the infections caused by coagulase negative *Staphylococci* were directly related to the intensity of line use. Of the catheters

Table 1.3. Micro-organisms isolated in 29 episodes of catheter related bacteraemia. Figures in brackets give the numbers of single isolates in individual episodes of infection

Micro-organism		No. of strains isolated
Coagulase-negative staphylococci		22 (1)
Staphylococcus epidermidis	12 (5)	
Staph. haemolyticus	3 (0)	
Staph. hominis	2 (1)	
Staph. warneri	1 (1)	
Staph. saprophyticus	1 (1)	
not speciated	3 (3)	
Staph. aureus		2 (2)
Stretptococcus pyogenes		1 (1)
Strep. faecalis		1 (0)
Strep. faecium		1 (0)
Strep. mitior		1 (0)
Strep. sanguis		1 (1)
Escherichia coli		5 (0)
Klebsiella oxytoca		2 (2)
Enterobacter cloacae		2 (2)
Ent. agglomerans		1 (0)
Acinetobacter calcoaceticus var anitratus		3 (0)
Candida glabrata		1 (1)
TOTAL		43 (20)

subjected mainly to light outpatient use, only 3/21 became infected. However, of those subjected to intensive use, with blood products, i.v. nutrition, and venesection occurring daily, then 17/19 eventually became infected. We did not find the degree of neutropaenia was playing a significant role in these staphylococcal infections.

These coagulase negative staphylococcal infections tended clinically to present as a low grade fever with minimal systemic upset and no physical signs. We did not find that external infection (tunnel or exit site) predicted for bacteraemia. Some patients experienced fever and rigors associated with line flushing. We left the lines in situ and gave at least 2 weeks' therapy with one or two antibiotics, depending upon the sensitivity of the organism(s) and whether or not neutropaenia was a factor. In general, we found vancomycin, flucloxacillin and netilmicin the most useful agents. However, this may simply reflect the local organism's sensitivities. *Table* 1.4 gives details of the success of this approach. Overall, we were able to eradicate 18/25 infections in which we could assess the results. The factor which we found played most part in predicting success was the number of different organisms infecting the line, either subtypes of *Staphylococci* or a separate species entirely. When only one organism was present, we eradicated 88 per cent of infection; when more than one, we were able to eradicate infection in only 38 per cent. Numbers were, however, small and this finding has yet to be confirmed. Whilst most of these infections are of low virulence, they do present a risk, particularly of endocarditis, hence they must be treated promptly and effectively. The consequences of removal of a catheter in a sick child at a difficult point in therapy can be serious; hence it is heartening to find that other groups[85] have found catheter-related infection treatable. Indeed, it should be unusual to be forced to remove a line due to uncontrolled infection. A reasonable policy is to administer a sensitive antibiotic for 72 hours and, if the patient is still bacteraemic at that point, consider taking out the line. Whether the newer totally implanted venous access systems such as the 'Portacath' will prove to be as free from infection as has been claimed[86] remains to be seen. It is possible that infection may be more difficult to clear once established. However, such evidence should emerge over the next years as their use expands.

The incidence of infection in Ommaya reservoirs is less than that associated with catheter use. However, a similar range of organisms is seen.[87] One problem may be to distinguish true infection from colonization of the reservoir. The presence of leucocytes and a clinical picture varying from mild headache to frank meningoencephalitis obviously will confirm infection. Again, the majority of these infections can be eradicated by antibiotic treatment without removal of the reservoir,[88] often utilizing intraventricular therapy.

Table 1.4. Success in eradication of catheter-related infection

	Total	Episodes Cure (%)	Failure
Single bacterial strain	17	15 (88)	2
Multiple strains	8	3 (38)	5
All episodes	25	18 (72)	7

The incidence of infection in both central lines and Ommaya reservoirs, whilst manageable by conventional antibiotic treatment, does represent a serious risk, particularly as inevitably systemic chemotherapy is likely to be interrupted. The organisms primarily responsible are skin commensals, and they gain access because of inadequate handling of the devices. The use of scrupulous aseptic technique when manipulating lines or injecting into reservoirs cannot be overemphasized. (It is no use training a group of highly motivated nurses to manage i.v. lines if the new resident does not wear gloves.) Medical staff are often the worst offenders. These lines or reservoirs may be a critical part of a patient's management and all staff using them must be briefed in their care. Once this is done, then the levels of infection seen are likely to be small and outweighed by the undoubted benefits of such devices.

GI PROBLEMS IN THE IMMUNOSUPPRESSED

The GI tract forms another vital physical barrier to micro-organisms which can be affected in a variety of different ways in children with malignant disease. The most common clinical picture resulting is that of diarrhoea and abdominal pain. It would be incorrect to ascribe this clinical picture to being always secondary to infection. Chemotherapeutic agents and radiation can damage the bowel mucosa; changes in liver function may produce alterations in bile salt concentrations. Secondary disaccharide intolerance and psychological factors are two non-infective causes to be considered.

The gut flora is profoundly altered by systemic antibiotic administration without necessarily systemic upset. There is some evidence that close monitoring of the predominant organisms in the gut and their sensitivity to antibiotics may predict future bacteraemias and be a useful guide to therapy.[19]

A more profound disturbance of bowel flora secondary to antibiotic use is that caused by the toxin of Clostridium difficile, giving rise, on occasion, to pseudomembranous colitis. This clinical syndrome of bloody diarrhoea, fever, abdominal pain with a characteristic membrane visible on sigmoidoscopy was first described mainly after clindamycin therapy.[89] It has emerged, however, as a far more widespread problem in not just the immunosuppressed but neonates[90] and in patients taking broad spectrum antibiotics for a variety of conditions. The situation has been complicated by the appearance of both the organism itself and its toxin in asymptomatic individuals.[91] There is no doubt, however, that sporadic cases and groups of cases of abdominal pain and diarrhoea, due to *Clostridium difficile* have occurred in the immunosuppressed. This has now been reported with a wide range of antibiotic combinations, despite an initial suggestion that clindamycin and broad spectrum cephalosporins may have been particularly potent inducers of the organism. The assessment of the role of this organism in a particular patient must be interpreted with caution in view of its now widespread occurrence in the asymptomatic. It is likely that only the new isolation of the organism and toxin in a patient previously known to be free of the organism will be accepted as a strong indicator of its role in pathogenesis. Treatment is usually by the oral administration of vancomycin, although metronidazole represents a cheaper alternative.

Two syndromes of GI infection are still widely feared; firstly, that of caecal inflammation termed 'typhilitis'; secondly, that of perianal cellulitis. Typhilitis characteristically presents as a severe right lower quadrant pain, profound shock and increasing signs of abdominal obstruction. The pathological process is a surgical cellulitis of the caecum which, if unchecked, leads to necrosis and perforation.[92] Once this stage has been reached, the situation is often beyond any hope of reversal. However, early aggressive non-surgical treatment with antibiotics and i.v. fluids is sometimes successful. A wide variety of organisms has been implicated, *P. aeruginosa* being common as well as anaerobes; hence these possibilities must be covered in any initial empiric therapy.

Most oncology units rightly place great emphasis on avoiding perianal sepsis. This process begins by organisms gaining entry to the perianal tissues through small perianal tears or fissures. Hence, the use of stool softeners and avoidance of suppositories and enemas are two widely used but important practices. Once perianal sepsis is established in a neutropaenic child, it rarely goes on to form an abscess; more commonly, a diffuse cellulitis, often with tissue necrosis, occurs. The organisms seen, not surprisingly, reflect the cross section of bowel flora and again, *Pseudomonas* and anaerobic species are well represented.[93] This is one area where many clinicians would resort quite rapidly to the use of granulocyte transfusions if a rapid response to appropriate antibiotics was not observed.

It should also be remembered that the syndrome of abdominal pain and diarrhoea may be caused by a host of conventional organisms as well as the more unusual examples given above. Again, a plea must be made to remember to perform the full range of microbiological and virological investigation required. Pathogenic *E. coli* and diarrhoea caused by *Candida albicans* overgrowth will be picked up by stool culture. A whole host of viruses, again common pathogens in childhood, such as rotavirus, CMV and enterovirus may all be seen and may require serology and electron microscopy to confirm them. Recently, *Cryptosporidium* has been responsible for GI disease in patients with AIDS[94] and also in patients immunosuppressed after chemotherapy.[95] This parasite may require special methods of identification[94] and treatment with spiramycin, although this is usually ineffective and the only way to control the diarrhoea is to interrupt chemotherapy. Overgrowth by other pathogens, such as *Giardia lamblia*, must also be excluded.

The situation following BMT may be more difficult to interpret. Acute graft versus host disease (GVHD) may have, as one of its manifestations, profound watery diarrhoea. Conversely, there is evidence that several viruses, particularly adeno- and rotaviruses, are more pathogenic in such circumstances, carrying a high mortality.[96] It is vital, in these circumstances, that the correct diagnosis is made as high dose steroids may well worsen any viral infection, yet would be the treatment of choice for GVHD. Other signs of GVHD, such as liver or skin involvement with, if necessary, biopsy should help to give the correct answer.

In summary, the GI tract is probably the most common system where the interaction between drugs, disease and its treatment come together, to give a similar clinical picture of abdominal pain and diarrhoea of varying severity. It is also the area where appropriate virological and microbiological investigation is likely to yield most dividends and to provide valuable directions for specific therapy.

CENTRAL NERVOUS SYSTEM INFECTIONS

The incidence of central nervous system infections is not greatly increased,[97] presumably because the meninges and blood brain barrier remain largely intact in most neutropaenic patients. Encephalopathic or thrombotic brain disease may be due to other causes than infection. The toxicity of cranial radiation in combination with methotrexate may cause quite acute brain syndromes[98] and the propensity of asparaginase to cause cerebral thromboses in some patients[99] is both well known, and needs distinguishing from infectious causes. Bacterial meningitis, though rare, will present with the same symptoms as in the non-immunosuppressed; however, the CSF cell reaction may not be as florid in a neutropaenic patient. Pneumococcal meningitis in post-splenectomy patients, *Cryptococcus neoformans* in patients with Hodgkin's disease and *Listeria monocytogenes* all feature quite predominantly in the organisms reported.[100] However, more common organisms are also seen.

The syndrome of focal brain disease, often presenting as seizures and a decreasing level of consciousness, raises the possibility of *Aspergillus* infection. This fungus, whose primary infection site is, in 90 per cent of cases, within the chest,[64] spreads haematogenously causing widespread infarction. The CT scan may provide useful information, but the poor inflammatory response in the neutropaenic patient often results in a negative scan in the early stages.[101] Cerebral *Aspergillus* is almost always fatal, only one possible survivor having been reported.[102]

Encephalitic brain disease is most often caused by viruses. *Varicella zoster* is now very effectively treated with acyclovir, but measles encephalitis still causes sporadic deaths, particularly in children with ALL on maintenance therapy.

The possibility of central nervous system infection should not be forgotten in a child with a febrile neutropaenia, and a low threshold to perform a lumbar puncture in such circumstances is to be encouraged. There are times, however, when the information from the lumbar puncture may be slightly misleading, the first being when the CSF cell count is done shortly following intrathecal chemotherapy (usually methotrexate); a pleocytosis, sometimes in conjunction with signs of meningism is not uncommon, and is caused usually by a chemical meningitis. The second instance is during the somnolence syndrome which follows cranial irradiation. A low grade fever is often part of this syndrome[103] and, if an LP is performed, a lymphoid response is sometimes seen in the CSF. The spinal fluid should be sent for routine culture, biochemistry and cytospin preparation. In addition, Indian ink preparations and specific viral,[104] bacterial and fungal serology should be considered as a valuable adjunct in certain infections.

SUMMARY

It is vital, when confronted with such an array of new drugs, new techniques and different environments, that all those concerned in the therapy of the immunosuppressed retain a critical attitude in the appraisal of their current practice and of reported new measures. Many of the measures mentioned earlier are time consuming, toxic and expensive and are likely to be applicable only to children undergoing very intensive therapy. Conversely, we should not be overcautious in applying proven measures to those groups of children who will benefit from them.

What problems remain in infection treatment and control? There are many in the areas of viral disease, and infection in the AIDS patient which are beyond the immediate brief of this chapter, but which are at present emerging as important areas. In the field of infection prophylaxis, the role of protected environments is well established, but we await a form of gut decontamination that is really acceptable to children. Research into more selective decontamination, with close surveillance of changing stool organisms may prove to be of benefit. Certainly, there is evidence that the stool flora may be of predictive value[19] in terms of subsequent bacteraemia. Other methods of prophylaxis, particularly using immunoglobulins, are likely to expand. The development of an antiserum against core gram negative proteins[39] will be an important advance if effective and free from side-effects. *Pseudomonas* septicaemia still kills a substantial number of adults and children and even if such antiserum does not prevent the infection, it would be an advance if the severity were reduced. Many childhood febrile neutropaenias are not due to bacteria and efforts to separate these from the significantly infected group are potentially attractive. To date, however, neither examining risk factors, nor biochemical parameters, such as C-reactive protein,[105] are sufficiently predictive in the individual child.

In the field of antibiotic usage, the search for a single agent suitable for empiric therapy will continue. Both ceftazidine and moxolactam[52] have been examined as single agents, but neither appears to be entirely satisfactory, and both have small but significant gaps in their antibacterial spectrum. The assessment of new agents is likely to become more difficult, the current regimens of a semisynthetic penicillin or third generation cephalosporin, in combination with an aminoglycoside, result in most infections being brought rapidly under control. Increasingly, the non-responders will be patients with early death due to overwhelming septicaemia, a situation in which assessment of an antibiotic's relative worth will be difficult.

Unfortunately, the same position is not true in fungal disease. There is an urgent need to develop new, effective, non-toxic antifungal agents and, additionally, the laboratory means to assess response to them. At present, evidence of invasive fungal disease is very difficult to assess and it is to be hoped that one of the newer serologic tests of fungal disease will eventually bring rewards. A similar situation also applies to the use of fungal prophylactic agents. While evidence of their effect on fungal colonization may be found, evidence for a decrease in invasive fungal disease and an increase in survival as a consequence is much more difficult. Many questions remain about the selection criteria for empiric antibiotics and fungal therapy, their optimum duration and the value of the results of surveillance cultures in predicting the organism isolated.

This chapter ends in a plea to remember the basics of clinical and microbiological methodology. There are many exciting advances in infection prophylaxis and treatment, yet they will only come to fruition when combined with sound microbiological practice. Cultures taken at the right time and in the right way, and liaison with experienced and interested staff—this is the basis on which future advances will be made.

REFERENCES

1. Bodey G. P., Buckley M., Sathe T. S. et al. (1966) Quantitative relationships between circulating leucocytes and infection in patients with acute leukaemia. *Ann. Intern. Med.* **64**, 328.
2. Pizzo P. A. (1981) Infectious complications in children with cancer. I. Pathophysiology of the compromised host and initial evaluation and management of the febrile cancer patient. *J. Pediat.* **98**, 341.
3. Duffy T. P. (1985) How much is too much high-dose cytosine arabinoside? *J. Clin. Oncol.* **3**, 601.
4. Wimperis J. Z., Brenner M. K., Prentice H. G. et al. (1986) Transfer of functioning humoral immune system in transplantation of T-depleted bone marrow. *Lancet* **i**, 339.
5. Noel D. R., Witherspoon R. P., Storb R. et al. (1976) Does graft versus host disease influence the tempo of immunologic recovery after allogeneic human marrow transplantation? An observation on 56 long-term survivors. *Blood* **51**, 1087.
6. Lange B. and Littman P. (1983) Management of Hodgkin's disease in children and adolescents. *Cancer* **51**, 1371.
7. Dickerman J. D. (1979) Splenectomy and sepsis: a warning. *Pediatrics* **63**, 938.
8. Francke E. L. and Neu H. C. (1981) Post splenectomy infection. *Surg. Clin. of North Am.* **61**(1), 135.
9. Pickering L. K., Anderson D. C., Choi S. et al. (1975) Leucocyte function in children with malignancy. *Cancer* **35**, 1365.
10. Cline M. J. (1974) Drugs and phagocytosis. *N. Engl. J. Med.* **291**, 1187.
11. Schimpff S. C., Young V. M., Greene W. H. et al. (1972) Origin of infection in acute non-lymphocytic leukaemia. Significance of hospital acquisition of potential pathogens. *Ann. Intern. Med.* **77**, 707.
12. Bodey G. P. (1979) Treatment of acute leukaemia in protected environment units. *Cancer* **44**, 431.
13. Yates J. W. and Holland J. F. (1973) A controlled study of isolation and endogenous microbial suppression in acute myelogenous leukaemia patients. *Cancer* **32**, 1490.
14. Dietrich M., Gaus W., Vossen J. et al. (1977) Protective isolation and antimicrobial decontamination in patients with high susceptibility to infection. A prospective co-operative study of gnotobiotic care in acute leukaemic patients. *Infection* **5**, 107.
15. King K. (1980) Prophylactic non-absorbable antibiotics in leukaemia patients. *J. Hyg. (Camb.)* **85**, 141.
16. Bodey G. P. and Johnston D. (1971) Microbiological evaluation of protected environments during patient occupancy. *Appl. Microbiol.* **22**, 828.

17. Pizzo P. A. and Levine A. S. (1977) The utility of protected environment regimens for the compromised host: a critical assessment. In: Brown B. (ed.), *Progress in Haematology*, p. 311.
18. Schimpff S. C. (1980) Infection prevention in patients with cancer and granulocytopenia. In: Grieco M. H. (ed.) *Infections in the Abnormal Host*. New York, Yorke Medical, p. 26.
19. Cohen M. L., Murphy M. T., Counts G. W. et al. (1983) Prediction by surveillance cultures of bacteraemia among neutropenic patients treated in a protective environment. *J. Inf. Dis.* **147**, 789.
20. Schimpff S. C., Greene W. H., Young V. M. et al. (1975) Infection prevention in acute non-lymphocytic leukaemia: laminar air flow room reverse isolation with oral non-absorbable antibiotic prophylaxis. *Ann. Intern. Med.* **82**, 351.
21. Rodriquez V., Bodey G. P., Freireich E. J. et al. (1978) Randomised trial of protected environment—prophylactic antibiotics in 145 adults with acute leukaemia. *Medicine* **57**, 253.
22. Pizzo P. A. (1983) Antimicrobial prophylaxis in the immunosuppressed cancer patient. In: Remington J. S. and Swartz M. N. (eds.) *Current Clinical Topics in Infectious Diseases*, Vol. 4, p. 153.
23. Levine A. S., Siegel S. E., Schreiber A. D. et al. (1973) Protected environments and prophylactic antibiotics. A prospective controlled study of the utility in the therapy of acute leukaemia. *N. Engl. J. Med.* **288**, 477.
24. Klastersky J., Debusscher L., Weerts E. et al. (1974) The use of oral antibiotics in protected environment units: Clinical effectiveness and role in the emergence of antibiotic resistant strains. *Pathol. Biol.* **22**, 5.
25. Nauseff W. M. and Maki D. G. (1983) A study of the value of simple protective isolation in patients with granulocytopenia. *N. Engl. J. Med.* **304**, 448.
26. Knittle M. A., Eitzman D. V. and Baer H. (1975) Role of hand contamination of personnel in the epidemiology of gram negative nosocomial infections. *J. Pediatr.* **86**, 433.
27. Hargadon M. T., Young M. T., Schimpff S. C. et al. (1981) Selective suppression of alimentary tract microbial flora as prophylaxis during granulocytopenia. *Antimicrob. Agents Chemother.* **20**, 620.
28. Hughes W., Kuhn S., Chaudhury S. et al. (1977) Successful chemoprophylaxis for *Pneumocystis carinii* pneumonia. *N. Engl. J. Med.* **279**, 1419.
29. Preisler H. D., Early A. and Hryniuk W. (1981) Prevention of infection and bleeding in leukaemia patients receiving intensive remission maintenance therapy. *Med. Pediatr. Oncol.* **9**, 511.
30. Watson J. G., Jamieson B., Powles R. L. et al. (1982) Co-trimoxazole alone for prevention of bacterial infection in patients with acute leukaemia. *Lancet* **i**, 5.
31. Pizzo P. A., Robichaud K. J., Edwards B. K. et al. (1983) Oral antibiotic prophylaxis in patients with cancer. A double blind placebo controlled trial. *J. Pediatr.* **102**, 125.
32. Wade J. C., De Jongh C. A., Newman K. A. et al. (1983) Selective antimicrobial modulation as prophylaxis against infection during granulocytopenia: trimethoprim-sulphamethoxazole vs. nalidixic acid. *J. Infect. Dis.* **147**, 624.
33. Gaya H., Glauser M., Klastersky J. et al. (1980) Double blind placebo controlled trial of prophylactic trimethoprim and sulphamethoxazole for the prevention of infection in granulocytopenic patients. *Proceedings of the 20th Interscience Conference on Antimicrobial Agents and Chemotherapy*. Abs. 331.
34. Weiser B., Lange M., Fialk M. A. et al. (1981) Prophylactic TMP-SMZ during consolidation chemotherapy for acute leukaemia: a controlled trial. *Ann. Intern. Med.* **95**, 436.
35. Zinner S., Gaya H., Glauser M. et al. (1981) Co-trimoxazole and reduction of risk of infection in neutropenic patients: a progress report. *Proceedings of the 21st Interscience Conference on Antimicrobial Agents and Chemotherapy*. Abs. 795.

36. Golde D. W., Bersch H. and Quan S. G. (1978). Trimethoprim and sulpha-methoxazole inhibition of haemotopoesis *in vitro*. *Br. J. Haematol.* **40**, 363.
37. Deeg C., Meyers J. D., Storb R. et al. (1979) Effect of trimethoprim/ sulphamethoxazole on haematological recovery after total body irradiation and autologous marrow infusion in dogs. *Transplantation* **28**, 243.
38. Winston D. J., Schiffman G., Wang D. C. et al. (1979) Pneumococcal infections after human bone marrow transplantation. *Ann. Intern. Med.* **91**, 835.
39. Ziegler E. J., McCutchan J. A., Fierer J. et al. (1982) Treatment of gram negative bacteraemia and shock with human antiserum to mutant *E. coli. N. Engl. J. Med.* **307**, 1225.
40. McCutchan J. A. and Ziegler E. J. (1983) Treatment with antigram-negative antibodies. *Lancet* **ii**, 802.
41. McClelland D. B. L. and Yap P. L. (1984) Clinical use of immunoglobulins. *Clin. in Haematol.* **13**(1), 39.
42. Graw R. E., Herzig G., Perry S. et al. (1972) Normal granulocyte transfusion therapy. Treatment of septicaemia due to gram-negative bacteria. *N. Engl. J. Med.* **287**, 367.
43. Darbyshire P. J., Williamson P. J., Pedler et al. (1983) Ceftazidime in the treatment of febrile immunosuppressed children. *J. Antimicrob. Chemother.* Suppl. A. **12**, 357.
44. Williamson P. J., Darbyshire P. J., Mott M. G. et al. (1984) Ceftazidime and tobramycin in the treatment of febrile immunosuppressed children. *J. Antimicrob. Chemother.* **14**, 671.
45. Meyers J. D. and Thomas E. D. (1981) Infection complicating bone marrow transplantation. In: Young L. S. and Rubin R. H. (eds.) *Clinical Approach to Infection in the Immunocompromised Host*, p. 507.
46. Pizzo P. A., Robichaud K. J., Wesley R. et al. (1982) Fever in the pediatric and young adult patient with cancer: a prospective study of 1001 episodes. *Medicine* **61**, 153.
47. Wade J. L., Schimpff S. C., Newman K. A. et al. (1982) *Staphylococcus epidermidis*: an increasing cause of infection in patients with granulocytopenia. *Ann. Intern. Med.* **97**, 503.
48. EORTC International Antimicrobial Therapy Project Group (1978) Three antibiotic regimens in the treatment of infection in febrile granulocytopenic patients with cancer. *J. Infect. Dis.* **137**, 14.
49. Tattersall M. H. N., Hutchinson R. M., Gaya H. et al. (1973) Empirical antibiotic therapy in febrile patients with neutropenia and malignant disease. *Eur. J. Cancer Clin. Oncol.* **9**, 417.
50. Gaya H. (1984) Rational basis for the choice of regimens for empirical therapy of sepsis in granulocytopenic patients. In: Prentice H. G. (ed.) *Clinic in Haematology*, Vol. 13, p. 573.
51. Ramphal R., Kramer B. S., Rand K. H. et al. (1983) Early results of a comparative trial of ceftazidime *vs* cephalothin, carbenicillin and gentamycin in the treatment of febrile granulocytopenic patients. *J. Antimicrob. Chemother.* Suppl. A, **12**, 81.
52. Fainstein V., Bodey G. P., Elting L. et al. (1983) A randomised study of ceftazidime compared to ceftazidime and tobramycin for the treatment of infection in cancer patients. *J. Antimicrob. Chemother.* Suppl. A, **12**, 101.
53. Morgan G., Hart C. A., Lilleyman J. S. (1983) Ceftazidime as a single agent in the management of children with fever and neutropenia. *J. Antimicrob. Chemother.* Suppl. A, **12**, 347.
54. de Pauw B. E., Kauw F., Muytjens H. et al. (1983) Randomised study of ceftazidime *vs* gentamycin plus cefotaxime for infections in severely granulo-cytopenic patients. *J. Antimicrob. Chemother.* Suppl. A, **12**, 93.
55. Barnes R. C., Winston D. J., Ho W. G. et al. (1982) Comparative efficacy and

toxicity of moxoloctam–pipericillin *vs* moxolactam–amikacin in febrile neutropenic patients. *Proceedings of the 22nd Interscience Conference on Antimicrobial Agents and Chemotherapy.* Abs. 66.

56. De Jongh C., Joshi J., Newman K. et al. (1982) Moxoloctam plus piperacillin or amikacin: empiric antibiotic therapy for febrile neutropenia cancer patients. *Proceedings of the 22nd Interscience Conference on Antimicrobial Agents and Chemotherapy.* Abs. 233.

57. De Jongh C. A., Wade J. C., Schimpff S. C. et al. (1982) Empiric antibiotic therapy for suspected infection in granulocytopenic patients. A comparison between the combination of moxoloctam plus amikacin and ticarcillin plus amikacin. *Am. J. Med.* **73**, 89.

58. Pizzo P. A. (1979) Infectious complications in children with cancer II. Management of specific organisms. *J. Pediatr.* **98**, 513.

59. Pizzo P. A., Robichaud K. J., Gill F. A. et al. (1979) Duration of empiric antibiotic therapy in granulocytopenic cancer patients. *Am. J. Med.* **67**, 194.

60. Ladisch S. and Pizzo P. A. (1978) *Staphylococcus aureus* sepsis in children with cancer. *Pediatrics.* **61**, 231.

61. Pizzo P. A., Commers J., Cotton D. et al. (1984) Approaching the controversies in antibacterial management of cancer patients. *Am. J. Med.* **76**, 436.

62. Pizzo P. A., Robichaud K. J., Gill F. A. et al. (1982) Empiric antibiotic and antifungal therapy for cancer patients with prolonged fever and granulocytopenia. *Am. J. Med.* **72**, 101.

63. Degregorio M. W., Lee W. M. F., Linker C. A. et al. (1983) Fungal infections in patients with acute leukaemia. *Am. J. Med.* **73**, 543.

64. Meyer R. D., Young L. S., Armstrong D. et al. (1973) *Aspergillus* complicating neoplastic disease. *Am. J. Med.* **54**, 6.

65. Sickles E. A., Young V. M., Greene W. H. et al. (1975) Pneumonia in acute leukaemia. *Ann. Int. Med.* **79**, 529.

66. Valdivieso M., Gil-Extramera B., Zornoza J. et al. (1977) Gram negative bacillary pneumonia in the compromised host. *Medicine (Baltimore)* **56**, 241.

67. Hughes W. T. (1984) Five year absence of pneumocystic carinii related penumonitis in a pediatric oncology centre. *J. Infect. Dis.* **150**, 305.

68. Darbyshire P., Eden O. B., Kay H. et al. (1985) Pneumonitis in lymphoblastic leukaemia. *Eur. Pediatr. Haematol. Oncol.* **2**, 141.

69. Shepherd V., Jameson B. and Knowles E. K. (1979) *Pneumocystis carinii* pneumonitis: a serological study. *J. Clin. Pathol.* **32**, 773.

70. Meyers J. D., Flournoy N. and Thomas E. D. (1982) Non bacterial pneumonia after allogeneic marrow transplantation: a review of ten years' experience. *Rev. Infect. Dis.* **4**, 1119.

71. Weiss R. B. and Muggia F. M. (1980) Cytotoxic drug induced pulmonary disease. *Am. J. Med.* **68**, 259.

72. Blacklock H. A., Griffiths P., Stirk P. et al. (1986) Cytotect treatment of cytomegalovirus pneumonitis after matched allogeneic bone marrow transplantation. *Proceedings of the 12th Meeting of European Bone Marrow Transplantation*, Abs. 22.

73. Ringden O., Lonnquist B., Gahrton G. et al. (1986) Experience using Foscarnet for treatment of severe cytomegalovirus infections in 20 allogeneic bone marrow transplant recipients. *Proceedings of the 12th Meeting of European Bone Marrow Transplantation*, Abs. 23.

74. Griffiths P. D. (1984) Rapid diagnosis of cytomegalovirus infection in immunocompromised patients by detection of early antigen fluorescent foci. *Lancet* **ii**, 1242.

75. Commers J. R., Robichaud K. J. and Pizzo P. A. (1984) New pulmonary infiltrates in granulocytopenic cancer patients being treated with antibiotics. *Pediatr. Infect. Dis.* **3**, 423.

76. Jaffe J. P. and Maki D. E. (1981) Lung biopsy in immunocompromised patients: one institution's experience and an approach to management of pulmonary disease in the compromised host. *Cancer* **48**, 1144.
77. Prober C. G., Whyte H. and Smith C. R. (1984) Open lung biopsy in immuno-compromised children with pulmonary infiltrates. *Am. J. Dis. Child.* **138**, 60.
78. Burt M. E., Flye M. W., Webber B. L. et al. (1981) Prospective evaluation of aspiration needle, cutting needle, transbronchial and open lung biopsy in patients with pulmonary infiltrates. *Ann. Thorac. Surg.* **32**, 146.
79. Hickman R. O., Buckner C. D., Clift R. A. et al. (1979) A modified right atrial catheter for access to the venous system in marrow transplant recipients. *Surg. Gynaecol. Obstet.* **148**, 871.
80. Ratherson R. A. and Ommaya A. K. (1968) Experience with the subcutaneous cerebrospinal fluid reservoir. Preliminary report of 60 cases. *N. Engl. J. Med.* **279**, 1025.
81. Darbyshire P. J., Weightman N. and Speller D. C. E. (1985) Problems associated with the use of indwelling central venous catheters. *Arch. Dis. Child.* **60**, 129.
82. Shapiro E. D., Wald G. R., Nelson K. A. et al. (1982) Broviac catheter-related bacteraemia in oncology patients. *Am. J. Dis. Child.* **136**, 679.
83. Reed W. P., Newman K. A., De Jongh C. et al. (1983) Prolonged venous access for chemotherapy by means of the Hickman catheter. *Cancer* **52**, 185.
84. Sanz M. A., Such M., Rafecas F. J. et al. (1983) *Staphylococcus epidermidis* infections in acute myeloblastic leukaemia patients fitted with Hickman catheters. *Lancet* **ii**, 1191.
85. Abrahm J. L. and Mullen J. L. (1982) A prospective study of prolonged central venous access in leukaemia. *J. Am. Med. Assoc.* **248**, 2868.
86. Gyves J., Emsminger W., Niederhuber J. et al. (1982) Totally implanted system for intravenous chemotherapy in patients with cancer. *Am. J. Med.* **73**, 841.
87. Bayston R. (1975) Serological surveillance of children with CSF shunting devices. *Dev. Med. Child Neurol.* Suppl. 17 **135**, 104.
88. Sutherland G. E., Palitang E. G., Marr J. J. et al. (1981) Sterilisation of Ommaya reservoir by instillation of vancomycin. *Am. J. Med.* **71**, 1068.
89. George R. H., Symonds J., Dimock F. et al. (1978) Identification of *Clostridium difficile* as a cause of pseudo-membranous colitis. *Br. Med. J.* **1**, 695.
90. Zedd A. J., Sell T. L., Schaberg D. R. et al. (1984) Nosocomial *Clostridium difficile* reservoir in a neonatal intensive care unit. *Ped. Infect. Dis.* **3**, 429.
91. Rogers T. R. (1981) Spread of *Clostridium difficile* among patients receiving non-absorbable antibiotics for gut decontamination. *Br. Med. J.* **283**, 408.
92. Shamberger R. C., Weinstein H. J., Delorey M. J. et al. (1986) The medical and surgical management of typhlitis in children with acute non-lymphocytic leukaemia. *Cancer* **57**, 603.
93. Schimpff S. C., Wiernik P. A. and Block J. B. (1972) Rectal abscesses in cancer patients. *Lancet* **ii**, 844.
94. Ma P. and Soave R. (1983) Three step stool examination for cryptosporidiosis in ten homosexual men with protracted watery diarrhoea. *J. Infect. Dis.* **147**, 824.
95. Lewis I., Hart C. A. and Baxby D. (1985) Diarrhoea due to cryptosporidium during maintenance treatment for acute lymphoblastic leukaemia. *Arch. Dis. Child.* **60**(1), 60.
96. Yolken R. H., Bishop C. A., Townsend T. R. et al. (1982) Infectious gastro-enteritis in bone marrow transplant recipients. *N. Engl. J. Med.* **306**, 1009.
97. Chernik N., Armstrong D. and Posner J. B. (1977) Central nervous system infections in patients with cancer. Changing patterns. *Cancer* **40**, 268.
98. Pochedly C. (1977) Neurotoxicity due to CNS therapy for leukaemia. *Med. Pediatr. Oncol.* **3**, 101.
99. Priest J. R., Ramsey N. K. C., Latchaw R. E. et al. (1980) Thrombotic and

haemorrhagic strokes complicating early therapy for childhood acute lympho-blastic leukaemia. *Cancer* **46**, 1548.

100. Hooper D. C., Pruitt A. A. and Rubin R. H. (1982) Central nervous system infection in the chronically immunosuppressed. *Medicine (Baltimore)* **61**, 166.

101. Enzmann D. R., Brant-Zawadzki M. and Britt R. H. (1980) CT of central nervous system infections in immunocompromised patients. *Am. J. Radiol.* **135**, 263.

102. Henze G., Aldenhoff P., Stephani U. et al. (1982) Successful treatment of pulmonary and cerebral aspergillosis in an immunosuppressed child. *Eur. J. Pediatr.* **138**, 263.

103. Houseman J. E., Johnston P. G. B. and Vore J. M. (1973) Somnolence after prophylactic cranial irradiation in children with acute lymphoblastic leukaemia. *Br. Med. J.* **4**, 523.

104. Klapper P. E., Laing I. and Longsom M. (1981) Rapid non-invasive diagnosis of herpes encephalitis. *Lancet* **ii**, 607.

105. Gozzard D. I., French E. A., Blecher T. E. et al. (1985) C-reactive protein levels in neutropenic patients with pyrexia. *Clin. Lab. Haematol.* **7**, 307.

2. Viral Infection

O. Caul and A. Roome

INTRODUCTION

In recent years, there has been a tendency towards more profound immunosuppression as a result of the introduction of newer, more successful chemotherapeutic agents to treat children with malignant disease. As a result, the need to protect children from exogenous virus infections is critical. Only a few viruses are commonly associated with life-threatening infections in the immunosuppressed patient. These include members of the herpes group (herpes simplex, varicella–zoster and cytomegalovirus)[1,2,3] and measles virus. Within the last few years, severe infections have been linked with other viruses which previously were not associated with serious disease (adenoviruses, parainfluenza viruses, rhinoviruses, enteroviruses and respiratory syncytial virus)[5,6] and these agents should be taken into consideration. The polyoma virus JC is recognized as a rare cause of central nervous system disease in immunocompromized patients, particularly in older age groups. More recently, infection has also been recognized in younger patients and in any BMT patient presenting with chronic progressive CNS disease, progressive multifocal leukoencephalopathy should be considered. Recent studies have associated the human polyoma virus BK with haemorrhagic cystitis in BMT recipients,[7] although these findings are not universally accepted.[8,9]

Within the herpes group, herpes simplex (HSV) and varicella–zoster (VZ) are a greater risk than cytomegalovirus (CMV) which rarely causes mortality until bone marrow transplantation, with its associated greater immunosuppression, is undertaken. The management of newly diagnosed childhood malignancy is partially dependent on the age of the patients at diagnosis and, consequently, their immune status whether by vaccination or naturally acquired infections. The important viruses in this context are measles and varicella.

Antibody testing at the time of diagnosis is mandatory, since levels may commonly drop to barely detectable values after induction therapy. History of previous vaccination is unacceptable without documented serological evidence of immunity, but if patients are known to be immune previously, dropping antibody levels following induction therapy are not a major concern, since serious exogenous re-infections are not a major problem until the intense immuno-suppression associated with bone marrow transplantation is reached.

SCREENING TESTS FOR ANTIBODY (PATIENTS)

A variety of assays are available for the detection of specific antibody (*Table* 2.1).

Table 2.1. Immunity screening on initial diagnosis

Virus	Serological method		
	Complement fixation	Indirect immune fluorescence	Latex agglutination
Measles	−	+	−
HSV	+	−	+
CMV	+	−	+
VZ	−	+	−
Mumps	+	+	−

Complement fixation (CF)

This assay has limited applications in immunity screening due to its lack of sensitivity. The exception to this general rule is antibody to cytomegalovirus (CMV) where excellent correlation between CF and other assays has been achieved in spite of the greater sensitivity of the enzyme-linked immunoassays in screening tests. CF has no value in immunity screening for VZ and measles virus, as more sensitive and rapid techniques are currently available.

Enzyme-linked immunosorbent assays (ELISA)

Currently, ELISA assays are highly sensitive[10] and specific and have been shown by numerous workers to be superior to the standard CF test[11] for immunity screening. The technique has the disadvantage of requiring several hours or overnight for completion and is more suited to batch testing than to one-off specimens.

Immunofluorescence (IF)

Various modifications to the standard indirect technique have been described. In our experience, this method is reliable, reproduceable and provides a rapid answer when urgency is paramount. When assaying for antibody to measles and varicella virus, excellent sensitivity and specificity have been found. However, care must be taken when screening for immunity to CMV and HSV because of false positive results due to Fc receptor sites in infected cells. It is, in our experience, essential to carry out such IF tests on pre-formed, infected monolayers. These techniques employ acetone-fixed preparations which can be stored at −20°C, allowing immediate retrieval for urgent specimens. Many workers have claimed increased sensitivity and specificity by using a membrane IF test on unfixed virus infected cells for determining specific antibody levels[12] although excellent sensitivity and specificity have been reported by others using acetone fixed preparations.[13] One drawback of the membrane IF test has been the need in the past for a continual supply of fresh virus infected cells; however, methods have now been described for the storage of such preparations in the wet state.[14]

Other serological methods are available, including radioimmune assay (RIA), biotin–avidin enhanced assays, and radial hemolysis for specific viruses. None of these would be the method of choice given that only single samples are commonly available to the laboratory.

SCREENING FOR ANTIBODY (STAFF)

Varicella

The standard procedure is to ask all new members of staff in the oncology department for a past history of chickenpox. Some 80 per cent of staff born in the UK, Europe, North America or Australasia give an affirmative history (sometimes with the help of their parents), and this, in our experience, correlates completely with the presence of antibody.

The 20 per cent who are either uncertain or respond negatively are tested by IF and half can be shown to be immune leaving only 10 per cent susceptible.[15]

The figures for immunity are different in overseas staff, and many more nurses and doctors from the Indian Sub-continent, South East Asia and the West Indies are susceptible to chickenpox [16,17] and this may pose infection control problems in the ward.

Measles

Previous history is unreliable but infection in staff is most unusual—

those under 25 will have immunity due to vaccination or natural infection and older staff will mostly have had measles in childhood.

In Northern Europe, most children have had measles by the age of 12 and infection in adults in the UK is extremely rare.[18] However, staff presenting with a measles like rash are removed from the unit and immunoglobulin given to those children in contact who are not known to be immune.

LIFE-THREATENING VIRUS INFECTIONS

Only two virus families can be commonly considered to present as life-threatening infections in childhood leukaemia. The first are members of the herpes group, namely HSV, VZ, CMV, and the second is measles. Infection with Epstein–Barr virus (EBV) is well documented as a serious complication of X-linked lymphoprolifera-tive syndromes and other inherited acquired immunodeficiency diseases.[19] However, it is not life-threatening in primary childhood leukaemias or solid tumours even after profound immunosuppressive therapy.

Measles

The rash, which can be extensive but more commonly limited, has no relationship to the severity of the principal life-threatening feature of measles in immunocompromized children. In severe measles infec-tion, it often presents as a fulminating giant cell pneumonia.[20]

Herpes simplex

The age of children presenting with leukaemia or solid tumours overlaps the age of first exposure to HSV, which may present as a primary infection. However, the immunosuppression produced either by the leukaemic state or by chemotherapy will be likely to reacti-vate a pre-existing latent infection. Usually these infections are mild and superficial but more severe disease with dissemination is recognized.[21,22] Manifestations of HSV infection may be more pro-longed with more persistent viral shedding. Disseminated infections are rare but have been documented and approximately 3 per cent of all bone marrow transplant patients die of HSV infection commonly presenting as pneumonia.[23] Following bone marrow transplantation, HSV infections appear during the first month after transplantation or after induction chemotherapy prior to transplantation.[24] Encephalitis is a rare and potentially fatal complication of primary or reactivated HSV infection[25] but immediate laboratory diagnosis is not essential, as clinical suspicion is sufficient for treatment with acyclovir.

Laboratory confirmation can be achieved retrospectively and no longer requires brain biopsy for diagnosis in view of the unacceptable risk associated with this procedure.

Varicella–zoster (VZ)

Although the severity and frequency of primary VZ infections in children undergoing treatment for Hodgkin's lymphoma, non-Hodgkin's lymphoma and lymphocytic leukaemia are well documented. In our experience, reactivations with this virus in children have been less frequent and milder in comparison.

In Bristol, 50 per cent of children newly presenting with malignant disease, mainly leukaemia, have serological evidence of immunity. Primary infection in susceptible children is a major life-threatening event requiring urgent measures for preventing or at least attenuating infection by post exposure administration of specific immunoglobulin. Alternatively, Japanese workers have described the use of vaccine-boosted immune whole blood transfusion (VIB) for prevention.[26] We would therefore stress the importance of immunity screening at the time of the initial diagnosis.

In contrast, VZ reactivations are a major problem in the bone marrow transplant unit where immunosuppression is much more profound. In a study reported by Atkinson et al.,[27] 65 per cent of a series of 140 bone marrow recipients had VZ infections with dissemination in approximately 6 per cent. Of the 92 infected patients, seven died (7·6 per cent) demonstrating the severity of infection in this group of patients.

Cytomegalovirus (CMV)

This infection is often contracted by intrafamilial and similar close contact such as in daycare nurseries.[28] In under-developed countries with lower standards of hygiene and overcrowding, acquisition of infection occurs at a younger age than in developed countries and approximately 90 per cent of teenagers are seropositive. In contrast, in countries with less crowding and higher living standards, infection is initially acquired later in life.[29,30] Other modes of transmission include blood transfusions in the immunologically normal individual[31–33] or in the immunosuppressed leukaemic child.[34] CMV is recognized as the most important pathogen leading to death following allogenic marrow transplantation with pneumonia as the terminal event. This highlights the need for the administration of CMV seronegative blood to seronegative recipients to avoid the risk of primary infection.[35] Seronegative blood is not required in seropositive patients where infection is due to reactivation and other methods such as prophylaxis with antiviral agents will be required.

Viral procedures during management of the oncology patient

The immune state of each patient with regard to the relevant members of the herpes group, as well as measles and mumps virus, would at this stage be known. This information should be linked via a databank to the ward and to the clinicians concerned. Furthermore, even in the absence of illness, it is of benefit to collect serum samples on a regular basis, preferably at 2–3 monthly intervals or when the patient is being bled for other purposes. This procedure has the advantage that these serum samples act as a baseline for any subsequent illness and is also useful for monitoring sub-clinical infections.

Laboratory methods

Antigen detection methods for vesicular rashes
The most important vesicular rashes are due to HSV and VZ infections. Generalized infections with these viruses are usually readily identified and are distinguishable by the clinicians as being due to one or the other virus. However, in oncology patients, these viruses may present atypically starting with a few spots and here rapid viral diagnosis is essential. Electron microscopy has a crucial role in these circumstances where rapid (within 15 minutes) identification is possible. All oncology units must have access to a 24 hour electron microscopy service. Reliance on electron microscopy should never be complete as occasionally it is necessary to supplement this technique with other antigen detection methods of which currently cell culture is still the most sensitive and widely available. Culture has the disadvantage of producing a retrospective diagnosis and other techniques which give a more rapid result are clearly needed. The use of monoclonal antibodies incorporated into enzyme-linked amplified assays or radioimmune assays[36] clearly has a role in the management of these patients. Monoclonal antibodies might be used to distinguish between the two viruses by immune electron microscopy or immune fluorescence from a scraping from the base of a vesicle. The differentiation of these two viruses would have implications in the control of infection measures to be adopted.

Respiratory infections

In our experience, either nasopharyngeal aspirates or post-nasal aspirates are excellent material for the detection of a wide range of respiratory pathogens. It can be expected that the immunosuppressed child excretes more virus and over a longer period than immunologically competent individuals. The advantages of collecting these specimens is that with the advent of monoclonal antibodies for the detection of RSV, adenovirus, influenza A and B and parainfluenza virus, a rapid diagnosis can be achieved down to a detection level of one infected cell as has been demonstrated for RSV.[37] These clinical specimens are also excellent sources for the detection of respiratory pathogens by either RIA or enzyme-linked immunosorbent assay techniques.[38-41] Such specimens can also be inoculated into cell culture for retrospective diagnosis. Although electron microscopy has been used for the direct detection of respiratory viruses in respiratory secretions[42], its low sensitivity argues against its routine use and our personal experiences support this view.

The role of DNA probes in diagnosis appears promising[43] but they require further evaluation to determine their sensitivity and usefulness in a variety of clinical settings. Although DNA probes have been described for the detection of adenoviruses in respiratory[44] and enteric[45,46] infections, it is more practical at present to utilize virus specific monoclonal antibodies of known sensitivity as a screening technique for a wide range of pathogens. The advantage of probes is that, if used at low stringency, they are able to detect different strains of the same virus. In the future, developments in this area will continue to be made but problems will still occur in the interpretation of positive probe signals in certain clinical settings. Clearly, the laboratory must be prepared for changes in technology, particularly in the areas of immunosuppression where early diagnosis is essential and antiviral therapy will be increasingly relevant.

Pyrexia of unknown origin

This clinical condition is the most common presentation of possible virus infection with an even greater number of non-viral causes. Since PUO can be associated with a wide range of viruses, a full screen is necessary. This involves collecting faeces, urine and respiratory samples as well as paired sera which should be examined by all the techniques described above, including cell culture propagation of those viruses which do not at present lend themselves to rapid diagnosis, i.e. picornaviruses.

Gastroenteritis

Viral causes of gastroenteritis are now well recognized. Rotaviruses are not a problem in these children as the majority of infections have already occurred prior to the onset of their malignancy. Rotavirus, astrovirus, small round virus, calicivirus and enteric adenovirus have been detected together in one patient[47] but this is the exception rather than the rule. The enteric adenoviruses have been associated with an outbreak in an oncology unit (personal observations) which was characterized by mild gastrointestinal symptoms with prolonged excretion of virus. Rapid diagnosis is easily obtained by electron microscopy and this allows appropriate barrier nursing.

Viral meningitis

The presence of lymphocytes in the CSF may not necessarily be due to viral infection but can be related to the leukaemic state or its treatment. However, it is important to investigate each presentation as fully as possible.

Electron microscopy has a limited role in the examination of CSF as there are not enough virus particles to make this a reliable technique. However, use of antibody coated grids increases the sensitivity of antigen detection and may have applications to the detection of picornaviruses. Specimens (CSF, faeces, throat swabs, urine) are inoculated into a range of cell cultures optimal for the detection of picornaviruses and mumps virus as well as for the rarer possibility of other agents.

Laboratory diagnosis of cytomegalovirus infections

As CMV can present in this group of patients as pneumonitis, although this is not common outside profound immunosuppression, the presence of this virus as a cause of infection should always be excluded. Urine samples should be collected and examined by electron microscopy which may occasionally give a rapid answer. The most sensitive technique currently available for the diagnosis of CMV infections is the detection of 'early' antigen in cell cultures previously inoculated with clinical samples using monoclonal antibody.[48] This detection system should be applied to respiratory specimens as well as fresh urine samples for optimal results. At the present time, monoclonal-based ELISAs are being developed for the rapid detection of CMV in urine but are currently hindered by interference with beta-microglobulin. This will be overcome in the near future making cell culture unnecessary for rapid diagnosis.

A summary of techniques available for the rapid diagnosis of the important virus infections in this group of patients is shown in *Table* 2.2.

VACCINATION IN IMMUNOSUPPRESSION

Measles

Due to the low uptake of measles vaccine in many parts of the United Kingdom (50–60 per cent),[49,50] there is a considerable risk of children

Table 2.2. Rapid techniques application to clinical material

| Clinical material | Technology | | | Viruses |
	Electron microscopy	Enzyme-linked immunosorbent assays	Monoclonal IF	Identified
NPA/post nasal aspirate	±	++	+++	Influenza Parainfluenza RSV, Measles Mumps, Adeno CMV
Vesicle fluid/ crust	+++	++	+	Herpes simplex Varicella zoster *Molluscum contagiusum*
Urine	±	+	+++*	CMV* BK/JC Papovavirus
Faeces	+++	+++	−	Rotavirus Adenovirus Astrovirus Calicivirus, SRSV,† Corona-like
Blood	−	++	−	μ-capture ELISA or indirect immunofluorescence IgM for CMV, mycoplasma pneumoniae, rubella, varicella zoster, hepatitis A, measles

* on cell culture grown virus using 'early' monoclonal antibody.
† SRSV—small round structured virus (Norwalk group).

being susceptible on initial diagnosis. In the UK, measles is thought to be the most important infectious risk to these children.[51] Antibody acquired by prior exposure to measles virus pre-diagnosis appears to be protective even when levels decline after induction therapy has been started. Measles vaccination is contraindicated in susceptible children post diagnosis and such children require close monitoring of any contact exposures and passive protection by immunoglobulin.[52]

Rubella vaccination programmes are currently under review and the proposal to use MMR (measles, mumps and rubella) vaccine in children of both sexes at 14 months should, with 'infilling' of children under 12, raise the level of herd immunity to those found in the United States. Eradication of measles virus would then reduce the risk of measles susceptible children presenting with malignant conditions enabling mortality due to this infection to attain the zero levels seen in the United States.

Varicella

In contrast to the situation with measles vaccine which cannot be given to immunocompromised patients, varicella vaccination of susceptible children with malignant disease is increasingly being shown to have an important role in VZ protection,[53] although this is not yet routinely available in the UK. It is safer to vaccinate children during remission and this can be done during maintenance therapy which need only be suspended for 2 weeks. Minimal illness consisting of a mild to moderate rash has been seen in children on maintenance therapy at the time of vaccination. It was shown that, whilst children with a rash developed higher antibody levels than those without, they did have a 10 per cent risk of transmitting the vaccine induced infection to others. Vaccinees were subsequently 80 per cent less likely than controls to develop chickenpox after a household contact and, if they did so, the illness was always mild.[54] It would appear unwise to vaccinate during severe immunosuppression where some uncommon cases of more severe reactions have been described.[55] Moreover, vaccination during induction therapy results in poor immune responses which has led to the suggestion that vaccination should not be done in the first year after diagnosis.[56] The Oka strain developed in Japan appears to be the best candidate vaccine developed so far.[57]

Recent retrospective studies by Brunell et al.,[58] using a live attenuated varicella vaccine (Oka strain), showed that 34 vaccinated children with acute lymphocytic leukaemia did not develop VZ infection over an approximately 6-year period. In contrast, 28 of 149 children who were not vaccinated developed zoster infections after natural varicella. The authors concluded that children who receive varicella vaccine are no more likely to acquire herpes zoster than children who get natural varicella infection.

Other workers have documented a low incidence of VZ in vaccinees compared with naturally infected controls[53] suggesting that vaccinees are less likely to acquire reactivated infections. Considerable data is still needed on the duration of protection after vaccination and the protective levels of immunity required during the decline of antibody induction therapy.

Clinical reinfections with VZ in patients who have pre-existing antibody levels are rare but well known.[59] A very small number of patients who had low levels of antibodies to fluorescent membrane antigen (FAMA) as a result of previous natural infection or vaccination developed mild chickenpox after a defined contact. It is not known yet, because of the small numbers involved, whether this is more common in vaccinated immunocompromised patients but it is not important enough to warrant changing policies on VZ immunity screening and vaccine immunization.

Influenza

Although influenza infections are not commonly a severe problem in children with malignant conditions, serious disease occasionally occurs and it has been our policy to promote annual vaccination in this group.

Antiviral chemotherapy

In the past, the use of antiviral compounds has been fraught with problems of toxicity resulting in arguable benefits to the patient. With the development of newer antivirals, the major problem of toxicity has been largely overcome and the prevention and treatment of some of the life-threatening virus infections, such as herpes simplex, is now highly effective. It is now possible for the first time to look to the future with confidence. A recent report of current trends in antiviral therapy summarizes these developments and the reader is referred to this excellent review.[60]

Herpes simplex

The advent of the anti-herpes drug, acyclovir, has revolutionized the chemotherapy and chemoprophylaxis of patients with malignant disease. Infections with herpes viruses comprise the major risk in the immunocompromised host and since acyclovir is effective in the early treatment of two members of this group (HSV and VZ) the low toxicity of this drug makes it eminently suitable for routine treatment. However, in contrast to early reports, it appears to have little effect in preventing cytomegalovirus infections in immunocompromised hosts.[61]

At the first signs of a vesicular rash, thought clinically to be due to a herpes virus, immediate administration of acyclovir is indicated. Studies have demonstrated that early acyclovir treatment shortens both symptomatology and lesions of mucocutaneous HSV infection in immunocompromised hosts and reduces the possibility of dissemination.[62] In patients known to be seropositive, maintenance doses of acyclovir administered intravenously or orally have been shown to prevent recurrences both during induction therapy and after transplantation.[63] Where immunosuppression is less intense, topical therapy with acyclovir cream may suffice if administered early in the illness.[61]

In suspected disseminated HSV infections, including encephalitis, the clinician should immediately administer acyclovir rather than await laboratory confirmation. Resort to brain biopsy is unacceptable when a drug known to have low toxicity and high specificity is available.[25] Studies have also confirmed the greater effectiveness of acyclovir in these situations in comparison with other anti-herpes drugs such as vidarabine.[64, 65]

Varicella zoster virus

It is now well established that acyclovir is the drug of choice in the treatment and prevention of disseminated infection in either primary or reactivated varicella zoster virus infections. Prober et al.[66] demonstrated that visceral dissemination was preventable following intravenous acyclovir treatment, whilst in placebo control 45 per cent of patients developed disseminated infection. In patients with sero-logical evidence of past exposure undergoing bone marrow trans-plantation, where reactivations are a life-threatening event, it is mandatory to treat prophylactically with intravenous acyclovir.[61]

Although vidarabine has been evaluated and shown to reduce new lesion formation, provided treatment is started within 72 h of onset,[67] this is not the drug of choice, particularly in view of its higher toxicity in comparison with acyclovir. A recent report compared FIAC with vidarabine and found it superior with relatively mild side-effects compared to vidarabine. However, it would seem more appropriate to have compared this antiviral agent with acyclovir.

Cytomegalovirus

In contrast to the situation in HSV and VZ infection, both prophyl-axis and treatment of CMV infections are at a much earlier stage on the road to routine successful chemotherapy. Therapeutic trials in Seattle[69, 70] have shown little benefit in CMV pneumonia using vidarabine, alpha interferon, acyclovir and combinations of these agents, although one author has reported more rapid improvement in a small series of immunocompromised patients with CMV infections who were treated with acyclovir.[71]

The acyclovir analogue DHPG 9 (1,3-dihydroxy-2-propoxy methyl-guanine) (also known as BW 759U) has been used to treat serious CMV infections in a group of patients mainly suffering from AIDS.[72] Whilst patients with CMV pneumonia responded poorly, there appeared to be improvement in patients with CMV retinitis and gastrointestinal disease although relapses occurred in most patients when treatment was discontinued. Early results from the UK show some promise in the early treatment of CMV pneumonitis after bone marrow transplantation[73] and joint European studies are in progress.

Foscarnet (trisodium phosphonoformate) has been found to be effective in CMV infections in immunocompromised patients although not in CMV pneumonitis in bone marrow transplant patients.[74] On the other hand, a preliminary report in two BMT patients with CMV pneumonitis is promising.[75] Another approach has been the use of CMV hyperimmune immunoglobulin, which resulted in a good response in a small series of immunosuppressed renal transplant patients with cytomegalovirus infections.[76] Similar benefit has been found in a group of BMT patients with CMV pneumonitis.[61] In CMV prophylaxis the most important single measure is the use of CMV negative blood products for CMV negative patients which has already been discussed. Most, but not all, reports on the use of passive immunization with high titred immunoglobulin are favourable as long as high antibody levels are attained.[77,78] Alpha interferon prophylaxis prevented CMV infection in a group of renal transplant patients with minimal toxic effects.[79]

Active vaccination, using the Towne strain, has been shown to attenuate (but not prevent) CMV infections in seronegative renal transplant recipients who were given kidneys from seropositive donors.[80] Recent studies in BMT patients suggest that there may also be beneficial results with live vaccine in this group of patients but the authors suggest caution.[61]

Influenza and respiratory syncytial virus

Influenza

It has been shown that amantadine hydrochloride is effective in reducing influenza A symptoms when given early in the illness.[81] In addition, maintenance doses of this antiviral will prevent clinical infection during an outbreak. The authors' policy following the recognition and laboratory diagnosis, by direct immunofluorescence from nasopharyngeal aspirates, of the index case, is to vaccinate contacts and treat with amantadine for 2 weeks to enable adequate levels of antibody to appear.

Respiratory syncytial virus (RSV)

The synthetic triazole ribavirin has been successfully used in the treatment of severe RSV infections, particularly in children with underlying heart and chest defects or in immunosuppression. The drug has been administered as an aerosol via a respirator and should be considered for use in severe RSV infections in this group of patients. It has the additional benefit of being active in severe parainfluenza infections.[82]

REFERENCES

1. Weller T. H. (1983) Varicella and herpes zoster. Changing concepts of the natural history, control and importance of a not-so-benign virus. *N. Engl. J. Med.* **309**, 1434–40.
2. Cory L. and Spear P. G. (1986) Infections with herpes simplex viruses. *N. Engl. J. Med.* **314**, 749–57.
3. Weiner R. S., Bortin M. M. and Gale R. P. (1986) Interstitial pneumonitis after bone marrow transplantation. *Ann. Intern. Med.* **104**, 168–75.
4. Ninane J. and Chessels J. M. (1981) Serious infections during continuing treatment of acute lymphoblastic leukemia. *Arch. Dis. Child.* **56**, 841–4.
5. Wood D. J. and Corbitt G. (1985) Viral infections in childhood leukemia. *J. Infect. Dis.* **152**, 266–73.
6. Kosmidis H. V., Lusher J. M., Shope T. C. et al. (1980) Infections in leukemic children—a prospective analysis. *J. Pediatr.* **96**, 814–19.
7. Arthur R. R., Shah K. V., Baust S. J. et al. (1986) Association of BK viruria with haemorrhagic cystitis in recipients of bone marrow transplants. *N. Engl. J. Med.* **315**, 230–4.
8. Koss L. G. (1987) BK virus and haemorrhagic cystitis. *N. Engl. J. Med.* **316**, 108.
9. Verdonck L. F., Dekker A. W., Rosenberg-Arska M. et al. (1987) *N. Engl. J. Med.* **316**, 109.
10. Supran E. M. (1984) Elisa: an update on the method and the interpretation of results—with apologies for the virological bias. Public Health Laboratory Service. *Microbiol. Digest* **1**, 36–43.
11. Booth J. C., Hannington G., Bakir T. M. F. et al. (1982) Comparison of enzyme linked immunosorbent assay, radioimmunoassay, complement fixation, anti-complement immunofluorescence, and passive haemaglutination techniques for detecting cytomegalovirus IgG antibody. *J. Clin. Pathol.* **35**, 1345–8.
12. Williams V., Gershon A. and Brunell P. A. (1974) Serological response to varicella zoster membrane antigens measured by indirect immunofluorescence. *J. Infect. Dis.* **130**, 669–72.
13. Cradock-Watson J. E. and Ridehalgh M. K. S. (1979) Specific immunoglobulin responses after varicella and herpes zoster. *J. Hyg. (Camb.)* **82**, 319–36.
14. Zaia J. A. and Oxman N. M. (1977) Antibody to varicella zoster virus induced membrane antigen: immunofluorescence assay using monodisperse glutaralde-hyde-fixed target cells. *J. Infect. Dis.* **136**, 519–30.
15. Heath R. B. (1981) New thoughts on chickenpox. *Hospital Update* **7**, 817–28.
16. Hastie I. R. (1980) Varicella zoster virus affecting immigrant nurses. *Lancet* **ii**, 154–5.
17. Gershon A. A., Raker R., Steinberg S. et al. (1976) Antibody to varicella zoster virus in parturient women and their offspring during the first year of life. *Pediatrics* **58**, 692–6.
18. Bottiger M. and Norrby E. (1983) The epidemiology of virus diseases. In: Lycke E. and Norrby E. (eds.) *Textbook of Medical Virology*. London, Butterworth, p. 202–12.
19. Rosen F. S. (1977) Lymphoma, immunodeficiency and the Epstein Barr virus. *N. Engl. J. Med.* **297**, 1120–1.

20. Morgan E. and Rapp F. (1977) Measles virus and its associated disease. *Bacteriol. Rev.* **41**, 636–66.
21. Hann I. M., Prentice H. G., Blacklock H. A. et al. (1983) Acyclovir prophylaxis against herpes virus infections in severely immunocompromised patients: randomized double blind trial. *Br. Med. J.* **287**, 384–8.
22. Jeffries D. J. (1985) Clinical use of acyclovir. *Br. Med. J.* **290**, 177–8.
23. Ramsey P. G., Fife K. H., Hackman R. C. et al. (1982) Herpes simplex pneumonia: clinical, virologic and pathologic features in 20 patients. *Ann. Intern. Med.* **97**, 813–20.
24. Saral R., Burns W. H. and Prentice H. G. (1984) Herpes virus infections: clinical manifestations and therapeutic strategies in immunocompromised patients. *Clin. Haematol.* **13**, 645–60.
25. Brett E. M. (1986) Herpes simplex virus encephalitis in children. *Br. Med. J.* **293**, 1388–9.
26. Takao H. (1984) Prevention of varicella in immunocompromised patients on unpredictable occurrence of the disease in a children's ward: vaccine boostered immune whole blood transfusion (VIB) method. *Biken J.* **27**, 137–41.
27. Atkinson K., Meyers J. D., Storb R. et al. (1980) Varicella zoster virus infection after marrow transplantation for aplastic anemia or leukemia. *Transplantation* **29**, 47–50.
28. Pass R. F., Hutto C., Ricks R. et al. (1986) Increased risk of cytomegalovirus infection among patients of children attending day care centers. *N. Engl. J. Med.* **314**, 1414–18.
29. Alford C. A., Stagnio S. and Pass R. F. (1980) Natural history of perinatal cytomegalovirus infection. *Excerpta Med. Ciba Foundation Sympos.* **77**, 125–47.
30. Krech U. H., Jung M. and Jung F. (1971) Mode of transmission. In: Karger S. (ed.) *Cytomegalovirus Infections of Man.* Switzerland, Basel, pp. 18–35.
31. Perham T. G. M., Caul E. O., Conway P. J. et al. (1971) Cytomegalovirus infection in blood donors—a prospective study. *Br. J. Haematol.* **20**, 307–20.
32. Caul E. O., Clarke S. K. R., Mott M. G. et al. (1971) Cytomegalovirus infections after open heart surgery. *Lancet* **i**, 777–81.
33. Adler S. P., McVoy M. and Baggett J. (1985) Transfusion associated cytomegalovirus infections in seropositive cardiac surgery patients. *Lancet* **ii**, 743–6.
34. Caul E. O., Dickinson V. A., Roome A. P. et al. (1972) Cytomegalovirus infections in leukaemic children. *Int. J. Cancer* **10**, 213–20.
35. Meyers J. D., Flournoy N. and Thomas E. D. (1986) Risk factors for cytomegalovirus infection after human marrow transplantation. *J. Infect. Dis.* **153**, 478–88.
36. Richman D. D., Cleveland P. H., Redfield D. C. et al. (1984) Rapid viral diagnosis. *J. Infect. Dis.* **149**, 298–310.
37. Freke A., Stott E. J., Roome A. P. C. H. et al. (1986) The detection of respiratory syncytial virus in nasopharyngeal aspirates: assessment, formulation and evaluation of monoclonal antibodies as a diagnostic reagent. *J. Med. Virol.* **18**, 181–91.
38. Sarkkinen H. K., Halonene P., Arstila P. P. et al. (1981) Detection of respiratory syncytial, parainfluenza type 2, and adenovirus antigens by radioimmune assay and enzyme immunoassay on nasopharyngeal specimens for children with acute respiratory disease. *J. Clin. Microbiol.* **13**, 258–61.
39. Hornsleth A., Brene E., Friss B. et al. (1981) Detection of respiratory syncytial virus in nasopharyngeal secretions by inhibition of enzyme linked immunosorbent assay. *J. Clin. Microbiol.* **14**, 510–15.
40. Hornsleth A., Friss B., Anderson P. et al. (1982) Detection of respiratory syncytial virus in nasopharyngeal secretions by ELISA: comparison with fluorescent antibody technique. *J. Med. Virol.* **10**, 273–81.
41. McIntosh K., Hendry R. M., Fahnestock M. L. et al. (1982) Enzyme linked immunosorbent assay for detection of respiratory syncytial virus infection: application to clinical samples. *J. Clin. Microbiol.* **16**, 329–33.

42. Doane F. W., Chatiyanouda K., McClean D. M. et al. (1967) Rapid laboratory diagnosis of paramyxovirus infection by electron microscopy. *Lancet* ii, 751.
43. Macrae M. A. (1984) DNA probes in diagnosis: practicalities and potential. *PHLS Microbiol. Digest* 1, 44–7.
44. Virtanen M., Palva A., Laaksonen M. et al. (1983) Novel test for rapid viral diagnosis: detection of adenovirus in nasopharyngeal mucus aspirates by means of nucleic acid sandwich hybridization. *Lancet* i, 381–3.
45. Kidd A. H., Harley E. H. and Erasmus M. J. (1985) Specific detection and typing of adenovirus types 40 and 41 in stool specimens by dot-blot hybridization. *J. Clin. Microbiol.* 22, 934–9.
46. Takiff E. H., Seidlin M., Krause P. et al. (1985) Detection of enteric adenoviruses by dot-blot hybridization using a molecularly cloned viral DNA probe. *J. Med. Virol.* 16, 107–18.
47. Christie I. L., Booth I. W., Kidd A. H. et al. (1982) Multiple faecal virus excretion in immunodeficiency. *Lancet* i, 282.
48. Griffiths P. D., Panjwani D. D., Stirk P. R. et al. (1984) Rapid diagnosis of cytomegalovirus infection in immunocompromised patients by detection of early antigen fluorescent foci. *Lancet* ii, 1242–5.
49. Eden O. B., Hann I. M., Glass S. et al. (1986) Measles exposure and the immunosuppressed child. *Lancet* ii, 283.
50. Noah N. D. (1982) Measles eradication policies. *Br. Med. J.* 284, 997–8.
51. Eden O. B., Glass S., Gray M. et al. (1986) Measles and the immunosuppressed child. *Lancet* ii, 691.
52. Kay H. E. M. and Rankin A. (1984) Immunoglobulin prophylaxis of measles in acute lymphoblastic leukaemia. *Lancet* i, 901–2.
53. Kimura M. and Takahasi M. (eds.) (1984) A live varicella vaccine (Oka strain). Symposium of the International Workshop on Live Varicella Vaccine, Osaka, Japan. *Biken J.* 27, 31–141.
54. Gershon A. A., Steinberg S. P., Gelb I. et al. (1984) Live attenuated varicella vaccine—efficacy for children with leukemia in remission. *JAMA* 252, 355–62.
55. Katsushima N., Yasaki N. and Sakamoto M. (1984) Effect and follow-up *Biken J.* 27, 51–8.
56. Brunell P. A., Taylor Wiedeman J., Shehab Z. M. et al. (1984) Administration of varicella vaccine to children with leukemia. *Biken J.* 27, 83–8.
57. Takahashi M., Otsuka T., Okuno Y. et al. (1974) Live vaccine used to prevent the spread of varicella in children in hospital. *Lancet* ii, 1288–90.
58. Brunell P. A., Taylor Wiedeman J., Geister C. F. et al. (1986) Risk of herpes zoster in children with leukemia: varicella vaccine compared with history of chickenpox. *Pediatrics* 77, 53–6.
59. Gershon A. A., Steinberg S. and Gelb L. (1984) Clinical reinfection due to varicella zoster virus. *J. Infect. Dis.* 149, 137–42.
60. Tyrrell D. A. J. and Oxford J. S. (eds.) (1985) Antiviral chemotherapy and interferon. *Br. Med. Bull.* 41, 307–405.
61. Prentice H. G. and Hann I. M. (1985) Antiviral therapy in the immunocompromised patient. *Br. Med. Bull.* 41, 367–73.
62. Bucker C. D., Clift R. A., Fefer A. et al. (1982) Bone marrow transplantation. In: Hoffbrand A. V. (ed.) *Recent Advances In Haematology,* 3rd edition. Edinburgh, Churchill Livingstone, pp. 144–59.
63. Corey L. and Spear P. G. (1986) Infections with herpes simplex viruses (2), *N. Engl. J. Med.* 314, 749–57.
64. Whitley R. J., Alford C. A. and Hirsch M. S. (1986) Vidarabine versus acyclovir therapy in herpes simplex encephalitis *N. Engl. J. Med.* 314, 144–9.
65. Skildenberg B., Fosgren M., Alestig K. et al. (1984) Acyclovir versus vidarabine in herpes simplex encephalitis. Randomized multicentre study in consecutive Swedish patients. *Lancet* ii, 707–11.

66. Prober C. G., Kirk L. E. and Keeney R. E. (1982) Acyclovir therapy of chicken-pox in immunosuppressed children—a collaborative study. *J. Pediatr.* **101**, 622–5.
67. Shepp D. H., Dandliker P. S. and Meyers J. D. (1986) Treatment of varicella zoster virus infections in severely immunocompromised patients. A randomized comparison of acyclovir and vidarabine. *N. Engl. J. Med.* **314**, 208–12.
68. Leyland-Jones B., Donnelly H., Myskowski P. et al. (1983) FIAC, a potent anti-viral agent: therapeutic efficacy against varicella zoster infections in immuno-suppressed patients and metabolism. In: Easmon C. S. F. and Gaya H. (eds.) *International Symposium on Infection in the Immunocompromised Host*, No. 60. London, Academic Press, pp. 39–42.
69. Meyers J. D., McGuffin R. W., Neiman P. E. et al. (1980) Toxicity and efficacy of human leukocyte interferon for treatment of cytomegalovirus pneumonia after marrow transplantation. *J. Infect. Dis.* **141**, 555–62.
70. Meyers J. D., McGuffin R. W., Bryson Y. J. et al. (1982) Treatment of cyto-megalovirus pneumonia after marrow transplant with combined vidarabine and human leukocyte interferon. *J. Infect. Dis.* **146**, 80–4.
71. Balfour H. H. Jr., Bean B., Mitchell C. D. et al. (1982) Acyclovir in immuno-compromised patients with cytomegalovirus disease. A controlled trial at one institution. *Am. J. Med.* **73**(1A), 241–8.
72. Collaborative DHPG Study Group (1986) Treatment of serious cytomegalovirus infections with 9 (1-3 dihydroxy-2-propoxymethyl) guanine in patients with AIDS and other immunodeficiencies. *N. Engl. J. Med.* **314**, 801–5.
73. Selby P., Poules R. C., Jameson B. et al. (1986) Treatment of cytomegalovirus pneumonitis after bone marrow transplantation with 9-[2 hydroxy-1-(hydroxymethyl)ethoxymethyl] guanine. *Lancet* i, 1377–8.
74. Oberg B. and Lernestedt J. O. (1983) Foscarnet, antiviral properties and clinical efficacy. In: Easmon C. S. F. and Gaya J. (eds.) *International Symposium on Infection in the Immunocompromised Host*, No. 60. London, Academic Press. pp. 43–6.
75. Apperley J. F., Marcus R. E., Goldman J. M. et al. (1986) Foscarnet for cyto-megalovirus pneumonitis. *Lancet* i, 1151.
76. Nicholls A. J., Brown C. B., Edwards N. et al. (1983) Hyperimmune immuno-globulin for cytomegalovirus infections. *Lancet* i, 532–3.
77. Bowden R. A., Sayers M., Flournoy N. et al. (1986) Cytomegalovirus immune globulin and seronegative blood products to prevent primary cytomegalovirus infection after marrow transplantation. *N. Engl. J. Med.* **314**, 1006–10.
78. Meyers J. D., Levzczynski J., Zaia J. A. et al. (1983) Prevention of cytomegalo-virus infection by cytomegalovirus immune globulin after marrow transplantation. *Ann. Intern. Med.* **98**, 442–6.
79. Hirsch M. S., Schooley R. T., Cosimi A. B. et al. (1983) Effect of interferon—alpha on cytomegalovirus reactivation syndromes in renal transplant recipients. *N. Engl. J. Med.* **308**, 1489–93.
80. Plotkin S. A., Friedman H. M., Fleisher G. R. et al. (1984) Towne vaccine induced prevention of cytomegalovirus disease after renal transplants. *Lancet* i, 528–30.
81. Galbraith A. L. L. (1985) Influenza—recent developments in prophylaxis and treatment. *Br. Med. J.* **41**, 381–5.
82. Editorial (1986) Ribavirin and respiratory syncytial virus. *Lancet* i, 362–3.

3.   Fungal Infection

D. Warnock

INTRODUCTION

Invasive fungal infections have become important causes of illness and death among immunosuppressed children. The organisms responsible for these infections can be divided into 2 groups: the pathogens and the opportunists. The former can produce deep infection after inhalation in non-immunosuppressed hosts, although the initial illness is often asymptomatic. These infections tend to occur in or near defined endemic regions in the Americas or the Tropics and include diseases such as histoplasmosis and coccidio-idomycosis. These infections have caused serious problems among immunosuppressed children in North America, but are seldom encountered in Europe.

The opportunist fungal infections include diseases such as aspergil-losis and candidosis and are most often seen in immunosuppressed patients. These infections have a global distribution. The organisms responsible often gain access to the host through the lungs, but the gastrointestinal tract and intravascular lines are other important sources of deep infection. These conditions often present difficult problems both of diagnosis and of subsequent management.

CANDIDOSIS

This is the most prevalent fungal infection among immunosuppressed children. *Candida albicans* is the most important cause of both superficial and deep forms of candidosis (candidiasis) in such patients, although the proportion of serious infections attributed to other members of the genus such as *C. tropicalis* and *C. parapsilosis* is rising.

Most *C. albicans* infections are endogenous in origin. This fungus is found as a commensal in the mouth and gastrointestinal tract of a substantial proportion of the normal population. It can be recovered from the mouth of around 10–30 per cent of normal children, but much higher rates have been recorded among immunosuppressed patients.

People colonized with *C. albicans* possess a number of defence mechanisms which prevent the fungus from establishing an infection. In the normal child, these anatomical and immunological mechanisms are sufficient to resist the fungus, but the balance between host and pathogen is a fine one. In the common, superficial forms of candidosis, trivial impairments of host defence are often sufficient to allow *C. albicans,* the most pathogenic member of the genus, to establish an infection. More serious impairment of the host can lead to lethal deep infection, often with less pathogenic species such as *C. tropicalis*.

Numerous predisposing factors have been associated with deep forms of candidosis. Neutrophil PMN cells form the earliest and most efficient host defence mechanism against deep *C. albicans* infection. Thus, low neutrophil counts and defects in neutrophil function because of disease or its treatment are important predisposing factors. Therapeutic procedures which damage anatomical barriers against infection are additional factors predisposing patients to candidosis. Thus, indwelling vascular catheters for drug administration or total parenteral nutrition have been associated with fungal sepsis. Administration of drugs that cause ulceration of the mouth or gastro-intestinal tract is an important predisposing factor because this site is the usual source of organisms that give rise to deep forms of candidosis. Oral and parenteral antibiotics are regarded as predisposing factors because their administration often has a profound effect on the microbial population of the gastrointestinal tract and can lead to proliferation of *C. albicans* in the intestinal contents.

Clinical manifestations and diagnosis of candidosis

In the immunosuppressed child, the mouth is often the initial site of *C. albicans* infection. Oral candidosis is a frequent problem in children undergoing treatment for cancer and is most prevalent in patients receiving drugs which lead to mucositis. Oesophagitis is a less frequent, but more serious, complication of such treatment; mucosal perforation can lead to haematogenous dissemination of the fungus. In most immunosuppressed children with deep *C. albicans* infection, more than one organ is affected.

Oral candidosis

This infection is most common in children with drug-induced oral mucositis. The characteristic white, raised lesions erupt on the buccal mucosa, tongue, gums and throat and can develop to become confluent. On removal, an eroded, bleeding surface is left. The lesions are often painless although erosion and mucosal ulceration can occur.

In some patients, oral candidosis is difficult to distinguish from drug-induced mucositis and it is important to confirm the diagnosis with isolation of the fungus in culture from smears or scrapings of lesions, and detection of fungus in wet-mount preparations or Gram-stained smears.

Oesophageal candidosis

This condition tends to occur in immunosuppressed patients with oral candidosis. It must be distinguished from herpetic oesophagitis which can give rise to similar symptoms and clinical and radiological findings.

The principal symptoms are dysphagia and retrosternal pain. On barium swallow examination, clusters of small, filling defects are outlined in the oesophagus. Endoscopic examination can confirm the diagnosis; the characteristic finding is white plaques adherent to hyperaemic, haemorrhagic mucosa. However, this procedure should be avoided in patients who are neutropenic and thrombocytopenic.

Gastrointestinal candidosis

The antemortem diagnosis of gastrointestinal tract infection with *C. albicans*, other than oesophagitis, is difficult. Most infections are asymptomatic, although infection of the bowel has sometimes been associated with abdominal pain, diarrhoea and rectal bleeding. Mucosal ulcerations, erosions and perforations are the most common lesions and can be the source of disseminated deep infection.

Candidaemia

The isolation of *C. albicans* or another member of the genus from the blood of an immunosuppressed child must be regarded as a potential indication of disseminated deep infection. Intravenous lines should be changed or removed, catheter tips should be cultured and blood cultures should be repeated. The patient should be examined for signs of disseminated candidosis such as macronodular skin lesions, retinal lesions, or candiduria. Antifungal treatment should be given if the child fails to improve after removal of intravenous lines, if blood cultures remain positive, or if there are other signs of deep candidosis.

Disseminated candidosis

In the immunosuppressed child, the most frequent manifestation of this condition is persistent fever which fails to respond to broad-spectrum antibacterial treatment. Other useful clinical signs that can assist the diagnosis include ocular lesions or visual loss, rash and muscular tenderness and pain. In some patients, oral or oesophageal infection with *C. albicans* will be apparent.

Ocular pain and visual loss have been recognized as frequent manifestations of disseminated *C. albicans* infection in patients receiving total parenteral nutrition. However, endophthalmitis is much less common in neutropenic individuals. Typical retinal lesions are white plaques with or without vitreous haze.

Characteristic skin lesions occur in some patients with disseminated candidosis. The lesions are discrete, erythematous nodules which can be single, multiple, localized or diffuse. Aspiration and culture of lesions will establish the diagnosis. Occasional patients with disseminated candidosis develop myositis. The patients complain of muscle tenderness and pain on palpation. Most of these individuals also have skin lesions.

Diagnosis of deep forms of candidosis

The diagnosis of deep infection with *C. albicans* is often difficult to establish because the clinical presentation is non-specific and the microbiological and serological findings are insufficient or confusing. The clinician should suspect deep candidosis if an immunosuppressed child develops persistent fever resistant to broad-spectrum antibiotic treatment, has mucosal candidosis or mucosal colonization with *C. albicans,* or infection with the fungus at a catheter insertion site.

If deep candidosis is suspected, repeated attempts should be made to recover the organism. Isolation of *C. albicans* from superficial sites such as the mouth, or from sputum or faecal specimens is seldom significant. The diagnosis of deep infection requires isolation of the fungus from blood, or from cerebrospinal, pleural, peritoneal or ascitic fluids, or from other closed sites, or from cutaneous lesions. Isolation of *C. albicans* from blood specimens is often unsuccessful in patients with deep infection. However, lysis-centrifugation and lysis-filtration methods can permit earlier diagnosis of infection. Isolation of the fungus from CSF specimens often requires repeated culture of large amounts of fluid. Isolation from urine is often an indication of serious infection, provided the child is not catheterized.

Serological tests can assist the diagnosis of deep candidosis in the immunosuppressed child. However, precipitins to certain antigens of *C. albicans* are often found in patients without significant infection. Nor is the detection of such precipitins a consistent finding in children with deep *C. albicans* infection. One positive serological test does not warrant the institution of antifungal treatment, although a high precipitin titre in conjunction with other findings might suggest serious infection. Serological tests should be repeated at frequent intervals and persistently high or rising titres regarded as suspicious.

Methods for detection of circulating *C. albicans* antigen have been devised and their usefulness has been demonstrated in an increasing number of immunosuppressed patients. GLC methods for detection of fungal products such as arabinitol also appear promising. The detection of antigen in a child with suspected candidosis should be regarded as an indication for antifungal treatment.

Histopathological demonstration of the fungus in tissue is diagnostic, but apart from cutaneous lesions, material is often difficult to obtain antemortem.

Treatment of candidosis

Most children with oral candidosis will respond to topical treatment. One ml of nystatin oral suspension (100000 u) should be placed in the mouth and 'swished' several times before swallowing. Treatment should be repeated at 4- to 6-hourly intervals. Nystatin oral suspension can also be used to treat mild oesophageal candidosis. Ingestion of 5 ml of suspension (500000 u) at 4-hourly intervals is recommended.

Oral and oesphageal lesions can be treated with miconazole oral gel. For best results, the gel should be retained in the mouth for as long as possible. Miconazole oral tablets can also be used; these should be allowed to dissolve in the mouth before swallowing. In children aged over 6, the recommended dose of oral gel is 5 ml at 6-hourly intervals; in children aged 2–6, 5 ml at 12-hourly intervals; and in children under 2, 2·5 ml at 12-hourly intervals. Treatment should be continued for 48 h after symptoms and signs have cleared.

If local treatment of oral or oesophageal candidosis fails, parenteral treatment with amphotericin B should be considered; a dose of 10 mg.d^{-1} for 1 or 2 weeks should be sufficient for oral lesions.

Amphotericin B remains the treatment of choice for deep infection with *C. albicans*. In most patients, a total dose of 1–2 g over 6–10 weeks is sufficient. Treatment should be continued until all symptoms and signs have disappeared.

Amphotericin B treatment should be initiated with a test dose of 1 mg of drug in 250 ml of 5 per cent dextrose solution given over 2–4 h. The patient's pulse rate and temperature should be recorded at half-hourly intervals during this infusion. If the test dose is tolerated, the dose can be increased in 5 or 10 mg increments up to a maximum of $0·6 \text{ mg.kg}^{-1}.\text{d}^{-1}$ if subsequent infusions are given at 24-hourly intervals, or $1·0 \text{ mg.kg}^{-1}.\text{d}^{-1}$ if given at 48-hourly intervals. The time required to reach full dosage will depend on the clinical condition of the patient. If the prognosis is bad, it is reasonable to attempt to administer sufficient drug to produce therapeutic concentrations within the first 24–48 h. If the condition of the patient is less critical, then a gradual escalation of the dose is preferable.

It is impossible to predict a patient's reaction to amphotericin B infusion. This can range from mild fever and nausea to high temperatures, rigors, vomiting, hypotension and delirium. Local thrombophlebitis at the infusion site is a further complication. Patients often show a threshold dosage above which side-effects are intolerable. If these cannot be eased with hydrocortisone or an antihistamine, antiemetic or sedative, then it is wisest to accept this threshold dosage as the highest that can be given.

Impairment of renal function occurs in almost all children treated with amphotericin B. Renal function tests should be performed twice per week during treatment. If the blood urea level rises higher than 17 mmol.l^{-1} or the serum creatinine level to higher than 100 nmol.l^{-1}, the drug should be discontinued until renal function returns below this level. Although nephrotoxic side-effects often limit the duration of amphotericin B treatment, the drug can be continued until the above limits of renal function are reached.

Amphotericin B is often used in combination with flucytosine (5-fluorocytosine) for the treatment of deep *C. albicans* infection. Unlike amphotericin B, flucytosine is well absorbed after oral administration and shows good penetration into the CSF, ocular and other fluids, and urine. However, emergence of resistance has been a frequent complication of treatment and flucytosine should not be used alone in children with deep candidosis.

If the combination regimen is used, the dose of amphotericin B can be reduced to 0·3–0·5 mg.kg^{-1}.d^{-1}. If renal function is normal, flucytosine is given at 150–200 mg.kg^{-1}.d^{-1} in 4 divided doses at 6-hourly intervals. Where there is impaired renal excretion of flucytosine, the interval between doses should be increased. Blood levels must be monitored and doses adjusted to maintain concentrations between 100 and 30 mg.l^{-1}. At blood concentrations greater than 100 mg.l^{-1}, the drug can cause bone marrow depression.

Miconazole is available as an intravenous preparation. It is better tolerated than amphotericin B, but penetration into the CSF and urine is poor. It is best regarded as a second choice drug in children with deep candidosis and should not be considered unless amphotericin B and flucytosine are not indicated or have proven toxic or unsuccessful. Miconazole has proved successful in patients with oesophageal candidosis. In children older than 12 months, the recommended dose is 20–40 mg.kg^{-1}.d^{-1}. Each infusion should not exceed 15 mg.kg^{-1}. The drug must be given diluted in 5 per cent dextrose solution or saline and infused over a period of at least

30 min. The duration of treatment will differ from patient to patient, but the drug should be continued until tests indicate that fungal infection is no longer present. Thrombophlebitis has been a common problem, but can be reduced by using a subclavian catheter or changing the infusion site at 48-hourly intervals. Nausea and vomiting can be mitigated with an antihistamine or antiemetic given prior to the infusion, or by reducing the dose, slowing the infusion, or avoiding administration near mealtimes. Pruritus has necessitated discontinuation of miconazole treatment in some patients.

Oral treatment with ketoconazole is not recommended for the treatment of deep forms of candidosis, but it can be considered for treatment of oral infection or oesophagitis. The recommended dose is $6 \text{ mg} \cdot \text{kg}^{-1} \cdot \text{d}^{-1}$.

ASPERGILLOSIS

Aspergillus fumigatus is the principal cause of the second most prevalent fungal infection among immunosuppressed children. Inhalation of spores of this ubiquitous saprobic fungus can give rise to a number of different clinical forms of aspergillosis, depending upon the immunological status of the host. In the non-compromised individual, *Aspergillus* can act as a potent allergen, or cause non-invasive lung infection. Invasive lung infection with haematogenous dissemination of the fungus occurs in the compromised host. This condition is often fatal even if diagnosed during life and treated. It must, however, be emphasized that with prompt diagnosis, successful treatment can often be achieved.

Invasive aspergillosis most often occurs in patients with haematological neoplasia, in transplant recipients, and in children with genetic defects of neutrophil PMN cell function. It is much less common in patients with solid tumours. Not all the factors that compromise the immunological response are as liable to predispose the host to *Aspergillus* infection. Defects of immunoglobulin production or of late complement components do not appear to be important risk factors. In contrast, more than 50 per cent of patients with invasive lung infection and more than 75 per cent with disseminated infection are neutropenic. It is common for *Aspergillus* infection to develop in leukaemic patients undergoing remission induction treatment, or during bone marrow transplantation.

A. fumigatus is often found in decomposing organic matter. Inhalation of spores that have been released into the air is the usual mode of infection in man. Clusters of *Aspergillus* infections have occurred among immunocompromised patients in cancer hospitals and transplant units and have been attributed to environmental

contamination of ventilation systems. Several interesting epidemiological investigations have demonstrated that release of spore-laden
dust during building renovation or reconstruction can lead to out-
breaks of nosocomial aspergillosis in immunosuppressed patients.

Clinical manifestations of aspergillosis

The clinical presentation of *Aspergillus* infection in the immunosuppressed child is varied and diagnosis is difficult. The typical patient
is neutropenic and has been receiving broad-spectrum antibiotic
treatment for proven or suspected bacterial infection. Fever and
cough are the most frequent clinical signs and pleuritic chest pain is
not unusual.

Chest radiological signs are often minimal or absent at the onset of
illness. The radiological presentation is varied, but homogenous,
diffuse infiltrates are uncommon. Focal lesions are normal. Multiple
lesions are common and tend to be peripheral in distribution. Large,
wedge-shaped infiltrates suggest aspergillosis although a similar
pattern is seen in bacterial pneumonitis and embolism with infarction.
The characteristic pathological finding is vascular invasion with
consequent thrombosis and ischaemic necrosis of surrounding lung
tissue.

Haematogenous dissemination of infection from the lung occurs in
a significant proportion of patients. In most children with CNS
involvement, lesions are found in the lungs although, on occasion,
direct spread from the nasal sinuses or ear can occur. The characteristic lesions in the brain consist of haemorrhagic infarction with
abscess formation. Meningeal involvement is uncommon. Confusion,
behavioural alterations, or declining consciousness (in particular if it
is coupled with the development of focal neurological signs or fits) in
an immunosuppressed child with lung changes suggest cerebral
progression of aspergillosis. The most common CSF findings are an
elevated protein and a normal glucose.

Gastrointestinal tract involvement in disseminated *Aspergillus*
infection is common. Oesophageal ulceration is the characteristic
lesion and bleeding (which can be fatal) is the most frequent manifestation. Aspergillus oesophagitis must be distinguished from viral
and other forms of oesophagitis.

Renal infection occurs in a few patients with disseminated
aspergillosis. Haematuria, proteinuria and pyuria are common. Renal
impairment developing during the treatment of aspergillosis may be
an indication of renal infection rather than a side-effect of amphotericin B treatment. This is a difficult situation as opposite changes in
treatment are indicated.

Cardiac involvement is unusual in patients with disseminated aspergillosis. Myocardial abscesses, myocarditis and pericarditis are the usual lesions. Aspergillus endocarditis is uncommon with disseminated infection.

Cutaneous lesions can occur in children with disseminated aspergillosis. Subcutaneous or cutaneous abscesses, pustules or maculopapular nodules can develop, often at multiple sites indicating haematogenous spread. In some leukaemic children, cutaneous *Aspergillus* infection has resulted from direct inoculation of the fungus at catheter insertion sites. Lesions can progress to ulceration and black eschar formation.

Diagnosis of aspergillosis

The diagnosis of aspergillosis is difficult. Isolation of the fungus is often sufficient reason for initiating antifungal treatment, but it is less than proof of infection. For this, histopathological confirmation is required. If treatment is initiated on suspicion, it should not be discontinued without good reason.

Isolation of *A. fumigatus* or *A. flavus* from sputum of an immunosuppressed child with fever that is not responding to antibacterial treatment, or with a lung infiltrate, should be regarded as an indication for prompt antifungal treatment. If the isolation of *Aspergillus* from sputum is ignored because of clinical improvement, remission of the underlying condition, or reduction in immunosuppression, or because the child does not have a lung infiltrate, the fact that the fungus has been isolated should be noted, in particular if further immunosuppression is planned.

If sputum investigation is unrewarding in an immunosuppressed patient with a lung infiltrate, transtracheal aspiration should be attempted. If this is unsuccessful, and the risk of fungal infection is great, then transbronchial or transthoracic methods can be considered, provided the patient can withstand the procedure. The method of choice will depend on local expertise. Nasal culture is a useful screening method, but must not be relied on for diagnosing aspergillosis.

Aspergillus is seldom isolated from blood, CSF or urine specimens from children with disseminated aspergillosis. If present, cutaneous lesions can be biopsied. Histopathological examination and culture will establish the diagnosis.

If *Aspergillus* precipitins are detected in an immunosuppressed patient with lung infiltrates, then the diagnosis of aspergillosis should be suspected and antifungal treatment should be considered. Testing serial blood specimens for precipitins is often useful, but it should be remembered that a substantial proportion of infected patients give negative findings. Methods for detection of circulating *Aspergillus* antigen have been devised, but recent work suggests that rapid host metabolism of fungal galactomannan could account for the frequent failure to detect this antigen in infected patients.

Treatment of aspergillosis

The successful management of aspergillosis in children with cancer is dependent upon prompt diagnosis and treatment of the infection and resolution of the underlying malignant condition. Success often depends on haematological remission.

Amphotericin B remains the drug of choice for the treatment of *Aspergillus* infection in immunosuppressed children. If this diagnosis is suspected in a deteriorating patient, fear of the nephrotoxic side-effects of the drug should not lead to hesitation in its use.

The dosage regimen of amphotericin B for aspergillosis is identical to that detailed earlier for candidosis. The amount of drug that should be administered and the duration of treatment will depend on the clinical and microbiological course of the individual patient. Adult patients have been cured of aspergillosis with 1–3 g of amphotericin B given over 6–8 weeks. If less than optimal dosage is used, more prolonged treatment may be advisable.

CRYPTOCOCCOSIS

Cryptococcus neoformans infection most often involves the central nervous system and lungs. However, bone and cutaneous infections, amongst others, are also seen. Cryptococcosis is not common in childhood. As with adult infection, meningitis is the most common clinical manifestation.

Cr. neoformans is found in soil, but is most abundant in pigeon habitats. Inhalation of fungal cells when dried droppings (or other contaminated matter) are disturbed is believed to be the most common mode of infection in man. It has been suggested that a significant proportion of normal individuals exposed to this fungus develop subclinical lung infection. However, this has still to be confirmed. Clinical infection with *Cr. neoformans* is seen in both normal and immunosuppressed individuals. In North America, almost 50 per cent of cases are found in normal hosts, but most British cases occur in predisposed subjects, often with underlying cell-mediated immunological defects.

Cryptococcosis is an infection of the lungs which can remain localized to that site or spread to other organs. It is more common for this infection to present with features of dissemination, such as meningitis, although there are often signs of accompanying lung involvement as well as signs of disseminated infection elsewhere.

Clinical manifestations of cryptococcosis
Infection of the lungs is the second most common clinical form of cryptococcosis. Symptoms include cough and fever, sputum production, chest pain, weight loss and haemoptysis. Radiological findings include alveolar or interstitial infiltrates, lobar consolidation, mass lesions, single or multiple nodules and pleural effusion. In normal hosts, *Cr. neoformans* infection often remains localized to the lungs and resolves without treatment. In immunosuppressed patients, dissemination is common.

Treatment is advisable where there are signs of dissemination, where the lung infection is prolonged, or where there is significant underlying illness. All patients should be investigated for signs of dissemination. This should include: full clinical examination; culture of blood, urine, sputum and CSF; and antigen tests on blood, CSF and urine.

CNS infection is the most common clinical form of cryptococcosis. Meningitis is the most frequent presentation. The illness is often insidious in onset, but rapid progression can occur in immunosuppressed patients. Frontal or temporal headache and mental changes, such as drowsiness and confusion, occur in most patients. Other symptoms include nausea, vomiting and neck stiffness. Fever is often absent or minimal, but on occasion may be marked. The eyes should be examined since papilloedema is common. Field defects or ptosis can also occur. However, unless focal lesions are present, specific central neurological defects are unusual.

The important steps in the subsequent management involve the establishment of the diagnosis and an assessment of the extent of infection and of complications, such as hydrocephalus. If available, a CAT scan of the head should be performed to detect mass lesions and hydrocephalus. Cultures of blood, urine, sputum and CSF should be performed, in addition to antigen tests on CSF, blood and urine. The CSF in *Cr. neoformans* meningitis should show one or more of the following abnormalities: raised opening pressure; elevated protein; lowered glucose; increased mononuclear white cell count; encapsulated yeast cells.

Cutaneous lesions occur in some patients with disseminated cryptococcosis. Subcutaneous swellings, raised granulomata, acneiform papules, nodules and ulcers have been described. Organisms are numerous in these lesions. Microscopic examination and culture of aspirated and biopsied material should establish the diagnosis.

Lytic bone lesions occur in some cases of disseminated *Cr. neoformans* infection. Bone pain and swelling and tenderness of adjacent tissue occur. Aspiration or bone biopsy is required for diagnosis.

Diagnosis of cryptococcosis

It is not as difficult to obtain positive cultures in *Cr. neoformans* infection as it is in aspergillosis. However, repeated lumbar puncture is sometimes required before a positive sample is obtained. The organism can also be found in blood, sputum or urine. The latter site is often neglected, but can be a useful indicator of widespread dissemination. The detection of encapsulated organisms in CSF or other specimens will establish the diagnosis, but the smears are often difficult to interpret. Histological demonstration of organisms in tissue is a rapid and reliable method of diagnosis.

The most useful serological method is the latex agglutination test for *Cr. neoformans* antigen. This is positive with CSF and blood specimens from most patients with cryptococcal meningitis. Occasional false positive reactions occur in patients with circulating or CSF rheumatoid factor, but this can be prevented if specimens are first treated with dithiothreitol. The antigen titre is often useful in determining the prognosis with high or rising titres reflecting progression of infection and declining titres indicating regression of infection and response to treatment.

Antibodies to *Cr. neoformans* are found in patients with localized infection, but not in individuals with meningeal or disseminated infection. Antibodies sometimes appear late in the course of treatment of infection.

Treatment of cryptococcosis

Combination treatment with amphotericin B ($0 \cdot 3$–$0 \cdot 5$ mg.kg^{-1}.d^{-1}) and flucytosine (150 mg.kg^{-1}.d^{-1}) is recommended for patients with meningeal or disseminated infection. The dosage regimen is identical to that outlined earlier for candidosis. Most patients will require at least 6 weeks' treatment, but this should be determined on the basis of clinical and CSF improvement and fall in antigen titre. Patients should be regarded as being in remission rather than cured. Follow-up is important.

If amphotericin B is used on its own, higher doses ($0 \cdot 8$–$1 \cdot 0$ mg.kg^{-1}.d^{-1}) will be required and may not be as well tolerated as the combination regimen. Local instillation of amphotericin B into the CSF may be indicated in a patient with meningitis who has failed to respond to combination treatment. Further information can be found in Hay (1982).

The use of intravenous miconazole is not well established in cryptococcosis and it should be reserved for combination regimen failures. In children, the usual dose is 25–40 mg.kg^{-1}.d^{-1} administered in three infusions. If there is no improvement, intrathecal treatment can be added.

Oral treatment with ketoconazole is not recommended.

MUCORMYCOSIS

This is an opportunistic fungal infection seen in immunosuppressed patients or diabetics. There are a number of clinical forms of mucormycosis, each associated with particular host defects. Diabetes mellitus and metabolic acidosis predispose to rhinocerebral infection, haematological neoplasia to infection of the lungs, wounds or burns to cutaneous infection and malnutrition and gastrointestinal tract lesions to gastrointestinal mucormycosis. Disseminated infection can occur as a complication of all of these conditions, but is most often seen in patients with haematological neoplasia.

The organisms responsible for this disease belong to the Order Mucorales. In the immunosuppressed patient *Absidia*, *Mucor* and *Rhizopus* are the most common pathogens. These fungi are widespread in nature, in soil and decomposing organic matter. Inhalation of spores is the usual mode of infection in man. In rhinocerebral mucormycosis spores are deposited on the nasal mucosa and the infection spreads into the sinuses and orbital structures, and then into the brain. Less commonly, infection follows ingestion of spores or direct inoculation through breaks in the skin.

Clinical manifestations and diagnosis of mucormycosis

One of the principal characteristics of mucormycosis is vascular invasion leading to thrombosis, ischaemic infarction and haemorrhagic necrosis.

Rhinocerebral mucormycosis

This is the most common clinical form of mucormycosis. It is most often seen in diabetic patients, but is becoming more common in leukaemic patients and transplant recipients. Three signs are characteristic of this condition; uncontrolled diabetes mellitus, orbital cellulitis and meningoencephalitis. Facial and ocular pain, nasal discharge, headache, fever and facial swelling with induration and discolouration are common presenting symptoms and signs. As the infection spreads to the cavernous sinus and frontal lobes of the brain, coma and hemiparesis develop. The course of infection from initial nasopharyngeal invasion to death is often rapid.

The diagnosis of this form of mucormycosis is not difficult once all the classical signs are evident. It is much more difficult to establish the diagnosis before there is obvious proptosis and encephalitis. Examination of the nasal mucosa and palate will often reveal a necrotic mucosal ulcer. Typical broad mycelia showing non-dichotomous branching can often be seen in material recovered from such lesions. This is the most reliable method of diagnosis as cultures from the nose or palate are often unsuccessful.

Sinus radiographs show opacification of involved sinuses and bone erosion in some patients. CAT scans are more useful in defining the extent of infection than establishing a diagnosis. The CSF is abnormal, but again non-specific. An increased white cell count with an elevated protein and normal or lowered glucose are common. The aetiological agent in mucormycosis has never been isolated from CSF.

There are no reliable serological tests at present for diagnosis of mucormycosis.

Pulmonary mucormycosis

This is the second most common clinical form of mucormycosis and is most often seen in patients with leukaemia, lymphoma or leucopenia. The clinical signs and symptoms are non-specific and similar to those seen with aspergillosis and a number of other conditions. For this reason, it is unusual for this often fatal form of mucormycosis to be diagnosed antemortem. Cough and fever that persist despite anti-biotic treatment are common findings. Haemoptysis and pleural pain are not frequent. Radiological findings include infiltrates, lobar consolidation, cavitation, fungus ball formation and pleural effusions. The characteristic pathological lesion is infarction with haemorrhagic bronchopneumonitis.

The aetiological agent is seldom recovered from sputum and culture of tissue specimens is often unsuccessful. Histological examination of lung tissue is the best method of diagnosis.

Disseminated mucormycosis

The disseminated form is found in patients with serious underlying conditions including leukaemia and lymphoma. The lungs are often the source of haematogenous dissemination. Liver, spleen and brain are often involved, but other organs can be affected. Again, vascular invasion is the predominant pathological finding and patients may present with acute liver failure, renal vein thrombosis or CNS dysfunction.

Cutaneous lesions occur in some patients with disseminated mucormycosis. These lesions can mimic the typical ecthyma gangrenosa lesion associated with *Pseudomonas* infection or appear as multiple non-ulcerative nodules. Aspiration of material for microscopic examination and culture can establish the diagnosis.

Treatment of mucormycosis

Mucormycosis in immunosuppressed patients is fatal if untreated. Moreover, if treatment is to be successful, a prompt diagnosis is required, infected and necrotic tissue must be removed, an antifungal must be administered, and the underlying illness or predisposing condition must be controlled.

Surgical debridement is an important component of treatment of rhinocerebral infection because vascular thrombosis will prevent antifungals from reaching involved tissue. Surgical debridement has seldom been attempted in patients with haematological neoplasia because mucormycosis tends to develop during haematological relapse.

Amphotericin B $(0 \cdot 8 - 1 \cdot 0 \text{ mg.kg}^{-1}.\text{d}^{-1})$ is the sole antifungal drug that is effective in mucormycosis. The dosage regimen is identical to that detailed earlier for candidosis. Treatment should be continued until there is no further clinical, radiological or histological sign of infection. The amount of amphotericin B that should be given and the duration of treatment will depend upon the individual patient's response. It is recommended that at least 2 g should be given.

OTHER UNUSUAL FUNGAL INFECTIONS

In addition to the major opportunistic fungal infections described in preceding sections of this chapter, other unusual fungal infections can occur in immunosuppressed children. *Geotrichum candidum, Petriellidium boydii, Trichosporon beigelii, T. capitatum, Fusarium moniliforme, F. solani,* and members of the genus *Penicillium* are among the unusual fungal pathogens that have caused deep infection in immunosuppressed individuals. Further information about these infections can be found in Warnock (1982).

It is often difficult to establish whether an unusual organism isolated from an immunosuppressed child is acting as a pathogen. There is a greater chance of it being significant if it can be isolated from infected organs under aseptic conditions; or identified in infected tissue; and if the patient has antibodies to the organism under investigation. Repeated isolation of an organism in the absence of other potential pathogens can help to establish a pathogenic role.

Amphotericin B is the drug of choice in the absence of prior experience. However, it is often helpful to determine the MIC to a range of antifungals.

PREVENTION OF FUNGAL INFECTION

Neutropenic patients are often treated with oral antifungals in an attempt to prevent infections such as aspergillosis and candidosis. Oral treatment with nystatin will often reduce oral and intestinal colonization with *C. albicans*. However, there has been no convincing demonstration that this prevents the development of either local or disseminated forms of candidosis. Several clinical trials have suggested that oral treatment with ketoconazole is superior to nystatin in reducing colonization with *C. albicans* and preventing candidosis in neutropenic patients. Other reports have been less encouraging and it is clear that ketoconazole offers no protection against *Aspergillus* infection. Prolonged prophylaxis with ketoconazole may lead to hepatic toxicity.

EMPIRICAL TREATMENT OF FUNGAL INFECTION

If a diagnosis of mycosis is suspected in a deteriorating neutropenic patient, empirical treatment with amphotericin B is indicated. If the patient responds to treatment and the diagnosis of fungal infection is confirmed, a full course of treatment should be given. If, however, the patient responds to treatment or the neutrophil count recovers without the diagnosis being established, treatment can be discontinued once the count exceeds $0.5 \times 10^9/l$.

FURTHER READING

Hay R. J. (1982) Clinical manifestations and management of cryptococcosis in the compromised patient. In: Warnock D. W. and Richardson M. D. (eds.) *Fungal Infection in the Compromised Patient*, Chichester, Wiley, pp. 93–117.

Hopwood V. and Warnock D. W. (1986) New developments in the diagnosis of deep fungal infection. *Eur. J. Clin. Microbiol.* **5**, 379–88.

Hughes W. T. (1982) systemic candidiasis: a study of 109 fatal cases. *Pediatr. Infect. Dis.* **1**, 11–18.

Salaki J. S., Louria D. B. and Chmel H. (1984) Fungal and yeast infections of the central nervous system. *Medicine* **63**, 108–32.

Seelig M. S. and Kozinn P. J. (1982) Clinical manifestations and management of candidosis in the compromised patient. In: Warnock D. W. and Richardson M. D. (eds.) *Fungal Infection in the Compromised Patient*, Chichester, Wiley, pp. 49–92.

Warnock D. W. (1982) Unusual fungal infections in the compromised patient. In: Warnock D. W. and Richardson M. D. (eds.) *Fungal Infection in the Compromised Patient*, Chichester, Wiley, pp. 217–28.

Warren R. E. and Warnock D. W. (1982) Clinical manifestations and management of aspergillosis in the compromised patient. In: Warnock D. W. and Richardson M. D. (eds.) *Fungal Infection in the Compromised Patient*, Chichester, Wiley, pp. 119–53.

Wilson R. and Feldman S. (1979) Toxicity of amphotericin B in children with cancer. *Am. J. Dis. Child.* **133**, 731–4.

Wong B. and Armstrong D. (1982) Clinical manifestations and management of mucormycosis in the compromised patient. In: Warnock D. W. and Richardson M. D. (eds.) *Fungal Infection in the Compromised Patient*, Chichester, Wiley, pp. 155–85.

4. Haematological Support

E. Simpson

INTRODUCTION

The use of aggressive chemotherapy in the treatment of childhood cancers has resulted in improved survival rates, but this improvement has only been made possible by advances in supportive care, particularly transfusion support and antibiotic therapy. It has been possible to ablate tumours totally with drugs and radiotherapy for many years, but at the expense of the normal cells, particularly the bone marrow, leaving the patient immunosuppressed, bleeding and anaemic, and with minimal chance of survival. Platelet concentrate transfusions only became routinely available in 1960; before that time, transfusions of fresh whole blood were the only way possible to attempt to stop bleeding for thrombocytopenia. In 1964, a study was reported on the cause of death of 414 patients with acute leukaemia at the National Cancer Institute, in the previous 10 years. Prior to the advent of platelet concentrate transfusions, 67 per cent died of acute haemorrhage; this fell to 37 per cent once platelet concentrates became available in 1960. The way was paved for increasingly aggressive therapy, with greater need for transfusion with the cellular components of blood, necessitating advances in the collection, preparation and storage of these blood products.

Bone marrow transplantation has an important part to play in the treatment of certain childhood cancers, particularly leukaemia, and the dependence on transfusion services continues to increase. Unfortunately, as more blood products are transfused to patients who survive their illness, new and unexpected problems related to the therapy given have caused considerable morbidity and mortality. Blood transfusions can pass on infections, and the transfusion-related viruses are a potent source of morbidity in the severely immuno-compromised patient undergoing treatment for cancer or post-bone marrow transplant. Alloimmunization to antigens on red cells, white cells and platelets causes reactions and eventual difficulties in finding compatible products for future transfusions; the risk of graft-vs.-host disease is also present, though yet to be fully evaluated. New techniques have had to be developed to attempt to prevent these complications, so that transfusion of blood products can be rendered safe for the recipient. However, it is wise to remember that blood is a drug, with known side-effects, and it should be used with all the respect and care due to a potentially toxic substance. The transfusion support required by a child with cancer can usually be predicted with reasonable accuracy, so blood products can be selected and given in such a way as to cause the least risk of future problems.

BLOOD PRODUCT SUPPORT

Red cells

The child with cancer may be anaemic at presentation because of marrow infiltration as in leukaemia or neuroblastoma, or because of bleeding, nutritional deficits, or chronic disease related to the tumour. There may be haemorrhage at the time of surgical operation, particularly when the tumour is vascular, but the most common reason for transfusion is marrow depression related to therapy, either chemotherapy, or radiotherapy, or a combination of the two. Whole blood is rarely indicated except in the treatment of massive acute haemorrhage, when it may have a place in treatment. Stored whole blood contains colloid and red cells but no functional clotting factors, leucocytes or platelets. It is an inefficient product, wasting the clotting factors and platelets which could have been harvested; and the non-functioning leucocytes and platelets left may actually be harmful to the recipient. 'Fresh' whole blood is never less than 24 hours old by the time the essential screening tests have been performed, and is usually 2–5 days old, when once again it contains little more than red cells and colloid. Plasma-reduced blood is the product of choice. In most transfusion centres in Britain, this is now produced by separating most of the plasma containing the relatively less dense platelets from the red cells, and resuspending the red cells in an 'optimal additive solution' containing saline, glucose, adenine and mannitol. Platelets can be separated, and the plasma can be processed to produce clotting factor concentrates, or packed and frozen as 'fresh frozen plasma'.

The special attributes of the optimal additive solution ensure that the flow-properties of the packed red cells are no different from those of whole blood, so that it can be given quickly and easily if required, and the glucose and adenine ensure that the red cells, stored at 4°C, remain in a healthy metabolic state during the period of storage. The lifespan, before irreversible metabolic change occurs, could be as long as 6 weeks, but as the transfusion services usually have a surplus of red cells, the units of blood are stored for 4 weeks only, with relatively little deterioration of red cell function. Not all white cells or platelets are removed in production, but the numbers are decreased, resulting in less antigenic stimulus from the leucocyte and platelet antigens.

With modern cross-matching techniques, including the use of the LISS (low ionic strength saline) techniques which will pick up weak antibodies during the cross-match, red-cell transfusion reactions should not be a problem. However, it is important, where possible, to prevent the development of such antibodies. When it can be predicted that a patient will require multiple transfusions, it is important that a full genotype is obtained, so that blood matched for the important antigens, particularly those of the Rhesus group, can be given. Patients with cancer on chemotherapy are immunosuppressed, and so are less likely to mount an antibody response to a foreign red cell antigen than a patient transfused for a non-immunosuppressive condition such as red-cell aplasia; however, if possible, the risk should be prevented, as once antibodies develop, the supply of compatible blood becomes increasingly difficult, sometimes necessitating the use of frozen cell panels.

The commonest form of transfusion reaction now seen is due to the reaction of leucocyte (HLA) antibodies with transfused leucocytes. A multiply transfused patient will have been exposed to white cells from many different donors and, eventually, most patients are sensitized to these antigens. The risk of alloimmunization is increased if products containing leucocytes are given; platelet concentrates prepared by the centrifuge method from donor blood are relatively heavily contaminated with leucocytes compared to plasma-reduced blood, and granulocyte transfusions, particularly from buffy coat preparations from random donors are most likely to cause alloimmunization. The reactions observed are allergic in nature and usually consist of a sudden rise in temperature accompanied by rigors. An urticarial rash may be seen, but wheezing and anaphylaxis are rare. Once antibodies are suspected, further blood product transfusions should be specially prepared to reduce the number of white cells given, or hydrocortisone and chlorpheniramine can be given intravenously at the start of a transfusion. A filter can be placed in the blood-giving line to remove some leucocytes, but a more effective filtration method can be performed by the transfusion service, under sterile conditions. Other centres will wash the red cells to remove the leucocytes, or will use frozen red cells (which have to be washed prior to use to remove the cryopreservative used), but this method tends to cause damage to the red cells and may reduce their *in vivo* survival once transfused. Units of blood treated in one of these ways become an infection risk as their integrity has been breached, and they must be transfused into the patient within 4–8 h.

Transfusions should be given for symptomatic relief of anaemia. If there is evidence of marrow recovery, or a good reticulocyte response to anaemia, transfusion may be withheld if the patient is asymptomatic. However, when the marrow depression is likely to be of longer duration, transfusion to 12–14 g/dl haemoglobin will be required regularly. A patient who presents with a very high white count should not be transfused to this level until the white cell count is under control, because of problems with hyperviscosity. Haemoglobin levels of 8–10 g/dl should be sufficient to prevent symptoms of anaemia in these children. A useful rule of thumb for transfusion in children is:

Desired rise in HB × Wt(kg) × 4 = volume of packed cells required

Clotting factors

Bleeding may be due to thrombocytopenia or deficiency in clotting factors. Very occasionally, this deficiency may be due to a hereditary coagulation disorder, but more often, the deficiency is secondary to the disease process. Massive transfusion for haemorrhage may deplete coagulation factors, and after transfusion of crystalloid and red cells equivalent to a complete exchange of blood volume, replacement of clotting factors and platelets should be considered, particularly if the bleeding continues. Primary or secondary malignant invasion of the liver may result in a decrease in the liver-produced factors, such as factors II, VII, IX and X. At levels of 30 iu or less (normal range 50–150 iu) bleeding may occur spontaneously, or haemorrhage may prove difficult to stop. The most common reason for depletion of coagulation factors in children undergoing treatment for malignant disease is disseminated intravascular coagulation (DIC). Certain tumours, predominantly found in adults, are known to precipitate a chronic form of DIC which may acutely decompensate and cause catastrophic bleeding. These tumours (colon, prostate and stomach) are rare in childhood, but acute promyelocytic leukaemia is associated with DIC, particularly at the start of treatment, and this form of leukaemia, though also rare, is found in children. DIC may be precipitated by many conditions common in cancer therapy; in particular, by severe infections, and it is infected patients who are at greatest risk of DIC. It may occur in the face of marrow depression, or with a completely normal marrow and response to infection.

Bacterial endotoxins cause vascular endothelial injury, which damages platelets and also has a direct effect on them. The result is microaggregation of platelets within the circulation, and release of tissue factors and platelet factors from the damaged endothelium and aggregated platelets. The intrinsic coagulation cascade is triggered, with concomitant stimulation of plasminogens and the fibrinolytic system. The fibrinolytic system is both faster acting, and with a greater reserve, so the net result of the process is consumption of coagulation factors and platelets, and increased fibrinolysis with evidence of fibrin degradation. The patient presents with bleeding, not thrombosis, although microthrombi in the circulation may have caused red cell fragmentation, seen on examination of the blood film, and may contribute to renal damage. DIC is described as compensated when there is laboratory evidence of increased fibrinolysis but no deficiency of clotting factors, or uncompensated when consumption of coagulation factors has exceeded production, and deficiencies particularly of fibrinogen, factors V and VIII, and platelets are evident. Clinical DIC is evidenced by massive bruising, purpura, oozing from venepuncture sites, and haemorrhage into organs. When platelets are low following chemotherapy, the assumption that bleeding is due to thrombocytopenia is a pitfall to be avoided, as platelet concentrate transfusion will be insufficient to treat the haemorrhage. It is important to suspect DIC, and obtain laboratory proof, by performing a coagulation screen, consisting of prothrombin time, partial thromboplastin time, fibrinogen, fibrin degradation products (FDPs) and blood film and platelet count. A sudden unexpected fall in platelets accompanied by red cell fragments on the blood film is suspicious of DIC. Prolonged prothrombin time and partial thromboplastin time, with reduced fibrinogen and increased FDPs is diagnostic. Other tests, such as fibrin monomer assays, and plasminogen assay are primarily research tools, and not required for the diagnosis. Treatment is aimed at the precipitating cause, usually broad spectrum antibiotics for a suspected infection, followed by replacement of platelets and clotting factors. This is best done by the use of platelet concentrates and fresh frozen plasma (FFP).

The volume of plasma recommended is 10–20 ml/kg, although this may need to be repeated, particularly if the cause of DIC continues. Problems are attached to the use of FFP, in particular the volumes required may be difficult in a child who is needing other intravenous fluid therapy, and may have renal impairment. Fresh frozen plasma is prepared in single donor packs of 100 or 200 ml and kept stored at $-40°C$. Once thawed, the activity of the coagulation factors reduces rapidly, so that for best effect, the volume required should be given over a maximum time of one hour after thawing. Despite this problem, freeze-dried concentrates made from large donor pools should be avoided, because of the known risks of transfusion viruses from these products. The concentrates are made in such a way that the coagulation factors are not left in the normal proportions, so it is difficult to replace all the factors depleted in DIC by the use of concentrates, and FFP remains the best-balanced product. Hypo-fibrinogenaemia requires large volumes of FFP to correct, and cryoprecipitate, a preparation which concentrates both F.VIII and fibrinogen, may be required. It is difficult to calculate the dose required accurately as units of cryoprecipitate vary greatly in volume and F.VIII and fibrinogen content, but 1 u (obtained from a single blood) donation) per 10 kg body weight would be adequate initially. Repeat clotting screens, as clinically indicated, should be performed, and further replacement therapy given until the bleeding has stopped, or coagulation tests improved and returning towards normal.

Platelets

Until 1960, it was only possible to correct bleeding from thrombocytopenia by the transfusion of fresh whole blood, given to the recipient within 4 h of donation. Once technology had advanced so that blood was collected into plastic bags, multipack systems could be used allowing for the preparation of platelet concentrates from whole blood by centrifugation. An early study on the effects of platelet concentrate transfusions was reported in 1965.[1] Patients studied were those with thrombocytopenia and active bleeding, rather than just bruising or purpura. It was found that if the platelet count was elevated by a maximum of $< 20 \times 10^9/l$, during the 24 h post-transfusion, 44 per cent of the patients stopped bleeding. If the maximum rise was $> 40 \times 10^9/l$, 75 per cent of patients stopped bleeding. The bleeding sites included nose, urinary tract and gastro-intestinal tract. If patients with melaena were excluded, the figures were 45 per cent and 100 per cent respectively. It was already known that there was a relationship between platelet count and bleeding episodes, which were rare at levels greater than $40 \times 10^9/l$. From this work, it was concluded that a rise of at least $40 \times 10^9/l$ was required to control bleeding. However, it was noted that the actual rise did not always match the expected rise, the *in vivo* recovery being less in the face of active infection. The recommended platelet dose was 8–10 u (1 u derived from 1 u of donor blood) per 100 lb body weight, a figure not dissimilar to present recommendations.

Platelets are still prepared in a very similar fashion, although improved plastics in the collection bags, more knowledge about correct centrifugation speeds and better methods of storage have improved the yield and shelf life of the platelets. They are now stored at room temperature, continuously agitated to prevent accumulation of lactic acid and fall in pH, and may be used up to 5 d after donation. These platelet preparations are heavily contaminated with donor white cells, and an adult would require 6–12 u/d (or more) for control of thrombocytopenic bleeding, so that alloimmunization to a wide range of donor leucocyte antigens is likely. Apheresis techniques,[2] using a cell separator, provide platelets from a single donor equivalent to 3 'normal' units of platelets, and by use of the 'surge' method, they are less contaminated with red and white cells, providing a less antigenic product. The prime indication for platelet transfusion is bleeding in the face of thrombocytopenia. No abnormal bleeding is likely to be encountered at platelet counts of greater than $100 \times 10^9/l$. Between $50-100 \times 10^9/l$, bleeding may occur, especially after trauma or at surgery, and platelets should be given to improve safety and operating conditions for the surgeon. At levels of $20-50 \times 10^9/l$, bruises and purpura may appear after minor trauma, but spontaneous bleeding is rare until platelet levels drop below $20 \times 10^9/l$. Most centres would give platelets prophylactically to prevent bleeding at levels of $< 20 \times 10^9/l$, until such time that the patient's own marrow resumed platelet production. Bleeding at higher platelet counts is increased when the patient is febrile, so during infectious episodes, the level for prophylactic platelets may be increased to $30-40 \times 10^9/l$.

The platelet dose recommended is 1 u obtained from 1 u of random donor blood (single donor platelets: 1 donation is equivalent to 3 random donor units) per 10 kg body weight. An alternative calculation is 4 u/m^2 surface area. However, as noted by early workers, response both clinically and by *in vivo* recovery is unpredictable, and a larger dose may be required for a clinical response. Rapid peripheral destruction of transfused platelets, resulting in poor response, may be caused by a number of factors, including infection, DIC, hypersplenism and active haemorrhage. These problems may be overcome by treating the cause, and temporarily increasing the number of units transfused. If the cause of peripheral destruction is alloimmunization to HLA antigens, a dose adjustment will not be adequate. In the presence of antibodies, 2–3 times the normal requirement of platelets may still be insufficient for control of bleeding, and will rapidly deplete available resources. HLA matched platelet transfusions become necessary, obtained from HLA matched single donors. The first source of such donors would be family members, unless the patient is to receive a bone marrow transplant from a matched sibling, in which case, family members should not be used as a platelet source, to prevent sensitization of the patient to family antigens. A panel of HLA typed donors is kept by the transfusion service, and HLA compatible (but not necessarily matched) donors can be selected from this panel. As red cells and plasma are returned to the donor, platelet pheresis can be undertaken 2–3 times in a week, or weekly for approximately 4 weeks depending on the donor, so a small number of donors will support the patient through a bleeding episode. Post bone marrow transplant it may be possible to use the marrow donor as a platelet donor, so avoiding alloimmunization, and perhaps boosting the graft.

If standard doses of platelets are not producing the required effect clinically, or producing inadequate increments, it is essential to identify the reason, remembering that in a severely ill, immuno-compromised patient, more than one mechanism may be effective. It has been found that the 1 h post-platelet transfusion increment is a valuable predictor of cause of rapid platelet destruction, a low 18–24 h increment[3] (following day level) being a non-specific indicator of peripheral platelet destruction. Patients undergoing induction therapy for leukaemia or intensive maintenance therapy were studied before and 1 h after transfusion with random donor platelets, and on a different occasion, before and after HLA matched single donor platelets. Lymphocytotoxicity tests to detect antibodies against a large panel of lymphocytes (HLA antibodies) were also done. It was found that the group of patients with strong, high levels of cytotoxic antibodies had 1 h increments of $< 10 \times 10^9/l$ with transfusions of random platelets, but significantly greater increments ($>10 \times 10^9/l$) with HLA matched platelets. Another group of patients, in whom no significant HLA antibodies were detected, had one hour post-platelet increments of $>10 \times 10^9/l$ after both random and HLA matched platelets. The incremental count was corrected for patient size and platelet dose, in order to standardize the results for statistical assessment as follows:

$$\frac{\text{Post-transfusion count} - \text{pre-transfusion count} \times SA\ m^2}{\text{No. platelets transfused}}$$

In practical terms, when the platelet count per unit transfused is not known accurately, and the dose given is related to patient size, the uncorrected 1 h increment can be used. Although this requires an extra blood test for the patient, the volume of blood required is small, and no specialized laboratory tests are needed. HLA antibodies can be identified in the laboratory by a microlymphocytotoxicity assay against a panel of lymphocytes, from up to 80 donors. Antibodies are graded by strength (percentage cell kill/well) and by the percentage of donor lymphocytes reacting with the antibodies. Gradings of 0 (no antibody detectable), to 4+ (75–100 per cent donors reactive) are made, grades from 2+ to 4+ being considered significant. This test is only available in specialized tissue-typing laboratories, but may be very helpful in the few cases where strong antibodies to a few HLA antigens are detected. Avoidance of these antigens, rather than full HLS matching, may make successful transfusion possible. Usually, antibodies are produced to a wide range of HLA antibodies, and HLA matching is required.

Once alloimmunization has occurred HLA matched platelets are necessary.[4] It would place too great a burden on resources to find HLA matched donors for every transfusion, so reliance is still on random platelet donors. Efforts should be made to minimize the risk of alloimmunization by use of single donors, and collection methods that reduce white cell contamination. Candidates for bone marrow transplant or long-term transfusion therapy should receive leucocyte depleted blood, from as few donors as possible, from the start of their illness.

HLA antibodies are the major immune cause for platelet destruction. Other immune causes may be present, which will not respond to HLA matching of donations. Drugs, particularly antibiotics, may alter and damage cells, resulting in the formation of immune complexes which are cleared from the circulation. Platelets also carry specific platelet antigens, and antibodies to these may develop. It would be extremely difficult to find HLA matched, platelet antigen matched donors, but the search may have to be made if the provision of HLA matched donors does not result in significant 1 h increments and reduction in bleeding.

Granulocytes

The good results following the use of platelet concentrates encouraged workers to believe that infectious problems in the immunocompromised would soon be solved by the use of granulocyte transfusions. This early optimism was not justified and the subject remains controversial, although it is now generally accepted that there is a small but clinically well-defined place for granulocyte transfusions. Most serious infections occur in neutropenic patients when the total neutrophil count is below $0 \cdot 5 \times 10^9/l$. It was also noted that many infections improve as the neutrophil count recovers following a period of marrow depression, and these observations resulted in the first trials of granulocyte therapy. In the early 1960s, the chosen donors had chronic granulocytic leukaemia (CGL), as it was easy to separate large numbers of granulocytes from the buffy coat of a unit of blood. Antibiotics did not provide the broad spectrum cover now offered, so it was not surprising that early results of granulocyte-transfused/antibiotic treated patients fared much better than those receiving antibiotics alone. Controlled trials in the 1970s were still in favour of granulocytes, but a trial in 1982 suggested no benefit from the procedure. Interpretation of the results is open to comment, particularly the fact that the dose of granulocytes used would now be considered inadequate.

Collection of granulocytes from normal donors is more difficult than the harvesting of platelets. In CGL, when the granulocyte count may be as high as $500 \times 10^9/l$, centrifugation of a unit of blood produced a wide band between red cells and plasma, the buffy coat. This can be removed, and red cells and plasma returned to the patient. It is possible to do this manually, but cell separators are available which will perform this by continuous vein–to–vein procedure, or by an intermittent cycle. It is possible to obtain donations of up to 2×10^{11} granulocytes from a single CGL donor. Normal donors have much lower granulocyte counts, but yields of up to 35×10^9 granulocytes can be obtained by continuous-flow centrifugation leucopheresis by the use of sedimenting agents such as hydroxyethyl starch (HES) to help separate red cells from white, and priming of the donor pre-pheresis with steroids. It is still necessary to process a large volume of blood (up to 10 l) to obtain this yield, which is time-consuming for the donor and for the operator of the machine. Intermittent leucopheresis is more efficient, but less blood can be processed in the same time, resulting in a lower yield (approx. 10–15 $\times 10^9$ granulocytes). In a normal adult, the rate of production of granulocytes is 10^{11}/day, and this can increase greatly in response to stress and infection. A granulocyte transfusion, prepared from a normal donor, is a small amount compared to the normal production, and is unlikely to produce a detectable rise in granulocyte count. In the trial concluding that granulocyte transfusions were of no benefit, the median dose given was 5×10^9 granulocytes, as donors were not primed with steroids, and the intermittent procedure was used, resulting in low yields. Other methods of granulocyte production are now not used. Gravity sedimentation was slow, and produced low yields. Filtration, in which granulocytes adhered to and were then removed from nylon fibres, produced cells which were found to be functionally impaired. The procedure also resulted in complement activation, causing some problems to the donor receiving back the red cells and plasma after the filtration. It may be easier to provide adequate doses of granulocytes for children from single donors, by the current techniques but even so, doses need to be given daily, and for at least 3–5 d. Granulocyte transfusions in septicaemic neonates have proved beneficial, and this may be because it is possible to obtain adequate doses easily. CGL donors, when available, are ideal. The yield of granulocytes is sufficiently high to make transfusions possible at 2–3 d intervals. It also provides a transfusion of precursor cells which, although they do not engraft, will divide *in vivo*, and prolong the beneficial effects of the granulocytes.

Risks for the donor from any apheresis technique, but particularly leucopheresis, are not inconsiderable. Blood is anticoagulated as it enters the centrifugation chamber, and during the processing of up to 10 l of blood, citrate toxicity may result. It is usually easily corrected with calcium supplements, but may be an unpleasant and frightening experience for the donor. Steroids, to boost the granulocyte count, have well-known side-effects, although minimized by the use of single large doses. HES is returned to the circulation, and if repeated leucopheresis is performed, may accumulate in the circulation. Complement activation was significant with filtration techniques, and could result in cramping abdominal pains, but is not a problem with the modern centrifugation methods. Donors should be carefully screened, and the indications for granulocytes clearly defined before leucopheresis is contemplated. Granulocytes should only be used as an adjunct to antibiotic therapy. At the first sign of infection in a neutropenic patient, cultures should be obtained, and broad spectrum antibiotics, chosen with the patient's known resistant flora, and the local bacterial sensitivities in mind, started immediately. Once the organism is identified, adjustments to dose and antibiotic used should be made to provide the maximum antibiotic cover. With this approach at least 80 per cent of patients should recover with antibiotics alone. However, it is possible to predict patients who may be slow to respond. These are the patients who are likely to have a prolonged period of marrow depression, i.e. those just after bone marrow transplantation, or immediately after intensive chemotherapy. Response to antibiotics may coincide with regeneration of the bone marrow, the minimal increase in peripheral granulocyte count being because of the migration of newly produced neutrophils to the site of infection. As treatment for leukaemia becomes more aggressive initially, remission is achieved more quickly, and the period of marrow depression is shortened in most patients. Paradoxically, therefore, in this group of patients, aggressive treatment may reduce the need for granulocyte transfusion, coupled with more effective prevention of infection by nursing and broad spectrum antibiotics, and more effective antibiotic therapy for established infections.

Side-effects have been reported with the use of granulocyte transfusions, particularly the incidence of pulmonary infiltrates and pulmonary symptoms. There have been reports that these are particularly serious in those patients also receiving amphotericin B infusions for systemic fungal infections. Damaged granulocytes can form microaggregates, which cause blockage to the pulmonary microvasculature, and the appearance of pulmonary signs. These reports were particularly prevalent when filtration collection methods, now known to damage white cells, were in use; but pulmonary complications are still reported in some recipients. Many patients receiving granulocytes have had multiple transfusions, and so are alloimmunized against HLA antigens, as previously described, or white cell antibodies may be transferred from multiparous female donors. Circulating white cells involved in antigen/antibody complexes will aggregate, and cause pulmonary infiltrates. It is vital, therefore, to select donors carefully to be HLA compatible with the recipient. Granulocytes also have granulocyte specific antigens, antibodies to which can be identified by leucoagglutination techniques. Ideally, a donor should be as well matched for HLA type as possible, but certainly HLA compatible as defined by cross-matching techniques, and also compatible for granulocyte antigens. If these criteria are followed, even when amphotericin B is also given, no excessive pulmonary complications are observed. A rapid increase in X-ray opacification may follow granulocyte infusion, as they migrate to infection sites in the lungs, but this should not be accompanied by a worsening of signs and symptoms, and is not an indication for withdrawal of granulocyte transfusions.

Prophylactic use of granulocytes in periods of prolonged neutropenia is being studied in various bone marrow transplant units. A decrease in the incidence of acquired infection was noted, but no difference in overall survival between transfused and untransfused patients. The study using random donors had an increase in alloimmunization, interfering with other transfusion support. Prophylactic granulocyte transfusion, at present, needs further research before it can be generally recommended.

In summary, there is a small but definite role for granulocyte transfusion. Adequate doses of HLA compatible granulocytes prepared by centrifugation from properly screened and primed donors should be given for 3–5 d, to severely neutropenic patients who fail to respond to adequate doses of antibiotics chosen specifically for the isolated causative organism, when the period of neutropenia is likely to be prolonged. These criteria will rarely be met in the treatment of acute lymphoblastic leukaemia, but may be present in non-lymphoblastic leukaemia, and in the context of bone marrow transplantation. Inadequate doses of granulocytes prepared from random donors are of no proven benefit if adequate antibiotics are employed. Amphotericin is not a contraindication to granulocyte transfusion.

IATROGENIC COMPLICATIONS OF INTENSIVE TRANSFUSION THERAPY

Transfusion-associated viruses

Infections can be passed on by transfusion, and the transfusion service attempts to exclude potentially infectious blood from the blood bank. Donors are asked about exposure to malaria, and if malaria carriage is possible, their red cells are not used for transfusion. All units of blood are routinely screened for syphilis, hepatitis

B and HIV, and the results of these tests known before blood is issued for transfusion. With the virtual exclusion of these infectious agents, other viral agents have become prominent as causes of post-transfusion morbidity and mortality.[5]

Non-A, non-B hepatitis (NANB) has been found in virtually all people receiving F.IX and F.VIII concentrates for the first time.[6] These are prepared from a large pool of random donors, who were apparently in good health. The incidence of NANB hepatitis after transfusion at cardiac surgery has been variously reported between 1·7–4 per cent of patients. Patients receiving multiple transfusions are also likely to develop hepatitis eventually, as shown by a transient rise in transaminases. NANB hepatitis is usually self-limiting, but has been known to cause chronic hepatitis, and may cause considerable diagnostic confusion in a severely ill child. As yet, no definite NANB marker has been discovered, so screening of donors is not possible. A suggestion that donors be screened for elevated ALT is not feasible, as this test is prone to false negatives and positives; and there are geographical variations in 'normal' ALT levels, making interpretation of results in a mixed population panel of donors difficult. Appropriate advice to those donors with elevated ALTs is difficult to provide. Human parvovirus infection was first identified following transfusion of blood from an infected donor, but this is not a major cause of transfusion associated infection.

Certain viruses are associated with transfusion of cellular elements of blood, and these present considerable risks to the immuno-compromised patient. Cytomegalovirus (CMV) infection has a significant mortality from pneumonitis in post-bone marrow trans-plant patients. The presence of CMV antibody, indicating past infection, does not protect against reactivation of the virus, although in general, primary infections are more serious than reactivations. There is no benefit in giving CMV antibody negative blood products to a seropositive patient, but efforts should be made to provide seronegative blood for a seronegative patient who is at risk. In Britain, the incidence of seropositivity in donors is between 50–60 per cent. It would not be possible to exclude these donors from the panel, but it is reasonable to screen for CMV seronegativity, and have a sero-negative panel available for use with post-transplant patients. CMV antibody does not necessarily mean that the blood carries infectious agents, but the carrier rate may be as high as 1 in 4. CMV antigen detection is possible but not reliable for detection of the infectious donors.

Epstein-Barr virus is similarly transmitted, but does not cause as many problems. About 90 per cent of donors have neutralizing anti-body circulating, and this may have a protective effect against possible infection from an infectious donor. Human T-cell lymphotropic virus

(HTLVI) is transmitted in cellular blood components, but the incidence of this virus in Britain is extremely low. Screening programmes have been introduced in Japan, where this virus is prevalent. HIV, the agent causing AIDS, is now known to be transfusion-transmitted by cellular components and plasma products. In Britain, donors are excluded by self-selection if in an at-risk category, and HIV antibody tests are a routine screen. It is possible that an antigen positive, antibody negative donor may escape detection, but in this country the risks are small.

Alloimmunization

Multiply transfused patients are likely to become sensitized to a wide range of HLA antigens, specific granulocyte antigens, and platelet antigens. The most important are the HLA antibodies, and these can cause reactions during transfusion, and refractoriness to transfusion, particularly platelet therapy. It is economically impossible to provide HLA matched transfusions for all recipients, and the use of random donors results in HLA antibody formation. When this occurs, HLA matched donations, or leucocyte-free red cell preparations, become essential. A small group of recipients can be predicted to need long-term intensive transfusion support and efforts should be made to provide leucocyte reduced products and single donor products from the start of the illness, in an attempt to delay the need for HLA matching. All granulocyte transfusions should be HLA compatible to reduce pulmonary complications.

Graft vs. host disease (GVHD)

Reports of this condition following blood transfusion are increasing recently. It has been reported in neonates, following intrauterine or exchange transfusion for severe haemolytic disease of the newborn, and has been attributed to the immaturity of the pre-term immune system. A severely immunocompromised patient is also at risk of engraftment by a non-matched leucocyte transfusion, and reports have included fatal GVHD following plasma, packed cells, platelets or granulocyte transfusion in patients with acute lymphoblastic leukaemia,[7] neuroblastoma and Hodgkin's disease,[8] as well as various immunodeficiency syndromes. Suggestions that all blood products should be irradiated before transfusion to immuno-compromised patients to prevent the occurrence of GVHD have been made but, at present, too little is known about the condition to justify this for all patients.[9] Most reports have been of fatal GVHD, sometimes only diagnosed post-mortem. Hepatitis, skin rashes, and diarrhoea are very common problems in severely ill patients and are often attributed to drug reactions, infections or chemotherapy side-effects. It is possible that GVHD is more common than realized, and that some of these complaints are caused by mild, self-limiting GVHD. A low radiation dose of 15 Gy is known to kill lymphocytes, preventing engraftment, while leaving platelets and granulocytes able to function normally; however, this is a costly procedure in terms of manpower and equipment and would radically alter present medical practice. Before irradiation of blood products becomes a routine, much more of the incidence and natural history of transfusion-induced GVHD needs to be known. Until this information is available, irradiated blood products should be reserved for the severely immunocompromised, such as patients with aplastic anaemia, those post-bone marrow transplant, and those receiving granulocyte transfusions.

Apheresis

Much has been said of the use of cell-separators in harvesting blood products from selected donors. They may also be used in a more direct therapeutic way. Leucopheresis may be useful to reduce the white cell count in a child with a very high white count in acute lymphoblastic leukaemia, when *in vivo* tumour lysis from chemotherapy could produce an unacceptable metabolic upset and renal load. It would only provide temporary benefit while other therapeutic measures were initiated.

Another important use is the harvesting and cryopreservation of leucocytes from patients with chronic granulocytic leukaemia. The optimum therapy for these patients now is a matched bone marrow transplant, while in chronic phase. However, not every patient has a suitable marrow donor available, and cryopreserved leucocytes can be used to engraft the marrow with a second chronic phase after intensive therapy for blastic transformation. If a matched bone marrow transplant does not graft, cryopreserved granulocytes could also be used as an insurance, as it should engraft readily, preventing death from marrow failure.

It is possible to cryopreserve platelets and granulocytes from patients in remission, for use in the event of relapse or transplant (particularly useful for those who are alloimmunized and for whom provision of bank products is difficult). However, it is not always easy to harvest and store enough products to provide cover for further intensive therapy, and this procedure is most appropriate for adult patients.

In summary, the advances in transfusion practice have made intensive chemotherapy a feasible approach to childhood cancer, but have also resulted in new iatrogenic problems, such as transfusion-associated viral infections, and graft vs. host disease. Careful planning and preparation of blood product therapy involving close links with transfusion services are needed to minimize the risks to the recipients.

REFERENCES

1. Alverado J., Djerassi I. and Farber S. (1965) Transfusion of platelets to children with acute lymphoblastic leukaemia. *J. Pediatr.* **67**, 13–22.
2. Robinson E. A. E. (1984) Single donor granulocytes and platelets. *Clin. Haematol.* **13**(1), 185–216.
3. Daly P. A., Schiffer C. A., Aisner J. et al. (1980) Platelet transfusion therapy. One hour post transfusion increments are valuable in predicting the need for HLA-matched preparations. *JAMA* **243**, 435–8.
4. Levy L. and Woodfield D. G. (1984) The transfusion of HLA-matched platelets to thrombocytopenic patients resistant to random donor platelets. *NZ Med. J.* **97**, 719–21.
5. Barbara J. A. J. and Tedder R. S. (1984) Viral infections transmitted by blood and its products. *Clin. Haematol.* **13**(3), 693–707.
6. Wick M. R. (1985) Non-A, non-B hepatitis associated with blood transfusions. *Transfusion* **25**(2), 93–101.
7. Weiden P. L., Zuckerman N., Hansen J. A. et al. (1981) Fatal graft vs. host disease in a patient with acute lymphoblastic leukaemia following normal granulocyte transfusion. *Blood* **57**, 328–32.
8. Dinsmore R. E., Strauss D. J., Pollack M. S. et al. (1980) Fatal graft vs. host disease following blood transfusion in Hodgkin's disease—documented by tissue typing. *Blood* **55**, 831–4.
9. Lind S. E. (Editorial) (1985) Has the case for irradiating platelets been made? *Am. J. Med.* **78**, 543–4.

FURTHER READING

Buckner C. D. and Clift R. A. (1984) Prophylaxis and treatment of the immuno-compromised host by granulocyte transfusions. *Clin. Haematol.* **13**(3), 557–72.
Dutcher J. P. (1984) Granulocyte transfusion therapy. *Am. J. Med. Sci.* **287**, 11–17.
Feusner J. (1984) Supportive care for children with cancer: guidelines of the Children's Cancer Study Group. The use of platelet transfusions. *Am. J. Pediatr. Hematol. Oncol.* **6**, 255–60.
Mayer K. (1984) Transfusion support for leukaemia and oncology patients. *Clin. Haematol.* **13**(1), 93–8.
Strauss R. G. (1984) Supportive care for children with cancer—guidelines of the CCSG. The role of granulocyte transfusion. *Am. J. Pediatr. Hematol. Oncol.* **6**, 247–53.

5. Metabolic Problems in Children with Leukaemia and Lymphoma

N. A. G. Coad and J. R. Mann

INTRODUCTION

Hyperuricaemia in association with leukaemia and lymphoma, occurring both before and after treatment, has been recognized for many years and its treatment with allopurinol was first described by Krakoff and Meyer in 1965.[1] The first recognized feature of the 'tumour lysis syndrome', originally described in Burkitt's lymphoma, was hyperkalaemia.[2] Later elevation of serum LDH and hyperphosphataemia with concomitant hypocalcaemia were observed[2-6] and similar post-treatment biochemical disturbances were described in children with acute lymphoblastic leukaemia (ALL).[7] A number of other metabolic problems have since been described and are detailed below.

PATIENTS AT RISK

Metabolic problems arise mostly in children with tumours which have a large growth fraction and extreme sensitivity to chemotherapy, i.e. certain patients with ALL and non-Hodgkin's lymphoma (NHL). The children at greatest risk[8] are those with:
1. T- or B-cell ALL.
2. Any ALL with white cell count (WCC) $>100 \times 10^9/l$.
3. ALL with pleural effusion, mediastinal mass or palpably enlarged kidneys.
4. T- or B-cell NHL with bulky mediastinal or unresected intra-abdominal disease and/or pleural effusion or ascites.
5. Children with elevated serum LDH.

Some of the features of the tumour lysis syndrome have also been described in adults with acute myeloid leukaemia[9] but we have not observed these in children.

PRE-TREATMENT PROBLEMS

These are principally the problems of renal failure, associated with hyperuricaemia and/or other factors. Patients with even mild renal insufficiency are at great risk of serious post-treatment metabolic problems[8,10,11] and are identified by finding elevated blood creatinine for age[12] (*Table* 5.1), the blood urea not being a reliable indicator of renal function. Oliguria (<200 ml/m^2/24 h) or anuria may be present but often there is renal insufficiency despite normal urine volume.

Lactic acidosis is also occasionally present,[13] due to the predominantly anaerobic glycolysis of lymphoblasts and may exacerbate the problems of renal failure.

Hyperviscosity of the blood in patients with very high WCC may lead to renal, cardiac and respiratory failure and stroke.[14]

Table 5.1. Normal values for plasma creatinine in childhood[12]

Age	μmol/l				
0–2 weeks	42–71				
2–26 weeks	33–61				
6–12 months	28–53				
2 years	30–51				
4 years	34–56				
6 years	36–65				
8–10 years		37–69			36–59
12 years		37–77			37–72
14 years	Boys	32–92	Girls		44–76
16 years		43–100			50–79
18–25 years		76–106			53–84

Aetiology of renal failure

This is multifactorial and the causes are shown in *Table* 5.2. In the series of 33 patients with NHL studied by Tsokos et al.[10] renal failure was most often associated with extensive abdominal disease.

Hyperuricaemia, presumed to be due to release of uric acid from spontaneously lysing lymphoblasts, may cause nephropathy when serum uric acid levels rise above 660 μmol/l.[15] Urate precipitates in the perivascular renal parenchyma, distal renal tubules, collecting system and more rarely the ureters. Renal parenchymal damage can be associated with perivascular inflammation, nephrosclerosis and pyelonephritis.

Hypercalcaemia is less common but occasionally occurs in children with ALL[16] and NHL[17,18] and is usually associated with extensive skeletal deposits.

Table 5.2. Causes of pre-treatment renal failure

Hyperuricaemia
Hypercalcaemia
Intravascular volume depletion
Malignant infiltration of kidneys
Obstruction of urine flow by tumour

Intravascular volume depletion leads to poor renal blood flow and 'pre-renal' renal failure. It may be caused by vomiting or haemorrhage or be associated with hypoproteinaemia or loss of fluid into ascites or pleural effusion. Hypoproteinaemia may be due to several causes, including protein loss into effusions, anorexia and hepatic impairment.[8]

Although in ALL renal failure from bilateral renal leukaemic infiltration is uncommon, 30–50 per cent of autopsied patients showed diffuse renal infiltration, while in NHL renal infiltration was usually nodular.[19] The diagnosis may be suspected if the kidneys are enlarged but they can be normal in size despite being infiltrated.

Obstructive uropathy should be considered, especially in patients with abdominal or pelvic disease where the degree of renal failure is not explained by other factors, and is confirmed by finding hydronephrosis, ureteric compression by retroperitoneal lesions or bladder compression by pelvic tumour. These findings emphasize the need for abdominal ultrasound in high risk groups.

POST-TREATMENT PROBLEMS

The principal metabolic problems which may follow treatment of ALL and NHL are shown in *Table* 5.3. With the exception of the drug-induced disorders described in Chapter 8 (for example, inappropriate ADH production due to vincristine, diabetes from asparaginase, renal tubular damage from aminoglycosides), they all result from the very rapid breakdown of lymphoblasts which occurs

Table 5.3. Metabolic problems after treatment

Renal failure
Hyperuricaemia
Hyperkalaemia
Hyperphosphataemia
Hypocalcaemia
Fluid overload
Drug-induced disorders (*see* Chapter 7)

after the start of cytotoxic therapy. Intracellular products are released into the circulation, notably nucleic acids, potassium and phosphorus. They are excreted by the kidneys, so that if renal function is compromised and/or the rate of their release exceeds the ability of the kidneys to excrete them, then an accumulation of urea, uric acid, potassium or phosphorus may occur and lead to serious complications including sudden death.[8,20]

Renal failure

This may be manifested by rising plasma urea and creatinine levels despite a good urine output, but some patients become oliguric or even anuric, despite prophylactic hyperhydration and other measures (*see* treatment section). Urgent measures are required to maintain urine flow and rarely peritoneal or haemodialysis are necessary. Because of the bulk of tumour products to be excreted, in some children serum urea and creatinine levels may not return to normal for over 2 weeks.[8,10,15]

Hyperuricaemia

While in many patients raised serum uric acid levels can be lowered before or during the first few days of chemotherapy by hyper-hydration, alkalinization of urine and allopurinol, in some children the levels continue to rise, particularly if oliguria or anuria occur.[8] At physiological pH urate is 95 per cent soluble, but when pH is < 5.5 urate is largely un-ionized and poorly soluble. Thus, if blood urate levels rise above 660 μmol/l precipitation of urate takes place particularly in the distal renal tubules and collecting systems, where the urine is acidified and concentrated,[15] and leads to further deterioration in renal function.

Hyperkalaemia

This is the principal cause of sudden death in patients with tumour lysis syndrome and can occur within 12 h of starting chemotherapy[8] (*Fig.* 5.1). In one of our patients with T-cell ALL and WCC 760 $\times$ 10^9/l who received just 15 mg prednisolone, fatal hyperkalaemia occurred after only 9 h. He had very mild renal dysfunction as judged by his serum creatinine level but, although total urinary potassium excretion increased, fractional excretion measurements revealed impaired tubular function and thus inability to handle the increased potassium load.

Hyperkalaemia is most likely to arise in children with T- and B-cell ALL, especially with high WCC, and in children with advanced B-

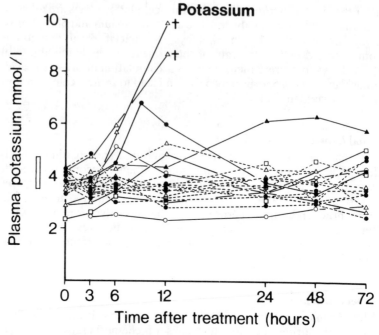

Fig. 5.1. Plasma potassium levels after treatment.
Key to symbols: □ 'common' ALL
△ T-cell ALL
▲ T-cell NHL
○ B-cell ALL
● B-cell NHL
• 'null' ALL
† patient died
   The solid lines indicate patients with impaired renal function. The dotted lines indicate patients with normal renal function.

cell NHL, particularly when renal function is even slightly impaired.[2,8,10,11] We have found that in T-cell ALL the rise of potassium is proportional to the initial WCC and may start as early as 3 h after the onset of chemotherapy.[8]

It is important to differentiate true hyperkalaemia from pseudo-hyperkalaemia[21] resulting from cellular lysis occurring during collection, clotting or storage of blood samples. This problem is especially likely when the WCC exceeds $50 \times 10^9/l$ or the platelet count exceeds $1000 \times 10^9/l$, or if blood is collected using narrow bore needles or by capillary sampling. Thus all samples for biochemical monitoring in these patients should be taken through wide bore needles or cannulae and the plasma should be separated immediately from the cells.

The potentially fatal cardiac effects of hyperkalaemia may be potentiated by co-existing acidosis or hypocalcaemia in patients with tumour lysis syndrome.

ECG monitoring is usually undertaken, but in our experience 3-hourly measurements of plasma potassium give earlier warning of potentially fatal hyperkalaemia than does the appearance of ECG changes, such as peaked T-waves, QRS complex widening, and arrhythmias.

Hyperphosphataemia

The onset of hyperphosphataemia is usually between 6 and 12 h after treatment. Levels tend to peak between 12 and 24 h except those with severe renal failure in whom levels tend to rise until renal function improves (*Fig.* 5.2). Hypocalcaemia is almost invariably associated and the majority of patients have hyperphosphaturia.[8]

Hyperphosphataemia results from rapid tumour breakdown with release of massive quantities of phosphorus into the circulation, but renal phosphorus retention is also a contributory factor[10,11] while drug-induced hypoparathyroidism[22] operates to a lesser extent. Lymphoblasts contain 4 times more phosphorus than mature lymphocytes[23] and the patients at greatest risk of hyperphosphataemia have T- or B-cell ALL or NHL, especially with high WCC,[7] large tumours or renal failure.[10,11]

Hyperphosphataemia may cause calcium phosphate deposition in the renal tubules and this, together with hyperuricaemia, are the major causes of post-treatment renal failure,[10] which leads to secondary renal phosphorus retention and perpetuates the cycle of metabolic deterioration.

Renal phosphorus retention does not usually take place until creatinine clearance has fallen to >25ml/min/$1\cdot73$m^2 but when there is a large phosphate load hyperphosphataemia may occur at more modest degrees of renal insufficiency.[5] When the calcium/phosphorus product exceeds $4\cdot8$, calcium phosphate crystals may be precipitated, causing tissue damage, renal tubular obstruction and hypocalcaemia.[25] Metastatic calcification may occur in the kidneys, skin, eyes, joints and lungs.

Hypocalcaemia

This is common following treatment of ALL[26] and NHL[10] in children and AML in adults.[9] In our series of 21 high risk children with ALL and NHL,[8] all had normal calcium levels before treatment whereas all but one developed hypocalcaemia in the immediate post-treatment period (*Fig.* 5.3). Onset was at 3 h with a nadir at 24 h and the fall was more pronounced in patients with renal failure. In half the patients hyperphosphataemia was not present, suggesting that mechanisms other than calcium phosphate precipitation were involved. Debilitation, septicaemia and hypoalbuminaemia may contribute in some patients but would be expected to produce pre-treatment abnormalities rather than the rapid fall *after* treatment. Other factors which may be important are steroid administration,[26]

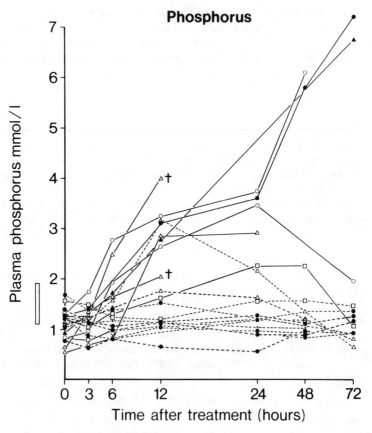

Fig. 5.2. Plasma phosphorus levels after treatment. Key as for *Fig.* 5.1. The block to the left of the vertical axis indicates the normal range.

cytotoxic or aminoglycoside-induced transient hypoparathyroid-ism[22,27] or hypomagnesaemia[28]—but the last did not occur in our patients.[8]

Despite its frequency, hypocalcaemia rarely causes symptoms in these patients and treatment is only required during the management of hyperkalaemia and in the rare event of tetany. Otherwise intravenous calcium salts should be avoided because of the risk of producing metastatic calcification in the presence of hyperphosphataemia.

Fluid overload

To correct the pre-existing metabolic problems and to prevent those which may arise after treatment, it is essential to establish a brisk diuresis in all high-risk patients. However, some patients have difficulty in excreting the fluid load due to renal functional impairment and therefore close monitoring of fluid balance and additional measures to promote diuresis and prevent cardiac failure from fluid overload may be required.

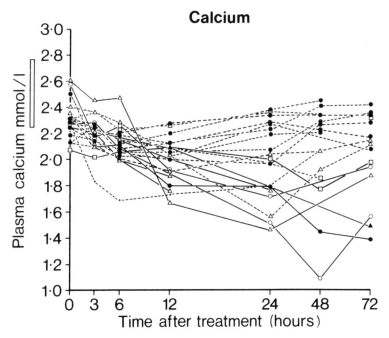

Fig. 5.3. Plasma calcium levels after treatment. Key as for *Fig.* 5.1. The block to the left of the vertical axis indicates the normal range.

ASSESSMENT BEFORE THERAPY

Clinical

Patients with ALL and NHL can be suspected to be at risk from the complications of tumour lysis if they have signs of massive tumour, superior vena caval obstruction, pleural effusion, ascites or acidosis. General anaesthesia can be dangerous in such patients and if possible, therefore, diagnostic procedures such as bone marrow aspirate, lumbar puncture and tapping of pleural effusion or ascites, should be undertaken with local anaesthesia. The patient's height and weight should be measured, his hydration assessed and urine output monitored.

Investigations

These should include chest X-ray to detect mediastinal mass and pleural effusion, blood count, plasma creatinine, sodium, potassium, calcium, phosphate, albumin and uric acid. Acid base balance should also be assessed, particularly if renal failure or signs of acidosis are present.

Lymphocyte marker studies on blood, bone marrow, effusion fluid or tumour biopsies are needed to confirm T- and B-cell malignancies.

Abdominal ultrasound examination and/or CT scans are valuable in assessing abdominal tumours and renal size. Intravenous urography may be needed if obstructive uropathy is suspected.

MANAGEMENT

Correction of pre-existing metabolic problems

Whenever possible, pre-existing metabolic problems should be corrected before cytotoxic chemotherapy is given. However, when life-threatening complications such as airway obstruction, superior vena caval obstruction and rapidly rising WCC are present, and in other patients with a massive tumour load, complete correction may be impossible. In all patients, a brisk diuresis must be achieved both to reduce already elevated plasma uric acid, calcium and creatinine levels and to facilitate the excretion of urates, potassium and phosphate after cytotoxic chemotherapy has been given. The recommended regimen is shown in *Table* 5.4.

The i.v. saline is given in a concentration of 0·45 per cent because such large volumes of more dilute saline are prone to cause hyponatraemia and water intoxication.

Table 5.4. Regimen to prevent metabolic complications of tumour lysis (and to correct existing ones)

---

1. Clinical and biochemical assessment (including measurement of blood count, creatinine, Na, K, Ca, PO_4, albumin, uric acid, acid-base).
2. Insert i.v. line and, if possible, a second cannula for venous blood sampling.
3. Hydrate with i.v. dextrose 5%, saline 0·45% at $3 l/m^2/day$, for minimum of 24 h before starting chemotherapy (unless rapidly rising WCC or SVC obstruction requires earlier intervention (*see* text) and continue after chemotherapy for at least 48 h, until biochemically stable.
4. Alkalinize urine to pH 7 to 7·5, starting with i.v. $NaHCO_3$ 3mmol/kg/day and increasing if necessary.
5. Replace fluid losses from vomiting, fever or diarrhoea with 0·9% saline in addition to the above.
6. Keep accurate fluid balance, measure all urine and weigh 12-hourly.
7. If fluid load is not adequately excreted, take additional measures (*see* text).
8. Give allopurinol $400mg/m^2/day$ orally or i.v. in 3 divided doses.
9. Aluminium hydroxide 5–10ml orally 6-hourly should be given if tolerated.
10. Monitor biochemical changes after the start of chemotherapy by taking venous blood for potassium and calcium at 0, 3, 6, 9 and 12 h. Then measure sodium, potassium, calcium, phosphate, creatinine, uric acid and albumin at 24 h and daily until stable.

The urine is alkalinized to prevent urates precipitating in the kidney at low pH.

If the patient is unable adequately to excrete the fluid load, give mannitol 1g/kg over 20 min, if necessary followed by frusemide (2mg/kg, repeated if necessary after 30–60 min). Hypoproteinaemia may cause hypovolaemia and poor renal perfusion resulting in oliguria. Therefore, hypoproteinaemia may need to be corrected by giving i.v. albumin or plasma to promote diuresis which should occur within 1 h of the above measures. If oliguria persists despite these measures, peritoneal or haemodialysis may have to be undertaken.

When renal function is inadequate, radiotherapy to the kidneys with 600–1000cGy has been advocated prior to definitive chemotherapy),[29,30] but may not always be appropriate. Obstructive uropathy usually responds rapidly to cytotoxic chemotherapy, with appropriate dose reductions for renally excreted agents, but in severe oliguria or anuria, urinary diversion or dialysis must be considered.

Allopurinol is a competitive inhibitor of xanthine oxidase, which converts xanthine and hypoxanthine to uric acid. Xanthine is more soluble than urates and less likely to be precipitated in the kidney, so xanthine nephropathy, though a potential hazard, is uncommon after allopurinol use.[31] Moreover, allopurinol suppresses purine biosynthesis and thus reduces the purine load. An alternative approach is to use urate oxidase, which converts urate to allantoin. This has been reported to be safer and more effective than allopurinol,[32,33] but further work is required and its use may be limited by hypersensitivity.

Oral aluminium hydroxide or calcium carbonate, if tolerated, will bind phosphorus in the gut and may help to reduce the blood phosphorus after chemotherapy but their effect is slow and unpredictable.

In patients with hyperviscosity due to high WCC, leucophoresis or exchange transfusion before cytotoxic therapy is given may be helpful to improve cardiac, renal and respiratory function and reduce the risk of stroke.[14]

A mediastinal or thymic mass may sometimes cause superior vena caval or tracheal obstruction in children with T-ALL or NHL. This may be rapidly progressive and constitutes a medical emergency. A tissue diagnosis should be obtained prior to treatment with emergency mediastinal radiotherapy or chemotherapy.[33]

Regimen to prevent complications after cytotoxic chemotherapy

Hydration, urine alkalinization and allopurinol are continued (*Table* 5.4), together with frequent clinical monitoring and assessment of fluid balance.

Blood should be taken for potassium and calcium at 0, 3, 6, 9 and 12 h after starting chemotherapy. Then monitor sodium, potassium, calcium, phosphate, creatinine, uric acid and albumin at 24 h and daily until stable.

The hydration regimen will be required for at least 48 h after the start of chemotherapy, and for much longer if renal complications occur. Allopurinol can usually be stopped after 7–10 days.

Hyperkalaemia

If the serum potassium rises above 6·0mmol/l initiate treatment as shown in *Table* 5.5. The mannitol and frusemide are given to promote

Table 5.5.   Treatment of hyperkalaemia (K > 6·0mmol/l)

1. Give mannitol 1·0g/kg i.v. over 20 min followed by frusemide 5mg/kg i.v. (maximum 100mg) by bolus.
2. Give 0·3ml/kg calcium gluconate i.v. slowly.
3. Give glucose and insulin, 0·3u/kg soluble insulin with 3g/kg glucose i.v. over 10 min (i.e. 6ml/kg of 50% glucose solution).
4. Correct acidosis if present.
5. Give calcium resonium 1g/kg orally or rectally and repeat 12-hourly as necessary.
6. Monitor ECG.
7. Repeat plasma K, Ca and glucose levels after 1 h.
8. Consider dialysis if no improvement.

further renal excretion of potassium, the calcium to stabilize the myocardium and the sodium bicarbonate to induce cellular uptake of potassium ions in exchange for hydrogen. The glucose and insulin also facilitate the uptake of potassium by cells.

Renal failure

If the measures already described to counteract oliguria (fluids, mannitol, frusemide and albumin) are ineffective and anuria, confirmed by bladder catheterization, supervenes, then measures to prevent fluid overload and for managing severe renal failure must be taken. Daily fluid intake is restricted to that required to replace insensible losses ($300ml/m^2/day$ allowing 10 per cent more for each $1°C$ of fever) plus gastrointestinal losses plus the volume of the previous day's urine output.

The majority of patients with renal failure can be managed conservatively, but peritoneal or haemodialysis may be needed in patients with anuria, plasma potassium above 7mmol/l or fluid overload and should be considered when uric acid levels are exceptionally high and if hypertension cannot be controlled.

Peritoneal dialysis is quickly available and effective but carries a risk of peritonitis in patients rendered neutropenic by cytotoxic chemotherapy.[8] Haemodialysis is 10–20 times more effective at removing urate than is peritoneal dialysis[15] but vascular access may be difficult in small children and haemodialysis is not readily available in all paediatric oncology units.

Hypocalcaemia

This is usually best left untreated unless hyperkalaemia or tetany occur, in which case give calcium gluconate slowly i.v. as described in *Table* 5.5.

Hyperphosphataemia

This is best treated by the methods already described for producing a diuresis and renal failure should be treated as described above. If tolerated, oral aluminium hydroxide will bind phosphorus in the gut and thus reduce the blood levels. Intravenous calcium salts should be avoided if possible to reduce the risks of metastatic calcification.

REFERENCES

1. Krakoff I. H. and Meyer R. L. (1965) Prevention of hyperuricemia in leukemia and lymphoma. *JAMA* **193**, 1–6.
2. Arseneau J. C., Bagley C. M., Anderson T. et al. (1973) Hyperkalaemia, a sequel to chemotherapy of Burkitt's lymphoma. *Lancet* **i**, 10–14.
3. Arseneau J. C., Cannellos G. P., Banks P. M. et al. (1975) American Burkitt's lymphoma: A clinico-pathological study of 30 cases. I. Clinical factors relating to prolonged survival. *Am. J. Med.* **58**, 314–21.
4. Brereton H. D., Anderson T., Johnson R. E. et al. (1975) Hyperphosphatemia and hypocalcemia in Burkitt's lymphoma. *Arch. Intern. Med.* **135**, 307–9.
5. Cadman E. C., Lundberg W. B. and Bertino J. R. (1977) Hyperphosphatemia and hypocalcemia accompanying rapid cell lysis in a patient with Burkitt's lymphoma and Burkitt cell leukemia. *Am. J. Med.* **62**, 283–90.
6. Siegel M. B., Alexander E. A., Weintraub L. et al. (1977) Renal failure in Burkitt's lymphoma. *Clin. Nephrol.* **7**, 279–83.
7. Zusman J., Brown D. M. and Nesbit M. E. (1973) Hyperphosphatemia, hyperphosphaturia and hypocalcemia in acute lymphoblastic leukemia. *N. Engl. J. Med.* **289**, 1335–40.
8. Coad N. A. G., Margerison A. C. F., Mann S. et al. Studies of metabolic problems associated with tumour lysis in children with lymphoblastic leukaemia (ALL) and non-Hodgkin's lymphoma (NHL). (In preparation.)
9. Mir M. A. and Delamore I. W. (1978) Metabolic disorders in acute myeloid leukaemia. *Br. J. Haematol.* **40**, 79–92.
10. Tsokos G. C., Balow J. E., Spiegel R. J. et al. (1981) Renal and metabolic complications of undifferentiated and lymphoblastic lymphomas. *Medicine* **60**, 218–29.
11. Cohen L. F., Balow J. E., McGrath I. T. et al. (1980) Acute tumour lysis syndrome. A review of 37 patients with Burkitt's lymphoma. *Am. J. Med.* **68**, 486–91.
12. Clayton B. E., Jenkins P., and Round J. M. (1980) *Paediatric Chemical Pathology.* Oxford, Blackwell Scientific Publications.
13. O'Regan S., Carson S., Chesney R. W. et al. (1977) Electrolyte and acid base disturbances in the management of leukemia. *Blood* **49**, 345–53.
14. Bunin N. J. and Pui C. H. (1985) Differing complications of hyperleukocytosis in children with acute lymphoblastic or acute non-lymphoblastic leukemia. *J. Clin. Oncol.* **3**(12), 1590–5.
15. Kjellstrand C. M., Cambell D. C., Hartitzsch B. et al. (1974) Hyperuricemic acute renal failure. *Arch. Intern. Med.* **133**, 349–59.
16. Stein R. C. (1971) Hypercalcemia in leukemia. *J. Pediatr.* **78**, 861–4.
17. Stapleton F. B., Lukert B. P. and Linshaw M. A. (1976) Treatment of hypercalcemia associated with osseous metastases and lymphoma *J. Pediatr.* **89**, 1029–30.
18. Speigel A., Greene M., McGrath I. et al. (1978) Hypercalcaemia with suppressed parathyroid hormone in Burkitt's lymphoma. *Am. J. Med.* **64**, 691–5.
19. Garnick M. B. and Mayer R. J. (1978) Acute renal failure associated with neoplastic disease and its treatment. *Semin. Oncol.* **5**, 155–65.
20. Leading article (1981) Tumour lysis syndrome. *Lancet* **i**, 849.
21. Kerr D. J., McAlpine L. G. and Dagg J. H. (1985) Pseudohyperkalaemia. *Br. Med. J.* **291**, 890–1.
22. Freedman D. B., Shannon M., Dandona P. et al. (1982) Hypoparathyroidism and hypocalcaemia during treatment for acute leukaemia. *Br. Med. J.* **284**, 700–2.
23. Rigas D. A., Dueist M. L., Jump M. E. et al. (1956) The nucleic acids and other phosphorus compounds of human leukaemic leukocytes: relation to cell maturity. *J. Lab. Clin. Med.* **48**, 356–78.

24. Goldman R., Bassett S. H., and Duncan G. B. (1954) Phosphorus excretion in renal failure. *J. Clin. Invest.* **33**, 1623–8.
25. Herbert L. A., Lemann J., Peterson J. R. et al. (1966) Studies of the mechanism by which phosphate infusion lowers serum calcium concentration. *J. Clin. Invest.* **45**, 1886–94.
26. Jaffe N., Kim B. S. and Vawter G. F. (1972) Hypocalcemia—a complication of childhood leukemia. *Cancer* **29**, 392–8.
27. Keating M. J., Sethi M. D., Boden G. P. et al. (1977) Hypocalcemia with hypoparathyroidism and renal tubular dysfunction associated with aminoglycoside therapy. *Cancer* **39**, 1410–4.
28. Brenton D. F. and Gordon T. E. (1984) Fluid and electrolyte disorders: magnesium. *Br. J. Hosp. Med.* **32**, 60–9.
29. Stoffel T. J., Nesbit M. E. and Levitt S. H. (1975) The role of radiotherapy in renal involvement in acute childhood leukaemia. *Radiology* **117**, 687–94.
30. Lundberg W. B., Codman E. D., Finch S. C. et al (1977) Renal failure secondary to leukemic infiltration of the kidneys. *Am. J. Med.* **228**, 271–6.
31. Leading article (1979) Acute renal failure, hyperuricaemia and myoglobinuria. *Br. Med. J.* **1**, 1233–4.
32. Kissel P., Manuary G., Royer R. et al. (1975) Treatment of malignant haemopathies and urate oxidase. *Lancet* **i**, 229.
33. Perez C. A., Present C. A. and VanAmberg A. L. (1978) Management of superior vena cava syndrome. *Semin. Oncol.* **5**, 123.

6.   Acute Medical Problems

A. Oakhill

INTRODUCTION

The commonest oncologic emergencies faced in the practice of paediatric oncology are related to infections and haematological complications, which are dealt with in the appropriate chapters in this book. The problems dealt with here are related to 'bulky' disease which may be the reason for the child's presentation as an emergency and warrant immediate action to reverse their life-threatening nature.

OBSTRUCTION TO THE SUPERIOR VENA CAVA

The superior vena cava, formed from the right and left jugular and innominate veins, may be obstructed in its course to the right atrium within the rigid structure of the mediastinum. This consists of 4 regions:

1. The *posterior* region which contains the aorta and oesophagus and lies behind the pericardium.
2. The *middle* region, which contains the heart, pericardium and the 2 main bronchi.
3. The *anterior* region, which contains the thymus and lies between the sternum and pericardium.
4. The *superior* region, which contains the thymus, great vessels, oesophagus and aorta and lies above the pericardium.

An anterior group of lymph nodes is closely associated with the SVC and aorta and has a major role in the development of SVC obstruction.

Knowledge of the anatomy of the mediastinum is important in helping to arrive at the causes of both SVC obstruction and mediastinal enlargement. The majority of children seen with these problems will have involvement of the anterior lymph node group due to non-

Table 6.1. Malignant causes of a wide mediastinum in childhood

Disease	Site
Non-Hodgkin's lymphoma	Anterior/superior
Hodgkin's lymphoma	Anterior/superior
T-cell ALL	Anterior/superior
Thymoma	Anterior/superior
Teratoma	Posterior
Primary tumours of the heart, pericardium and great vessels, e.g. rhabdomyosarcoma	Middle
Neuroblastoma	Posterior

Hodgkin's lymphoma (NHL), Hodgkin's disease and T-cell acute lymphoblastic leukaemia (*Table* 6.1).

The clinical presentation of the SVC syndrome may be due to compression of the trachea and main bronchi as well as the SVC. Patients complain of the development of difficulty in breathing, wheezing, orthopnoea and a change of voice (due to involvement of the phrenic nerve). A rapid onset is more suggestive of NHL or T-cell ALL than Hodgkin's disease.

On examination, the patient may look very ill with a decreased level of consciousness due to cerebral oedema. The face, neck and upper thorax may be plethoric and oedematous. Distended jugular veins and collateral veins on the chest wall are usually obvious.[1]

Cyanosis, tachypnoea, wheeze and stridor occur with airway obstruction and the patient is usually more comfortable sitting up. A hoarse voice, due to vocal cord paralysis and occasional Horner's syndrome, may be found. This constellation of symptoms and signs requires urgent investigation and treatment, but great care must be taken to prevent a respiratory catastrophe.

A chest X-ray should be performed which, in most cases of SVC obstruction, will show a mass in the anterior–superior mediastinum. Other investigations are directed at coming to a tissue diagnosis but should not preclude emergency treatment if deemed necessary. A full blood count may reveal the presence of lymphoblasts. A bone marrow aspirate and lymph node biopsy may both be possible under local anaesthetic. Tissue from the mass will usually be necessary, however. Consultation with anaesthetist and surgeon, on the safety of the procedure, is of paramount importance and then a decision must be made on an approach by mediastinoscopy, cervical mediastinal exploration or thoracotomy. The presence at biopsy of a pathologist, so that 'touch preparations' can be performed, may allow a more rapid diagnosis.

The desirability of a tissue diagnosis is due to the difference in treatment of NHL and Hodgkin's disease. It may be that time will not allow this distinction and emergency treatment will be necessary. The treatment of both NHL and T-cell ALL can lead to profound metabolic problems. Intravenous fluids should be given, preferably into a foot vein as the veins draining into the SVC may bleed profusely or be thrombosed. The volume of fluid given needs to be carefully assessed as the patient may have cerebral oedema as well as being dehydrated. Allopurinol should be given and the patient alkalinized.

Having attempted a tissue diagnosis and instituted pre-emptive treatment of metabolic problems, radiotherapy is the treatment of choice. Prior to this, steroids in high dose should be given to prevent oedema and increasing obstruction from the initial effect of radiotherapy. Steroids alone, particularly in NHL and T-cell leukaemia may cause shrinkage of the mediastinal mass.

If it is considered that the patient's life is threatened by transporting him to the radiotherapy department (and this may need the accompaniment of an anaesthetist), alternative treatment would be cytoreductive chemotherapy. A combination, such as the 'CHOP' regimen (cyclophosphamide, adriamycin, vincristine and prednisone), using a high dose of steroids, would be appropriate and effective against both NHL and Hodgkin's disease.[2]

SPINAL CORD COMPRESSION

Paralysis due to spinal cord compression is often permanent without rapid diagnosis and prompt treatment. In children, it occurs with epidural, intradural and intramedullary tumours and rarely because of subdural haematomas and vertebral subluxation.

The presenting symptoms and signs will depend on several factors, including the site of the lesion, type of tumour and the age of the child. Unlike adults and adolescents, weakness of the legs is more common than either local or radicular pain. When the latter does occur, it is often accentuated by coughing, spinal percussion and straight leg raising. Autonomic and sensory abnormalities will also occur and, again, will depend on the site of the tumour. In simple terms, lesions in and above the thoracic cord will lead to symmetrically decreased sensation and power, spastic bladder and constipation. Lesions below the thoracic cord will often have asymmetric decreases in power and a large, easily palpable bladder with incontinence.

The most difficult dilemma is if cord compression is a presenting feature of an undiagnosed malignancy (*Table* 6.2). The likeliest reasons for this presentation would be the diseases listed under epidural, intramedullary and vertebral subluxation sites in the table.

Table 6.2. Causes of spinal cord compression

Site	Cause
Epidural	Neuroblastoma Lymphoma Soft tissue sarcoma (Ewings and rhabdomyosarcoma)

Intradural	Metastases from ependymoma,
	  medulloblastoma and primitive
	  neuroectodermal tumour (PNET)

Intramedullary	Astrocytoma and ependymoma of cord
Subdural	Haematoma (following lumbar puncture in thrombocytopenic patients)
Vertebral subluxation	Histiocytosis X Acute lymphoblastic leukaemia

Neuroblastoma may arise in the paravertebral ganglia and grow through an intravertebral foramen to give cord compression (the so-called 'dumb bell' tumour). This presentation often has a good prognosis as it typically occurs in young children who have not developed metastases. Lymphomas and soft tissue sarcomas also extend through the intravertebral foramina.

Metastases from ependymomas, medulloblastomas and PNETs are now rarer, due to the treatment of the whole craniospinal axis with radiation following diagnosis of the primary brain tumour.

Astrocytomas of the cord often have a long history and appear in older children. Subdural haematomas subsequent to lumbar punctures are thankfully rare, as thrombocytopenic patients with acute leukaemia will usually have platelet transfusion prior to the procedure.

Vertebral erosion, due to histiocytosis X and ALL are frequently seen. It is unusual to proceed to collapse and, when this occurs, is often planar rather than wedged with occasional subluxation. If this does happen, it may involve the cervical (which is extremely dangerous) or thoracic vertebrae.

Following careful clinical assessment, the diagnosis of cord compression will be made through radiological evaluation. A plane X-ray of the spine will reveal both epidural and vertebral causes. Most patients will require a myelogram, however, and this should be performed in a neurosurgical centre. The recent introduction of Nuclear Magnetic Resonance may, in the future, replace unpleasant and dangerous myelography.

Other investigations will be aimed at diagnosing the underlying malignancy and should include a full blood count, urinary catechol-amines, chest X-ray and skeletal survey.

Attempts at a tissue diagnosis should be made, but taking into consideration the urgency of treating the cord compression. Needle aspiration may sometimes be possible but laminectomy and biopsy is still necessary in some patients. Although laminectomy is diagnostic and therapeutic, it is associated with damage to the vertebrae. Dexamethasone, at a dose of 50mg/m^2 i.v. bolus, followed by 10mg/m^2 q.d.s. should be given prior to any other treatment. This will decrease the oedema around the tumour and also prevent swelling due to radiotherapy. Unfortunately, steroids make the diagnosis of lymphoma difficult by dissolving the tumour prior to biopsy.

A decision now needs to be made regarding therapeutic radiation and/or laminectomy. This will depend on the necessity for biopsy and the degree of cord compression. An alternative is to use cytoreductive chemotherapy in a similar way to that suggested for SVC obstruction. A combination of ifosfamide, adriamycin and vincristine (with the prescribed dexamethasone) would be appropriate for the majority of diseases listed in the table which are highly sensitive to treatment.

RAISED INTRACRANIAL PRESSURE

The symptoms and signs of raised intracranial pressure will usually have a gradual onset allowing the cause to be elicited before life-threatening problems occur. This will be particularly true in primary tumours of the central nervous system (CNS). An acute presentation may, however, be seen and rapid treatment and diagnosis must be initiated.

Raised intracranial pressure is a rare complication at presentation of ALL with a high white cell count. This is due to stasis in small intracerebral vessels (and occasionally sagittal sinus thrombosis) and the problem may be accentuated by the presence of CNS disease at diagnosis. This stasis, combined with thrombocytopenia, is extremely dangerous and a fatal intracerebral bleed is a common outcome. Management is controversial and must take into consideration the metabolic sequelae of treating high white cell count disease. Present considerations include urgent brain irradiation and leucopheresis.

Much commoner will be the symptom complex that occurs with raised intracranial pressure in established disease. This will usually be due to infection, haemorrhage or metastatic disease. In children who have a ventricular peritoneal shunt, blockage is a common complication.

Cerebral abscesses are seen particularly in children with leukaemia and post bone marrow transplantation. *Aspergillus* (usually secondary to lung infection) is an important cause and is fatal in the majority of patients. In severely immunosuppressed patients, gram-positive, gram-negative and anaerobic organisms, either singly or mixed, may cause abscess formation. Other infectious agents, such as *Crypto-coccus,* may cause basal meningitis and acute hydrocephalus.

Intracerebral and subdural haemorrhage is rare in childhood cancer, but may be seen at presentation of high white cell count ALL, severe thrombocytopenia, DIC (as in acute promyelocytic leukaemia) or due to a bleed into a metastasis.

Consequent on the improved survival of solid tumours, intracranial metastases have become more common. Leptomeningeal disease is much more frequent than single intracerebral metastases. Relapsed acute leukaemia, retinoblastoma, neuroblastoma and rhabdomyo-sarcoma may present with raised intracranial pressure and an acutely decompensating patient. Seventy per cent of patients with ALL prior to the use of prophylactic nervous system treatment developed CNS disease. This has now fallen to between 3 and 5 per cent. Relapse in the CNS occurs in head and neck rhabdomyosarcoma, particularly if there is cranial nerve involvement (this does not include orbital rhabdomyosarcoma). In the hope of preventing CNS disease, prophylactic intrathecal chemotherapy and radiation fields, including the base of the brain, are now incorporated into protocols treating head and neck tumours.

Metastatic neuroblastoma primarily involves the bones of the skull and rarely extends through the dura. When the skull base is involved, CNS sequelae do, however, occur.

When retinoblastoma presents with orbital disease or extends along the optic nerve, CNS disease is common and usually fatal.

Intracranial neoplasms, particularly medulloblastoma and ependymoma, may also metastasize within the CNS.

As with ALL, the intention should be to prevent CNS disease, as cure is unlikely once it has occurred. Prophylaxis is, therefore, an important component in the treatment of ALL, head and neck rhabdo-myosarcoma, retinoblastoma, ependymoma and medulloblastoma.

The signs and symptoms of raised intracranial pressure are both subacute and acute, the subacute form being typical of meningeal relapse in ALL. Here, early morning headaches with nausea and effortless vomiting soon progress to neck stiffness. A sixth cranial nerve palsy may occur as a false lateralizing sign. Facial nerve palsies are also a feature.

The acute signs and symptoms are due to cerebral herniation. There are 3 clinical syndromes associated with this problem: uncal, central and tonsillar herniation.[3]

Uncal herniation will be seen with masses in the temporal lobe or subdurally, both situations being rare in childhood cancer. Apart from the typical headache and vomiting, there are often ipsilateral neurological features, such as third nerve palsy and hemiparesis which may appear before coma.

In *central herniation* (particularly relevant to leptomeningeal disease and acute hydrocephalus), the diencephalon is forced downwards. Headache is associated with increasing drowsiness and the development of Cheyne-Stokes respiration. There are rarely lateralizing signs, but small reactive pupils may be seen prior to fixed pupils. Dysconjugate eye movements and odd postures are also seen.

Tonsillar herniation is seen when there is a mass in the posterior fossa and, therefore, likely at the presentation and relapse of medulloblastoma. Headache, vomiting and hiccoughs occur early. There is then progression to a stiff neck and even opisthotonus. Loss of consciousness is associated with irregular respiration and apnoea. Arterial hypertension is a further complication and a variety of ophthalmic signs, including skew deviation, occur.

With such rapid and life-threatening progression, treatment and diagnosis must go hand-in-hand. If abnormal respiration and loss of consciousness ensue, the patient should be intubated and perhaps hyperventilated to reduce carbon dioxide tension to around 23 mmHg.

To reduce pressure, mannitol should be given to produce a rapid osmotic diuresis. An initial dose of 1g/kg would be appropriate.

Although dexamethasone takes several hours to be effective, it should be given early. A high dose should be given initially (1mg/kg) and reduced in subsequent doses.

When the patient is in a stable condition, an emergency CT scan should be performed which should reveal the underlying aetiology of the cerebral herniation. Appropriate neurosurgical approaches should then be considered aimed at decompression (the Ommaya reservoir is useful both diagnostically and therapeutically) and CSF analysis for malignant cells and infectious organisms.

In an acutely decompensating patient, lumbar puncture should never be attempted without prior thorough investigation.

REFERENCES

1. Bowen R. J. and Kiesawitter W. B. (1977) Mediastinal masses in infants and children. *Arch. Surg.* **112**, 1003.
2. Halpern S., Catten J., Meadows A. T. et al. (1983) Anterior mediastinal masses: anaesthesia hazards and other problems. *J. Paediatr.* **102**, 407–10.
3. Plum F. and Posner J. B. (1972) *Diagnosis of Stupor and Coma.* Philadelphia, Davis.

FURTHER READING

Gilbert R. W., Kim J. H. and Posner J. B. (1978) Epidural spinal cord compression from metastatic tumour. *Ann. Neurol.* **3**, 40–51.

7. Chemotherapy: Problems and Precautions

S. Siddall

Before the administration of chemotherapy, several checks are required by doctors, pharmacists and nurses to ensure that the patient receives optimal treatment with minimal toxicity.

The correct doses of cytotoxic drugs are ascertained from relevant protocols based on body surface area, taking into account any dosage adjustment required due to low white cell count or renal impairment. Route of administration is often dependent on protocols with suggested method and time of administration given and compatible fluids listed, and these factors must be carefully considered before treatment commences.

Personnel prescribing, checking and giving chemotherapy should be aware of any potential side-effects before administration since it may be possible to avert or reduce these with appropriate drug treatment or fluid/electrolyte replacement. Cytotoxics given intravenously may be vesicant and steps should be taken before use to reduce the possibility of thrombophlebitis or extravasation. Danger of anaphylaxis or hypersensitivity is also a problem.

Preparation of cytotoxic drugs presents a health hazard to personnel handling them which should be considered before use to avoid exposure of hospital personnel to possible carcinogens.

Data on reconstitution, storage and stability are readily available for individual drugs on package inserts, data sheets or in-hospital procedure manuals. *Tables* 7.1 and 7.2 have been designed as checklists to assess, prevent and manage any problems arising with chemotherapy and should be used in conjunction with local protocols. Methods of administration have been specifically chosen for paediatric use.

The following checklist is suggested for reference before and during chemotherapy:

Clinical checklist
1. Has the patient's current weight and surface area been checked?
2. Is the oncology treatment part of a protocol and, if so, have all the drugs required been prescribed?
3. Is a test dose necessary?
4. Is the route of administration appropriate and safe, and is extravasation likely? Are nursing staff familiar with reconstitution, administration, and extravasation policies?
5. Is the drug compatible with prescribed i.v. fluids—will it be administered before the drug expires?
6. Are you aware of all possible side-effects and problems with drug treatment?
7. Are there any other drugs or fluids required to counteract toxicity?
8. Has the patient had any previous adverse reaction to chemotherapy?
9. Have antiemetics been prescribed and is time of administration correct?
10. Monitor blood count and electrolytes. Identify cause of any change in electrolytes.
11. Has the patient any pre-existing problems, e.g. hypertension, hepatic or renal impairment?
12. Are any prophylactic antibiotics required?
13. Will any other drugs prescribed affect the toxicity of any cytotoxics?

SIDE-EFFECTS OF CYTOTOXIC DRUGS

Many adverse effects of cytotoxic drugs can be predicted since tumour cells are not selectively destroyed. Rapidly proliferating cells such as those in the bone marrow, gastrointestinal tract, oral mucosa and hair follicles are all affected, resulting in adverse and often dose-limiting toxicity. The severity of these side-effects is dependent on dose and frequency of administration and recovery time allowed between treatment courses. Other side-effects such as cardiotoxicity, renal or pulmonary toxicity are specific to individual drugs but may present dose-limiting problems. Previous radiation may also increase the toxicity of certain drugs.

Bone marrow depression
Most cytotoxic drugs induce bone marrow depression leading to

Table 7.1. Side-effects of cytotoxic drugs

1) Low occurrence side-effects
2) More severe side-effects
3) Severe side-effects or dose-limiting

	Amsacrine	Asparaginase	Azacytidine	Bleomycin	Busulphan	Chlorambucil	Cisplatin	Cyclophosphamide	Cytosine	Dactinomycin	Daunorubicin	Doxorubicin	Etoposide	Ifosfamide	Melphalan	Mercaptopurine	Methotrexate	Mitozantrone	Procarbazine	Teniposide	Thioguanine	Vinblastine	Vincristine	Carboplatin	Epirubicin
Renal excretion	✓		✓	✓	✓	✓	✓	✓	✓	✓	✓	✓	✓	✓	✓	✓	✓	✓	✓	✓	✓	✓	✓	✓	
Hepatic metabolism	✓	✓	✓	✓	✓	✓		Activation	✓		✓	✓	✓	Activation	✓	✓	✓	✓	✓	✓	✓	✓	✓		✓
Bone marrow depression	3	1	3		2	3	2	3	3	3	3	3	3	3	3	2	3	2	3	3	3	3	1	3	2
Nephrotoxicity		1					3		2														1	2	
Hepatotoxicity	2	2	1	1	1	1	1	1	1		2	2	1	1		2	2	1		1	1	1			2
Neurological symptoms	1	2	1	1	1	1	1	1	1		1	1	1	1	1		1	1	2	1	1	1	3	1	
Cardiac symptoms	1	1					1	1			3	3						1				1			2
Pulmonary symptoms				3	1			1			1		1	1	1	1	1		1	1		1			
Anaphylaxis/hypersensitivity	3		3	3			2	1	1	1		2	2	1	1	2	1	1	1	2	1	1			2

Fever/chills	1	2	1	2	1				1	1	1	1	1		1			1	1				1	1	1
Hypotension			1	1							2					2									
Alopecia		2	1	1	2	2	2	2	3	2	1		2	1	1	1	2	2	1		1	1	1	1	3
Urological toxicity				1	3	1		2	3	3		1	1	1											
Pancreatitis	1																								
Hyperuricaemia			2		1	1	1	1						1						1					
Mucosal ulceration	1	2		1	1	1	2	1	1	1		1	2	1		1	1	1			1				1
Gastrointestinal + Nausea + vomiting	2	3	1	1	3	2	2	2	3	2	2	1	1	1	2	1	1	2	1	1	3	2		2	2
Hyperglycaemia	1																								
Skin rash/erythema	1	1	2	1	1	1	1	1		1	1	1									1	1			
Tissue irritation	2	1				3	3	3		1				1						3	3				3
Ototoxicity				3																					1
Electrolyte abnormalities	1		2		1																				2
Paralytic ileus																							1	1	
Cerebral symptoms				1																					
Photosensitivity						1													1						

Table 7.2. Common chemotherapeutic agents

Drug	Strength available	Routes of administration	Methods of administration	Compatible fluids	Pharmaceutical precautions	Clinical problems (see also Table 7.1)
Amsacrine (Amsidine or M-Amsa)	75mg/1·5ml + 13·5ml Lactic acid diluent	i.v. infusion	Reconstituted solution contains 5mg/ml. Further dilute in at least 100ml fluid and infuse over 60–90 min.	Glucose 5%	Amsidine reacts with plastic syringes so glass syringes must be used. Solutions containing up to 2mg/ml are stable for up to 8 h at room temperature, protected from sunlight. Flush line before and after administration with glucose since amsacrine may precipitate with sodium chloride solutions.	Higher infusion rates lead to thrombophlebitis and pain at the infusion site. Monitor liver enzymes. Transient ↑ in liver enzymes and hyper-bilirubinaemia. Monitor for cardiotoxicity (mild and rare). Monitor b.m.d. nadir of w.b.c. 8–16 d.
Asparaginase (Erwinia)	Vials: 10 000 units	i.m. i.v. slow bolus	Add 2ml sod. chlor. 0·9% Add 2ml sod. chlor. 0·9%	Glucose 5% Sod. chlor. 0·9%	Use within 15 min to avoid denaturation and avoid contact with rubber cap. Discard any cloudy solutions.	Administer an intradermal test dose of 50 u to exclude primary hypersensitivity. Give by slow bolus by doctor if i.v. because of risk of anaphylaxis.

Drug	Preparation	Route	Method	Diluent	Stability	Monitoring
Azacytidine	Vials: 100mg	i.v. bolus	Add 19·9ml water for injection to 100mg to give 5mg/ml.	*Glucose 5%* or *Hartmann's* solution	Use reconstituted solution within 30 min and infuse within 3 h.	Monitor b.m.d. nadir of w.b.c. 14–28 d. Monitor liver enzymes and albumin level. Monitor BP and temp. Monitor phosphate levels.
		i.v. infusion	Further dilute in 100ml fluid and administer over 2 h.			
		s.c.	Not usually recommended. Painful and may cause skin discoloration			
Bleomycin	Ampoule: 15mg	i.m.	Dissolve in up to 5ml of sod. chlor. 0·9% or 2ml of lignocaine 1%.	*Sod. chlor.* 0·9% *Glucose 5%*	Stable for 24 h after addition to infusion.	Avoid extravasation. Monitor temperature. Monitor pulmonary function and monthly chest X-rays. Monitor renal function. A test dose is advised for patients receiving the drug for the first time and monitor for anaphylaxis.
		i.v. bolus	Dissolve in 5ml sod. chlor. 0·9% to give 3mg/ml and give slow bolus.			
		i.v. infusion	Usual method of administration. Dissolve in 5–200ml of sod. chlor. according to age and fluid requirement.			
Busulphan	Tablets: 0·5mg 2mg	Oral	Usually single daily dose.			Monitor b.m.d. nadir 14–28 d. Monitor pulmonary function and electrolytes on long-term treatment.

Table 7.2. (continued)

Drug	Strength available	Routes of administration	Methods of administration	Compatible fluids	Pharmaceutical precautions	Clinical problems (see also Table 7.1)
Carboplatin	Vials: 150mg	i.v. infusion	Add 15ml w.f.i. or sod. chlor. 0.9% to give 10mg/ml. Further dilute and infuse over 15–60 min. 24-h infusions have also been used.	Sod. chlor. 0.9%	Stable for 8 h. Do not use administration sets or needles including aluminium.	Monitor b.m.d. nadir 14–28 d. Nephrotoxicity, neurotoxicity and ototoxicity are rare unless patient has previous renal damage. Monitor renal function and caution with other nephrotoxic drugs. Monitor serum electrolytes, particularly Mg, K and Ca. Monitor liver function.
Chlorambucil	Tablets: 2mg 5mg	Oral	Usually single daily dose.		Store in a fridge.	Monitor b.m.d. which is cumulative. Monitor liver function before therapy and at 3-monthly intervals.

Cisplatin					
Neoplatin powder	10mg 50mg	Short i.v. infusion	Reconstitute powder with w.f.i. to give 1mg/ml solution. Over 30 min with adequate pre- and post-hydration.	*Glucose 5% Sod. chlor. 0·9% Hydration* solution (*see* next column)	Stable 20 h when added to compatible fluid. Protect from light. Do not refrigerate. Do not use administration sets containing aluminium. Prehydration over 4–12 h required. High-dose cisplatin must be accompanied by concurrent hydration for at least 24 h (*see* individual protocols). Suggested hydration: 3000ml/m² glucose 2·5% + sod. chlor. 0·45% + 20mmol/litre KCl + 70ml/litre mannitol 20%.
Cisplatin powder	10mg 25mg 50mg				
Cisplatin solution 1mg/ml	10mg 25mg 50mg	24-h infusion	Add to hydration fluid or compatible fluid. Add cisplatin to one 24-h infusion bag if possible to ensure total dose is given.		
Platinex solution 0·5mg/ml					

Check creatinine clearance before each course and do not administer unless in normal range. Renal damage takes approx. 1 week to develop with ↑ BUN ↓ creatine clearance and ↑ serum creatinine. Irreversible renal tubular damage may occur with repeated courses. Nephrotoxic antibiotics may ↑ tubular damage. Monitor b.m.d. nadir 18–23 d. Monitor neurotoxicity and ototoxicity. Audiometry tests suggested before treatment and then every 3 months. Observe for anaphylaxis/hypersensitivity. Monitor liver function every 3 months. Monitor serum electrolytes, particularly Mg, K and Ca.

Table 7.2. (continued)

Drug	Strength available	Routes of administration	Methods of administration	Compatible fluids	Pharmaceutical precautions	Clinical problems (see also Table 7.1)
Cyclo-phosphamide	Tablets: 10mg 50mg Vials: 100mg 200mg 500mg 1000mg	Oral	Taken in the morning so adequate fluids can be taken and the bladder voided. Reconstitute to 20mg/ml with w.f.i. Inject into the tubing of a fast-running infusion.	Sod. chlor. 0·9% Glucose 5% Glucose/saline	Use reconstituted solutions within 24 h.	Doses > 500mg/m^2 are usually accompanied by 3000ml/m^2 hydration for 24 h to avoid haemorrhagic cystitis, or concurrent use of mesna. Monitor b.m.d. nadir 5–10 d. Monitor liver function. Monitor electrolytes, particularly sod. and observe for water retention. May potentiate cardio-toxicity of daunorubicin/doxorubicin.

Drug	Presentation	Route	Reconstitution/dilution	Compatible fluids	Storage	Precautions/monitoring
Cytosine (Cytarabine)	Ampoule: 40mg/2ml 100mg/5ml Vial: 100mg + dil. 500mg + dil.	i.v. bolus	Use reconstituted solution or add 5ml of special diluent to 100mg vial (20mg/ml) or 10ml to 500mg vial (50mg/ml)	Sod. chlor. 0·9% Glucose/saline Glucose 5%	Store reconstituted solutions at room temp.—stable for 48 h. Discard any solution in which a haze develops.	Monitor b.m.d. nadir of w.b.c. 5–7 d. Monitor serum uric acid. Monitor temperature. Monitor liver function.
		i.v. infusion	Further dilute in sod. chlor. 0·9% or glucose saline and administer over 1–24 h according to protocol.			
		s.c.	Reconstitute 100mg vial with 1ml of diluent.			
		i.t.	DO NOT use diluent or solutions containing preservative. Reconstitute 100mg vial with 5ml w.f.i.			
		i.m.	Not usually recommended due to poor absorption.			
Dactinomycin (Actinomycin D)	Vials: 500µg	i.v. bolus (preferred)	Add 1·1ml w.f.i. to give 500µg/ml. Inject into tubing of a fast-running infusion and flush after.	Sod. chlor. 0·9% Glucose/saline Glucose 5%	DO NOT use any other solvents since precipitation may occur. Use reconstituted solutions immediately.	Avoid extravasation. Monitor b.m.d. nadir 14 d. Monitor hepatic function. Monitor renal function. ↑ incidence of side-effects following irradiation.
		i.v. infusion	Add to compatible fluid.			

Table 7.2. *(continued)*

Drug	Strength available	Routes of administration	Methods of administration	Compatible fluids	Pharmaceutical precautions	Clinical problems (see also Table 7.1)
Daunorubicin	Vials: 20mg	i.v. bolus	Reconstitute with 4ml sod. chlor. 0·9% (5mg/ml). Further dilute to 10–20ml and inject into tubing of a fast-running infusion, and flush well.	Sod. chlor. 0·9%	Reconstituted solutions stable at room temp. for 48 h. Protect from light. Incompatible with heparin.	Avoid extravasation. Monitor b.m.d. nadir 10–14 d. Monitor cardiac function. Maximum cumulative dose 20mg/kg. Monitor hepatic function ↓ dose if impaired. Monitor temp. Colours urine red.
Doxorubicin	Vials: 10mg 50mg	i.v. bolus	Reconstitute with w.f.i. or sod. chlor. 0·9% to give 2mg/ml. Inject into tubing of fast-running infusion over 2–3 min and flush well.	Sod. chlor. 0·9% Glucose 5% Glucose/saline	Reconstituted solutions stable for 24 h room temp. or 48 h in fridge. Protect from light.	Avoid extravasation. Monitor b.m.d. nadir 10–15 d. Monitor cardiac function. Maximum cumulative dose 450mg/m² in children. ↓ dose in hepatic failure. Monitor for hypertensive crisis immediately after injection. Colours urine red.

Drug	Form	Route	Preparation	Diluent	Stability	Problems and precautions
Epirubicin	Vials: 10mg 20mg 50mg	i.v. bolus	Reconstitute with w.f.i. or sod. chlor. 0·9% to give 2mg/ml solution. Administer via tubing f a fast-running infusion over 3–5 min. Further dilute according to protocol.	*Sod. chlor.* 0·9% *Glucose* 5% *Glucose/saline*	Stable for 24 h at room temp. or 48 h in fridge. Protect from light.	Avoid extravasation. Monitor liver function and ↓ dose in liver disease. Monitor b.m.d. nadir 21 d. Monitor for cardiac toxicity.
		i.v. infusion				
Etoposide (VP16)	Caps: 100mg Amps: 100mg/5ml	Oral	Absorption poor and twice the i.v. dose is usually given.	*Sod. Chlor.* 0·9%	Stable for 6 h at concentrate of 0·25–0·5mg/ml. Observe for precipitation.	Rapid infusion may cause hypotension. Monitor b.p. Monitor b.m.d. nadir 8 d. Monitor serum uric acid. Monitor liver function. Monitor for hyper-sensitivity.
		i.v. infusion	Dilute in appropriate volume (*see* Pharmaceutical Precautions) and administer over ½–4 h depending on protocol.			
Ifosfamide	Vials: 500mg 1 g 2 g	i.v. bolus	Reconstitute as follows to give 80mg/ml. 500mg—add 6·5ml w.f.i. 1 g—add 12·5ml w.f.i. 2 g—add 25ml w.f.i. Further dilute to less than 40mg/ml for i.v. bolus.	*Sod. chlor.* 0·9% *Glucose/saline* *Glucose* 5%	Stable for 24 h at room temp.	Administer with mesna to avoid urothelial toxicity (*see* mesna section). Ensure adequate hydration—3l/m². Monitor b.m.d. nadir 5–10 d. Monitor liver function.
		i.v. infusion (preferred)	Infuse in glucose/saline over ½–24 h according to protocol. Use with mesna in same fashion or separately.			

Table 7.2. (continued)

Drug	Strength available	Routes of administration	Methods of administration	Compatible fluids	Pharmaceutical precautions	Clinical problems (see also Table 7.1)
Mercaptopurine	Tabs: 10mg 50mg (scored) Susp: various strengths	Oral	Take before food as a single daily dose.		Suspension prepared in special base with 6-month expiry in fridge. Ensure dose is measured accurately.	Reduce dose to ¼ if given with allopurinol. Monitor b.m.d. Monitor liver function every 3 months and more frequently initially.
Mesna	Amps: 200mg/2ml 400mg/2ml	Oral	Use injection solution mixed with orange juice.	*Sod. chlor.* 0·9%	Open amps. immediately before required, and discard remainder. Stable for 24 h. Protect from light.	Oral dose—give 40% of cyclophosphamide/ ifosfamide dose at 0, 4 and 8 h (total 120%).
		i.v. bolus	Used when ifosfamide or cyclophosphamide given as bolus. Administer over 15–30 min.	*Sod. chlor.* 0·9% + Ifosfamide.		Bolus dose—At 0, 4 and 8 h give 20% of ifos. or cyclo. dose as mesna (total 60%).
		i.v. infusion	Usually use 24 h concurrent infusion with ifosfamide. Followed by 12 h infusion of mesna only, or 3 bolus doses at 28, 32 and 36 h.			Infusion dose—give 20% of ifos. dose as bolus then 100% of ifos. over 24 h then 60% of ifos. dose over 12 h (total 180%). Regimes vary according to protocol.

Methotrexate	Tabs: 2·5mg 10mg (both scored) Oral solution various strengths)	Oral		Single weekly dose taken before food.	Solution prepared using injection solution diluted in special base— 1 month expiry. Suggest dispensing in oral syringes to ensure accurate doses.	Monitor b.m.d. nadir 10–14 d. Monitor liver function. Ensure adequate hydration with high doses to avoid haemorrhagic cystitis and ensure urine is > pH 6·5 to prevent precipitation. Alkalinize with sodium bicarbonate or acetazolamide (*see* protocols). Ensure folinic acid rescue with high doses. Commence 24 h after MTX starts, giving at least 10 doses at 6-hourly intervals. Monitor MTX level until $< 10^{-7}$M. Monitor renal function prior to each i.v. course. Warn patient of photosensitivity.
	Amps: 2·5mg/ml Inj: 25mg/ml various sizes available from 1–200ml	i.t. i.v. bolus i.v. infusion	*Sod. chlor. 0·9% Glucose 5% Glucose/saline Hartmann's*	Contains no preservative therefore suitable i.t. Low dose boluses may be given into tubing of a fast-running infusion.	Avoid aspirin and issue aspirin warning card. Methotrexate is highly protein bound and other protein bound drugs should be avoided, e.g. tetracycline, phenytoin and chloral hydrate. Alcohol may potentiate hepatotoxicity. Infusions stable for 24 h protected from sunlight.	
Mitozantrone	Vials: 20mg 25mg 30mg (2mg/ml)	i.v. bolus i.v. infusion	*Sod. chlor. 0·9% Glucose 5% Glucose/saline*	Administer via tubing of fast-running infusion over 5 min. Dilute to at least 50ml and administer over 30 min.	Stable for 24 h at room temp. Incompatible with heparin.	Monitor b.m.d. Monitor cardiac function particularly if previously exposed to anthracyclines. Monitor hepatic function. Monitor renal function.

Table 7.2. (continued)

Drug	Strength available	Routes of administration	Methods of administration	Compatible fluids	Pharmaceutical precautions	Clinical problems (see also Table 7.1)
Procarbazine	Caps: 50mg	Oral	Divided daily doses to reduce nausea.		Weak MAOI inhibitor. Counsel patients, but foods may restart 24 h after discontinuing drug. Avoid tricyclic anti-depressants and sympathomimetics, and observe caution with CNS depressants. Avoid alcohol.	Monitor b.m.d. nadir 14–28 d.
Teniposide (VM26)	Amp: 50mg/5ml		Dilute in appropriate volume (see Pharmaceutical Precautions) and infuse over ½–4 h.	Sod. chlor. 0·9%	0·5–2mg/ml stable for up to 4 h at room temp. 0·1mg/ml stable for up to 8 h. Observe for precipitation.	Rapid infusion may cause hypotension. Monitor b.p. Monitor b.m.d. Avoid extravasation. Monitor liver function. Monitor for hyper-sensitivity.
Thioguanine	Tabs: 40mg (scored) Susp: various strengths	Oral	Usually given once daily for a short course.		Suspension prepared in special base with 3-month expiry in fridge. Ensure dose is measured accurately.	Monitor b.m.d. Monitor liver function every 3 months.

Vinblastine	Vial: 10mg with 10ml diluent (1mg/ml)	i.v. bolus	Inject into the tubing of a fast-running infusion over 1–2 min and then flush well.	*Sod. chlor.* 0·9% *Glucose* 5%	If special diluent is used solution is stable up to 30 d in a fridge.	Avoid extravasation. Monitor b.n.d. nadir 5–10 d. Monitor for signs of neurotoxicity. Pain may occur at tumour site which is harmless. Monitor hepatic function and ↓ dose if impaired.
Vincristine	Vial: 1mg 2mg } + 10ml diluent 5mg 1mg/ml	i.v. bolus	Inject into the tubing of a fast-running infusion over 1–2 min, then flush well.	*Sod. chlor.* 0·9% *Glucose* 5%	If special diluent is used solution is stable for 14 d in a fridge.	Avoid extravasation. Monitor signs of neurotoxicity. Monitor mild b.m.d. Monitor hepatic function and ↓ dose if impaired. Monitor constipation or paralytic ileus. Monitor serum sodium to check for hyponatraemia. Monitor serum uric acid. Maximum recommended dose of 2mg.
Notes:					Stability times may be extended in some circumstances if full aseptic precautions are taken—refer to manufacturers.	b.m.d. = bone marrow depression w.f.i. = water for injection

SECTION V

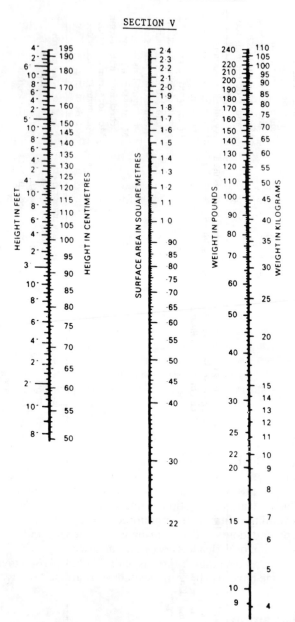

Fig. 7.1. Nomogram showing the relationship between weight and height and body surface area. A line connecting the height with the weight intersects the middle line at the corresponding surface area. (Reproduced by kind permission of Eli Lilly & Co. Ltd.)

leucopenia, thrombocytopenia and, less commonly, anaemia. Stem cells which produce leucocytes, platelets and erythrocytes are killed by cytotoxics, but since circulating blood cells are not affected and it takes several days for these cells to die naturally, bone marrow depression does not occur immediately. Thrombocytopenia occurs 7–14 days after chemotherapy as platelets die and are not renewed. Erythrocytes have a longer lifespan of about 4 months, so drug-induced anaemia is not apparent until later in treatment.

The rate or degree of bone marrow depression varies with different drugs. The nadir of bone marrow depression is approximately 5–10 d for cyclophosphamide and 14–28 d for azacytidine. Bleomycin, however, has no effect on bone marrow and vincristine, cisplatin, teniposide and methotrexate with folinic acid have relatively little effect when used alone.

Gastrointestinal toxicity

Cells lining the gastrointestinal tract are continually dividing and are therefore very susceptible to damage by cytotoxic drugs. This causes severe stomatitis and mucosal damage in the oesophagus, small intestine and colon resulting in abdominal pain, diarrhoea and haematemesis on occasions.

Most cytotoxics also produce nausea and vomiting within a few hours of administration, the most emetogenic drugs being cisplatin and doxorubicin. This side-effect should be predicted and appropriate antiemetics started before treatment with frequent review. Anorexia and a change in perception of taste buds may also occur.

Cardiotoxicity

Cardiotoxicity from the anthracycline drugs is usually cumulative and may range from ECG changes to cardiomyopathy. Epirubicin appears to be less cardiotoxic than its counterparts, daunorubicin and doxorubicin. Cardiac function, using echo cardiography or isotope heart scanning, should be monitored throughout each course of treatment and doses reduced in patients receiving radiation in the thoracic region or with a history of cardiac disease.

Amsacrine, asparaginase, cisplatin, cyclophosphamide and mitozantrone have also been associated with cardiac toxicity.

Pulmonary toxicity

Bleomycin selectively localizes in the lung producing pulmonary toxicity in some patients, usually of a cumulative nature. Respiratory function should be closely monitored during bleomycin treatment, particularly if thoracic radiation has been given. CO transfer factor is the most sensitive measurement of damage. The dangers of using hyperbaric oxygen at operation should also be pointed out to anaesthetists and surgeons.

Neurotoxicity

Neurotoxicity is the usual dose-limiting effect of vincristine, but is less severe with vinblastine. Liver damage or biliary obstruction may potentiate neurotoxicity. Suppression of the Achilles' tendon reflex is the earliest sign of vincristine toxicity and subsequent doses should be reduced or omitted until recovery occurs. Further neurotoxicity results in muscle weakness, sensory impairment and incoordination with possible seizures or mental changes. Recovery from these reactions is slow and only partial in some cases.

Vincristine also has an autonomic effect resulting in constipation and occasionally paralytic ileus.

Asparaginase may affect cerebral function resulting in somnolence and lethargy and high doses of cytarabine have produced motor incoordination, muscle weakness and slurred speech. High doses of procarbazine may also have some central effect producing dizziness, hallucinations and occasional convulsions.

Urological toxicity

Many cytotoxics are excreted by the kidney and dose reduction is essential if renal function is impaired, so it is particularly important to check renal function before each course of chemotherapy. Methotrexate is excreted mainly unchanged by the kidneys requiring dosage adjustment in renal impairment, and with high doses alkalinization of the urine with oral/i.v. sodium bicarbonate or acetazolamide plus adequate hydration to prevent precipitation of methotrexate in the renal tubules. Renal damage with cisplatin is cumulative and the dose may need reducing for each course depending on creatinine clearance. Hydration and an osmotic diuretic such as mannitol help reduce this nephrotoxicity. Serum Mg, Ca and K may also be depleted by cisplatin and must be monitored and replaced if necessary. Carboplatin has been shown to produce significantly less nephrotoxicity but dose reduction is still essential if renal damage is apparent.

The bladder mucosa may be damaged by cyclophosphamide or more commonly by ifosfamide, leading to haemorrhagic cystitis. Adequate pre- and post-dose hydration is essential to prevent this damage with concurrent mesna in susceptible patients or those receiving high doses. Mesna prevents urothelial toxicity by reacting with the causal metabolite, acrolein, but must be given during and for 8–12 h post treatment to give continued protection.

Hepatotoxicity

Hepatic function should be monitored before chemotherapy, and doses of drugs metabolized by the liver reduced if liver impairment is present. Many drugs, however, have mild effects on the liver shown by transiently raised serum transaminases.

Long-term methotrexate and mercaptopurine may occasionally lead to hepatic fibrosis and cirrhosis, whilst asparaginase has direct hepatotoxicity. Several drugs are metabolized by the liver and dose reductions considered in patients with hepatic dysfunction.

Other side-effects

Many other side-effects have been attributed to individual drugs including alopecia, fever, anaphylaxis, hypersensitivity, hypotension, pancreatitis, hyperglycaemia, ototoxicity and photosensitivity. *Table* 7.1 shows the relative incidence of these side-effects and whether these are dose-limiting. Gonadal dysfunction is of particular concern to patients and parents, and its severity depends on total drug dose, radiation and patient's age at time of treatment. Most cytotoxic drugs produce azoospermia in males and amenorrhoea, due to primary ovarian failure, in females. Increasing survival from chemotherapy has also led to an increased risk of secondary malignancies developing, but this has yet to be quantified.

ADMINISTRATION OF IRRITANT AND VESICANT DRUGS

Local tissue reactions to cytotoxic drugs may result from the vesicant properties of the drug itself, from insufficient dilution of the drug, from choosing the wrong injection site or from poor administration technique. Extravasation occurs when a drug reaches interstitial tissue outside the vein and leads to intense tissue inflammation and pain. Young children are particularly at risk because they cannot communicate pain and extravasation is not always immediately visible.

Drugs which commonly produce tissue necrosis are actinomycin D, amsacrine, dacarbazine, doxorubicin, etoposide, mithramycin, mitomycin C, teniposide, vinblastine, vincristine and vindesine. Erythema, tenderness and pain are the first signs which may be followed by skin ulceration and damage to tendons resulting in loss of limb function.

Prevention

The following techniques are suggested to avoid extravasation.
1. Use a central venous access line if possible or alternatively a newly sited i.v. line, butterfly needle or cannula inserted in one attempt. Teflon catheters are preferred to steel needles and the tubing should be taped distal to the cannula taking care not to obscure the injection site.
2. Choose the administration site carefully avoiding, if possible, areas with poor venous circulation, sites previously exposed to radiation, the wrist, antecubital fossa or bruised, sore areas. The site chosen should be supported well.
3. Dilute the drug adequately to avoid high tissue concentrations.
4. Test for backflow of blood.
5. Irrigate the line with a compatible fluid before and after treatment.
6. Observe for signs of infiltration, erythema or pain during administration.

Treatment

Management of extravasation is controversial with little published data and regimes varying from hospital to hospital. It is important, however, to draw up some basic guidelines so that treatment may be instituted as soon as possible to minimize damage. A basic treatment plan is as follows:
1. Stop the injection immediately, keeping the needle *in situ*.
2. Withdraw approximately 5ml of blood to aspirate any drug remaining, then remove the needle.
3. Aspirate the subcutaneous tissue to remove as much drug as possible.
4. Instil hydrocortisone 50–100mg intradermally or subcutaneously to reduce inflammation around the outer area of extravasation. Ethyl chloride spray may be useful to reduce pain around the site.
5. Apply hydrocortisone cream 1 per cent and continue applying q.d.s. until the redness completely subsides.
6. Apply an icepack to the area and keep in place for 24 h if possible.

Specific antidotes, such as sodium bicarbonate, sodium thiosulphate or hyaluronidase have been suggested for certain drugs but their use remains unproven. Heat has been advocated for vincristine to aid diffusion, but may lead to maceration of the area, and cold compresses are generally preferred to constrict the vein and reduce the extent of damage.

HAZARDS OF HANDLING CYTOTOXIC DRUGS

Many cytotoxic drugs can cause local tissue damage if spilt on the skin, inhaled or splashed in the eye. Experimental studies have also shown that cytotoxic drugs could produce mutagenic, carcinogenic or teratogenic effects in personnel handling them. The extent of this risk is undetermined but does pose an occupational hazard and safe handling precautions must be observed by pharmaceutical, nursing and medical staff. Skin contact may occur from spillage during preparation or administration of the drug or by leakage from infusion tubing, syringes or needles, and inhalation may arise from aerosol formation on puncturing a vial or opening an ampoule. Handling urine or faeces from patients undergoing chemotherapy also poses a health hazard to staff, since some drugs are excreted unchanged.

Guidelines on handling cytotoxic drugs have been produced in many countries and, in Great Britain, advice has been given by the Pharmaceutical Society, ASTMS and the Health and Safety Executive. Limits for safe levels of cytotoxic exposure do not exist and depend on the drug, length of exposure and individual susceptibility, so it must be kept to a minimum and documented. Procedure manuals should be available locally with specific guidelines on reconstitution and administration, also covering designated personnel, preparation area, training, protective clothing, techniques, labelling, spillage and disposal.

A centralized designated area should be used for preparation of cytotoxic drugs by nominated personnel, excluding pregnant women. A pharmacy aseptic unit is preferable for preparation, using a Class II microbiological safety cabinet with vertical laminar air flow, conforming to BS5726 for operator protection and BS5295 for microbiological protection. If aseptic facilities and cabinet are not available, a designated side room of a ward or clinic should be used, with easily cleaned work surfaces, running water and suitable disposable clothing provided.

Protective clothing, including PVC gloves, surgical mask, goggles/glasses, apron and armlets are recommended and drugs should be prepared in a disposable tray to contain spillage. Special devices used to eliminate aerosol formation during reconstitution should be considered and ampoules covered in gauze when opening. Luer lock syringes and fittings are used as an additional safety measure. Any spillages should be dealt with immediately wearing protective clothing, using soap and water for spillages on the skin/work surface and saline irrigations in the eye as immediate measures, with later reference to any individual drug recommendation. Preparation equipment, clothing and drugs should be disposed of in a suitable sharps container with cytotoxic hazard warning and care in administration of cytotoxics and handling of urine and faeces should be observed by medical and nursing staff.

Reconstituted drugs may not always be given immediately and should be clearly labelled with content, storage and expiry and an indication that it is a cytotoxic drug.

Cytotoxic tablets, capsules and powders also present a health hazard and special counting or measuring equipment should be reserved for their use. Suspensions should be prepared in a designated area using protective clothing.

Finally, patients or relatives should be counselled about handling their drugs carefully and storing them safely for their own protection, but without causing undue alarm.

FURTHER READING

Chemotherapy Instruction Manual, 3rd edition (1986) Leeds, Cookridge Hospital.

Dorr R. T. and Fritz W. L. (1982) *Cancer Chemotherapy Handbook.* London, Kimpton.

Fahey M., Oakley P. A. and Sims K. (1984) Prescription monitoring and the oncology patient. *Prescribers J.* pp. 483–5.

Guidelines for the Handling of Cytotoxic Drugs (1983) Pharmaceutical Society Working Party Report. *Prescribers J.* pp. 230–1.

Katcher B. S., Young L. Y. and Koda-Kimble M. A. (1983) *Applied Therapeutics— The Clinical Use of Drugs.* 3rd edition. Spokane, Applied Therapeutics Inc.

Perry M. C. and Yarbo J. W. (1984) *Toxicity of Chemotherapy.* New York, Grune & Stratton.

8. Antiemesis

P. Ward

INTRODUCTION

Intensive combination chemotherapy has become an integral part of the modern management of cancer and leukaemia in childhood and has contributed greatly to the improving prognosis of many of these conditions. One of the penalties, however, has been the emergence of severe nausea and vomiting as a direct consequence of the administration of cytotoxic drugs. The magnitude of this problem should not be underestimated. Adults receiving chemotherapy frequently regard post-chemotherapy nausea and vomiting as one of the most dreaded side-effects of cancer treatment.[1]

The consequences of post-chemotherapy vomiting are rarely directly life-threatening; the quality of life, however, may be seriously impaired. Physical consequences may include dehydration, electrolyte disturbance, haematemesis and even pathological fractures. Mental suffering may be severe. Anxiety and fear of side-effects may result in poor compliance, undesirable delays between courses of treatment, and even refusal to continue with potentially life-saving chemotherapy.

Poorly controlled vomiting has adverse effects on staff and parents as well as children. The sight of a child vomiting may provoke feelings of misery and guilt in parents who have consented to chemotherapy. Medical and nursing staff, especially those in training, may feel guilty about contributing to their patients' distress. If the staff's only experience with oncology patients is on the ward, they may lose confidence in the value of chemotherapy and these feelings may be transmitted to patients and their parents.

It is vital, therefore, that chemotherapy-induced nausea and vomiting be managed aggressively right from the beginning of chemotherapy. Only in this way can the confidence of patient, parents and staff be assured and, hopefully, the enormous problem of anticipatory vomiting be avoided.

Antiemetic therapy attracted little attention until the early 1970s and even today there is a paucity of information concerning the control of chemotherapy-induced nausea and vomiting in children. However, the last decade has seen a proliferation of publications, stimulated by the development of potent but highly emetic cytotoxic drugs such as cisplatin. At present, the majority of this research has been conducted in adults and much is still needed in children. This chapter attempts to describe the methods by which cytotoxic drugs produce nausea and vomiting and reviews the treatments available to prevent and alleviate these distressing side-effects.

NEUROPHYSIOLOGY OF VOMITING

The control of chemotherapy-induced nausea and vomiting is vital to the proper management of childhood malignant disease and yet few paediatricians have a systematic understanding of the neurophysiology of vomiting or of the action of antiemetics. Borison and Wang have been conducting animal studies into drug-induced nausea and vomiting since 1949 and have greatly contributed to the present knowledge of the subject.[2] Many of their findings are relevant to the problem of chemotherapy-induced emesis.

Vomiting is one of the most primitive protective functions of the body and may occur in many different situations. It is often one of the principal signs of drug toxicity irrespective of the route of administration. The act of vomiting may be considered in 3 phases which may occur in sequence, separately or in any combination. The first phase, nausea, is the unpleasant, subjective awareness of the need to vomit and is accompanied by the autonomic expressions of pallor, cold-sweating, pupillary dilatation, bradycardia and gastric stasis. The second stage is retching during which rhythmical contractions of the respiratory muscles generate negative intrathoracic pressure and facilitate the regurgitation of gastric contents into the lower oesophagus. In the final stage, forceful and sustained contraction of the abdominal muscles and elevation of the diaphragm transmit positive pressure to the thorax resulting in expulsion of gastric contents through the mouth. It is clear that vomiting is a highly co-ordinated sequence of events, involving respiratory, abdominal and bulbar muscles and must, therefore, be under the direction of the central nervous system.

Vomiting is believed to be controlled by the vomiting centre, situated deep in the lateral reticular formation of the medulla oblongata near to the respiratory centre. Some authors have postulated that nausea, retching and vomiting may be controlled by separate discrete centres. The vomiting centre is not itself accessible or sensitive to emetic substances but functions reflexly in response to inputs from the chemoreceptor trigger zone (CTZ) and vestibulo-cerebellar, vagal, spinal visceral and cortical afferents.

The CTZ is a specialized area of the brain situated in the area postrema of the floor of the 4th ventricle. It is accessible from blood and cerebrospinal fluid and thus functionally lies on the circulatory side of the blood–brain barrier. Emetic substances impinge upon receptors in the CTZ and messages are transmitted to the vomiting centre. Evidence for the existence of the CTZ in humans is provided by the observation that following surgical ablation of the area postrema, patients with intractable vomiting have fewer symptoms and can be shown to have an elevated threshold to the emetic effect of intravenous apomorphine.[3] Apomorphine is a highly emetic drug which possesses dopamine agonist activity. The CTZ is richly endowed with dopamine receptors and antiemetic drugs which block dopamine receptors, for example chlorpromazine, have a protective effect against the emetic action of apomorphine. Unfortunately, the CTZ also contains receptors to substances other than dopamine, since some drugs will produce vomiting despite dopamine receptor blockade. Furthermore, some substances, such as pilocarpine, when administered intravenously, will initiate vomiting even when the CTZ has been surgically ablated. It seems, therefore, that there may be other centres in the central nervous system which are accessible from blood and cerebrospinal fluid and contain receptors sensitive to emetic substances.

It is known that emetic chemicals may cause vomiting by routes independent of the CTZ. In cats, intragastric copper sulphate produces vomiting even when the CTZ has been surgically ablated. However, division of the vagus and visceral sympathetic nerves prevents copper sulphate-induced vomiting in the presence of an intact CTZ. Copper sulphate, mercuric chloride and zinc sulphate may be regarded as examples of peripherally-acting emetics, their effect being mediated via peripheral chemoreceptors and visceral afferents in the vagus and sympathetic nerves. Yet other substances may act at more than one receptor site. Digitalis glycosides, for example, are believed to have a central site of emetic action in the CTZ and to a lesser extent a local effect on the gastrointestinal tract.

Afferent inputs from the vestibular apparatus, whilst of obvious importance in motion sickness, are not thought to be involved with chemotherapy-induced nausea and vomiting. However, afferents from higher centres within the central nervous system are undoubtedly of importance, being involved with vomiting in response to the sights, sounds, smells and procedures associated with chemotherapy, culminating in the development of anticipatory vomiting prior to the administration of cytotoxic drugs. It has been postulated that these higher, cortical centres modulate the activity of the medullary vomiting centre by messages sent 'downstream'.

It seems, therefore, that inputs from any or all of at least 4 sources—the CTZ, gastrointestinal tract, cerebral cortex and vestibular apparatus—may initiate vomiting via the vomiting centre. All but the last of these inputs are believed to be involved in the initiation of chemotherapy-induced nausea and vomiting.[4]

SITES OF EMETIC ACTIVITY OF CYTOTOXIC DRUGS

Although it is well recognized that cytotoxic drugs are commonly associated with nausea and vomiting, surprisingly little is known about the sites of emetic activity of these drugs. It seems very probable that different cytotoxic drugs act at different sites and that a single cytotoxic drug may have more than one site of emetic activity. The conscious perception of nausea is a cerebral function, as must be the phenomenon of anticipatory or conditioned vomiting. Experimental evidence suggests that cytotoxic drugs may possess central emetic activity at the CTZ and/or peripheral action at peripheral receptors associated with the gastrointestinal tract.

Experimental work in dogs suggests that the CTZ is important in the emetic action of mustine (mechlorethamine). CTZ ablation abolishes the vomiting caused by both mustine and radiotherapy. In cats, however, visceral afferent pathways from the upper abdomen are more important. CTZ ablation in cats has been shown to provide protection against cisplatin-induced vomiting. The vomiting response to cytotoxic drugs is commonly delayed in comparison to the classical emetics such as apomorphine. This delay suggests that secondary products of drug metabolism or tissue breakdown contribute to the emetic response.

Whilst the majority of research has concentrated on the central mediation of drug-induced vomiting, research has also been conducted into the effect of emetic and antiemetic drugs on the gastrointestinal tract. Normal co-ordination of gastrointestinal motility involves proximal pacesetter potentials which generate action potentials spreading distally, i.e. away from the mouth, thus co-ordinating orderly, smooth muscle contraction and hence peristalsis. However, if a pacesetter potential is artificially generated distally, for example in the duodenum, proximal propagation of action potentials may occur, resulting in retrograde peristalsis and regurgitation of duodenal contents into the stomach. Emetic drugs may alter gastrointestinal motility by modifying the frequency and direction of pacesetter and action potentials. It is not clear how emetic drugs exert this effect but it may be due either to direct action on the smooth muscle of the gut or it may be mediated directly or indirectly via central and peripheral neural pathways. Experiments in dogs injected intravenously with cisplatin demonstrated, after a lag phase of 90–120 min, action potential burst patterns distally in the jejenum which were propagated proximally through the duodenum and stomach. These episodes were immediately predictive of the onset of vomiting.

A number of neurotransmitters has been implicated at both the CTZ and in gut neurons. Dopamine, known to be important in the CTZ, is also a neurotransmitter in the peripheral autonomic nervous system. Drugs possessing dopamine receptor blocking activity have been found to be useful antiemetics. Metoclopramide is a potent dopamine blocker. Prior administration of intravenous metoclopramide to dogs, subsequently given intravenous cisplatin, prevents disruption of gastrointestinal electrical activity and prevents vomiting.

In summary, cytotoxic drugs may exert their emetic activity at more than one site in the body and different drugs may act at different sites. Not only the drug itself but also its metabolites and the products of tissue breakdown may contribute to the total emetic effect. Modern chemotherapy regimes commonly employ a number of different cytotoxic drugs used in combination. Given the complexity of the aetiology of chemotherapy-induced nausea and vomiting, it is not surprising that prevention and control may be extraordinarily difficult.

RELATIVE EMETIC ACTIVITY OF DIFFERENT CYTOTOXIC DRUGS

Not all cytotoxic drugs are of equal emetic potency. Some drugs, such as vincristine, rarely cause vomiting whereas others, such as cyclophosphamide, usually do. Although it is possible to draw up a rough 'league table' of relative emetic activity, such a listing is necessarily very imprecise. Children vary enormously in their susceptibility to cytotoxic-induced nausea and vomiting. It is our impression that younger children tolerate chemotherapy better than older children and teenagers. The emetic response is influenced by the mode of administration of the drug. Cisplatin probably enjoys the most evil reputation for producing severe nausea and vomiting. When administered in a single large dose, e.g. $100mg/m^2$ with mannitol diuresis, vomiting is virtually inevitable. However, if the same total dose is administered in 3 divided doses on 3 consecutive days, although vomiting may occur on the first day, antiemetics may not even be necessary on the second and especially the third day. The whole issue is further complicated by the variability in patient

Table 8.1 Relative emetic activity of different cytotoxic drugs

---

Very high emetic incidence (>90%)
   Cisplatin
   Dacarbazine

High emetic incidence (60–90%)
   Cyclophosphamide/Ifosfamide
   Actinomycin D
   Lomustine (CCNU)
   Carmustine (BCNU)
   Procarbazine

Moderate emetic incidence (30–60%)
   L-asparaginase
   Daunorubicin (daunomycin)
   Doxorubicin (adriamycin)
   Azacytidine

Low emetic incidence (10–30%)
   Bleomycin
   Cytosine arabinoside
   Etoposide (VP16)
   6 Mercaptopurine
   Methotrexate
   Vinblastine

Very low emetic incidence (<10%)
   Thioquanine
   Corticosteroids
   Vincristine

(Reproduced from Borison & McCarthy, 1983.)

populations, disease types and activities, and the use of multiple-drug chemotherapy regimes. Finally, there is no universally agreed method of quantifying the emetic activity of drugs and even though the number of vomits and volume of vomitus can be objectively recorded, there is no really reliable way of quantifying nausea, especially in young children. Notwithstanding these difficulties, *Table* 8.1 represents an attempt to list commonly used cytotoxic drugs in groups according to their relative emetic activity. No attempt has been made to list them in order within the groups.

ANTICIPATORY NAUSEA AND VOMITING

Before discussing the management of post-chemotherapy vomiting it is pertinent to mention the problem of anticipatory nausea and vomiting. This is the phenomenon whereby children may suffer nausea and/or vomiting prior to administration of cytotoxic drugs. One of our patients, for example, would begin vomiting when a drip stand was wheeled into her cubicle; another unfortunate child used to start vomiting when travelling in the family car on the way to the hospital. The boy was not subject to motion sickness at other times.

Studies of adult chemotherapy recipients have described prevalence rates of 18–45 per cent for anticipatory nausea and 9–38 per cent for anticipatory vomiting. Adults who experience anticipatory nausea and vomiting also usually suffer more severe symptoms following cytotoxic administration. These patients are likely to be receiving chemotherapy combinations of greater emetic potency than those not suffering anticipatory symptoms. Anticipatory nausea and vomiting in adults usually develop following two to four cycles of chemotherapy.

Dolgin et al. surveyed 80 consecutive children, aged from 2 to 14 years, suffering from various malignant diseases and attending an outpatient chemotherapy clinic.[5] Twenty-eight per cent were currently experiencing anticipatory nausea and 20 per cent anticipatory vomiting at the time of the survey. A further 1 per cent had experienced anticipatory nausea or vomiting in the past but not currently. The majority of affected children had developed anticipatory symptoms within the first 4 months of chemotherapy. Some, however, had started within the first month of treatment and others had begun as late as 4 years after commencing cytotoxic therapy. During individual episodes, nausea generally began 2–4 h before chemotherapy but in 3 children began 12–24 h before treatment. The intensity of the nausea progressively increased as the time for treatment drew nearer and was maximal in the final hour. Anticipatory vomiting generally began within the 2 h preceding chemotherapy and was maximal at the time of administering the cytotoxic drugs. By performing stepwise multiple regression analyses the authors demonstrated that the most significant predictor factors for the development of anticipatory nausea and vomiting were the intensity of nausea and vomiting following chemotherapy, the emetic potential of the chemotherapy regime, the presence of cyclophosphamide in the drug schedule, the time elapsed since diagnosis and the level of parental anxiety. Children with and without anticipatory symptoms showed no significant differences in age, sex or ethnic groups.

The aetiology of anticipatory nausea and vomiting has been thought of in terms of classical conditioning, whereby previously neutral stimuli such as the sites, smells and tastes associated with chemotherapy, become associated with post-chemotherapy emesis. A parallel example is the development of food aversions. Certain foods eaten shortly before receiving chemotherapy become associated with post-chemotherapy nausea and vomiting and the children subsequently demonstrate an aversion to those particular foods.[6,7] This phenomenon may contribute to the anorexia commonly seen in children receiving chemotherapy.

Adults suffering from anticipatory nausea and vomiting have been shown to be more anxious and depressed than those who do not and they seem to have a more negative view of both their treatment and their future. Children and parents questioned about their beliefs concerning the cause of their anticipatory symptoms mainly gave psychological reasons including treatment-related anxiety and preoccupation with and expectations of distressing adverse effects.[5] A few children or parents mentioned specific stimuli as being causative. These included the odour of the clinic and particular tastes experienced during drug infusion. Of even greater interest are the reasons given by children or parents for the disappearance of anticipatory symptoms where they had previously existed. In 4 of 9 cases, symptoms ceased following the withdrawal of a specific cytotoxic drug from the chemotherapy regime. Three children improved following formal or informal behavioural therapy and in 2 children, no explanation was apparent.

The management of anticipatory nausea and vomiting is discussed below.

THE MANAGEMENT OF CHEMOTHERAPY INDUCED NAUSEA AND VOMITING

The maxim that 'prevention is better than cure' is never truer than when applied to the control of chemotherapy-induced nausea and vomiting. Once the patient has experienced severe symptoms, the problem is likely to become increasingly severe in subsequent cycles with the ever-growing possibility that anticipatory nausea and vomiting may develop. It therefore behoves the clinician to make every effort to minimize nausea and vomiting right from the start of treatment.

It should not be assumed that nausea and vomiting following treatment are always the direct consequences of chemotherapy. If symptoms continue unabated for more than 18–24 h it may be necessary to search for an alternative explanation. Raised intracranial pressure, intestinal obstruction, uraemia, hepatic dysfunction and infection may need to be considered, depending on the clinical picture.

The aetiology of chemotherapy-induced vomiting is complex and involves numerous different stimuli. From the foregoing discussion, it is apparent that anxiety and stress associated with chemotherapy exacerbate nausea and vomiting and it is important to try to keep these to a minimum. It follows that the environment in which cytotoxic drugs are to be administered should be as agreeable and non-threatening as possible. The ward, clinic and treatment rooms should be made welcoming and attractive and they should be free of unpleasant chemical odours. Whether children receiving cytotoxic drugs should be nursed alone in cubicles or on open wards with similar patients is debatable. Whilst it is desirable to avoid feelings of isolation, the sight and sound of a child suffering from poorly controlled chemotherapy-induced emesis may precipitate an 'epidemic' of vomiting amongst other patients on the ward. Different conditions are likely to suit different children and a flexible approach should be adopted.

The staff caring for children with cancer play a vital role in reducing the anxiety surrounding chemotherapy. They should adopt a warm, confident and optimistic attitude tempered with sympathy and honesty. A high degree of technical expertise is essential. Many children are more frightened of repeated venepunctures than they are of the cytotoxic drugs themselves. It is important that the operator should not persevere for too long. A useful 'house rule' is that no more than 3 unsuccessful attempts at a practical procedure should be permitted before summoning someone else to help. In one study of the use of tunnelled central venous catheters for blood sampling and administering cytotoxic drugs, an unexpected benefit was a reduction in the incidence of anticipatory nausea and vomiting.[8] Once chemotherapy has been administered, much can be achieved by distraction. Watching video films or playing computer games may be helpful and the services of an enthusiastic and imaginative playleader can be invaluable. Some children who have been given sedative antiemetic drugs may be too somnolent to benefit from distraction but even they will find comfort in discovering a parent at the bedside during moments of lucidity.

PHARMACOLOGICAL CONTROL OF CHEMOTHERAPY-INDUCED NAUSEA AND VOMITING

Most children receiving intensive combination chemotherapy will be nauseated and may vomit unless they are given antiemetic medication. Even then, emesis may commonly occur although, hopefully, it will be less severe. When initiating chemotherapy, antiemetics should be administered right from the start unless the cytotoxic drugs to be given are known to be of very low emetic potential. Some children, however, may eventually decline antiemetic therapy, preferring to endure nausea and vomiting rather than experience any adverse effects of the antiemetics. In particular, some patients dislike the sense of loss of control produced by the sedative action of some antiemetics. As the child becomes more experienced, it is wise to pay heed to his views.

No single antiemetic is likely to produce satisfactory results in all children on every occasion. It may be necessary to try several different antiemetics or combinations to achieve the best control. It is useful to keep a record of antiemetics used and results obtained for reference in subsequent treatment cycles.

When prescribing antiemetic drugs, it is important to give thought to the route and scheduling of administration. Most intensive chemotherapy regimes require intravenous access and this route can also be used for antiemetics, at least initially. Ideally, the child should have an effective blood level of an antiemetic drug before the first cytotoxic drug is administered. A suitable regime might involve giving the first antiemetic 1 h before chemotherapy, followed by subsequent doses 2–4 hourly afterwards depending on the individual drugs used. Mandatory doses should be given for the first 12 h or so with 'as required doses' thereafter.

The route and scheduling of antiemetics may need to be altered for children being treated as outpatients. It is usually possible to give the first few doses intravenously but a supply of an appropriate oral or rectal drug should be provided for the child to take home. It is prudent to try to avoid excessive sedation in outpatients, particularly in the last few hours before discharge as the child may face a long car journey with only one adult—the driver—in attendance.

CHOICE OF ANTIEMETICS

For a number of years, the control of chemotherapy-induced nausea and vomiting was a Cinderella subject and received little attention. Recently, however, the introduction of highly emetic cytotoxic drugs such as cisplatin has stimulated the quest for more satisfactory emetic control and a plethora of publications has followed. The overwhelming majority of clinical trials have been conducted in adults and relatively few have been conducted in children. Many trials have been unsatisfactory for methodological reasons and the immense number of variables involved makes comparison between trials difficult. The current view is that antiemetic drug trials should preferably be randomized, double blind, crossover trials comparing the trial drug with either a placebo or an established treatment. Patients entered into the trial should all have the same diagnosis, should receive identical chemotherapy and should not have received chemotherapy prior to entering the trial.[9] Few trials conform to these ideals. The assessment of efficacy is fraught with difficulty. Whilst the number and volume of vomits can be objectively quantified, these may not be the most important criteria for the patient. It is helpful to try to obtain some indication of the subjective experiences and

Table 8.2 Classification of antiemetics by pharmacological groups and postulated sites of action

Antiemetic	Site of action
Antihistamines	VC, cerebral cortex
Anticholinergics	VC
Dopamine antagonists	
phenothiazines	CTZ
butyrophenones	CTZ
metoclopramide	CTZ, periphery
domperidone	CTZ, periphery
Cannabinoids	Cerebral cortex
Miscellaneous agents	
corticosteroids	Unknown
lorazepam	Cerebral cortex

VC = vomiting centre, CTZ = chemoreceptor trigger zone.

preferences of the patients and their parents. For many years phenothiazines have been the mainstay of antiemetic therapy, but they have now been joined by a variety of new compounds, some of which seem to be more effective. *Table* 8.2 lists some of the antiemetics in current use and relates them to their presumed sites of action. In the following sections, individual drugs will be discussed with reference to reviews of trials conducted in adults and specific reference will be made to experience in children where this exists.

Phenothiazines

The phenothiazines are the best known antiemetic drugs and have been in medical usage since 1950. Their antiemetic properties have been known since 1953 when chlorpromazine was first used in patients with cancer. The role of phenothiazines and related drugs in the control of chemotherapy-induced nausea and vomiting has been reviewed by Wemplar.[10]

Phenothiazines are believed to exert their antiemetic action by blocking dopamine receptors in the CTZ. Unfortunately, dopamine receptor blockade is also responsible for the extrapyramidal reactions which may occur, especially in children. The basal ganglia are richly invested with dopamine receptors, thus making the antiemetic and extrapyramidal actions of phenothiazines inseparable. Other adverse effects include autonomic reactions such as dry mouth, constipation and hypotension, hypersensitivity reactions—the commonest being cholestatic jaundice and endocrine effects, especially galactorrhoea. In practice, the commonest adverse reaction is sedation which may be marked with some members of the group. Extrapyramidal reactions are usually successfully treated by withdrawing the drug and giving diphenhydramine or anti-Parkinson agents, such as benztropine, by intravenous injection. Hypotension, which is particularly common with chlorpromazine because of its anti-adrenergic effects, usually responds to simple measures such as raising the foot of the bed and administering intravenous saline.

Wemplar,[10] reviewing a number of published trials in adults, concluded that phenothiazines are more effective than placebo in controlling mild to moderate chemotherapy-induced emesis but were less effective than some of the newer antiemetics, such as cannabinoids and high-dose metoclopramide, particularly with highly emetic cytotoxic regimes involving cisplatin. Few adult patients, asked to express a preference, chose phenothiazines despite a higher incidence of side-effects with the novel antiemetics.

Chlorpromazine and prochlorperazine are the most widely used of the phenothiazine antiemetics. Wemplar feels that there is little to choose between them in terms of antiemetic efficacy and the choice should be made on the balance of side-effects. Chlorpromazine is more sedating, but extrapyramidal reactions are not generally prominent at the doses required for full antiemetic action. Prochlorperazine is less sedative, but severe dystonic reactions sometimes occur, especially in children.

Chlorpromazine may be diluted in saline and be given by slow intravenous injection over 10–15 min. A suitable dose is 0·5mg/kg body weight (maximum 25mg), 3–4 hourly. It is also available as an elixir (25mg/5ml). Prochlorperazine may be given orally as an elixir (25mg/5ml) or rectally as suppositories (5mg and 25mg).

Butyrophenones

The butyrophenones are a group of compounds structurally related to the phenothiazines and they possess a range of activities and side-effects similar to chlorpromazine. Clinical trials of haloperidol and droperidol in adults suggest that they are at least as effective as the phenothiazines in controlling cytotoxic-induced nausea and vomiting.[10] There is very little information about the use of these compounds in children.

Metoclopramide

Metoclopramide is believed to exert its antiemetic effect by blocking dopamine receptors in the chemoreceptor trigger zone. It also appears to have a peripheral site of action since it is able to inhibit nausea and vomiting caused by the ingestion of copper sulphate.

Metoclopramide is known to enhance gastrointestinal motility.

Early clinical trials using metoclopramide in patients receiving chemotherapy employed low doses ($0 \cdot 15$–$3 \cdot 0$mg/kg) and the results were not promising. However, the introduction of cisplatin stimulated further research into metoclopramide resulting in the development of high-dose regimes.[11]

Randomized, double-blind, crossover, comparative trials in adults receiving cisplatin 120mg/m^2 as a single dose have shown high-dose metoclopramide to be superior to placebo, prochlorperazine and tetrahydrocannabinol. The dose of metoclopramide used in these trials was 2mg/kg body weight administered as an intravenous infusion over 30 min $0 \cdot 5$ h before and $1 \cdot 5$, $3 \cdot 5$, $5 \cdot 5$ and $8 \cdot 5$ h after giving cisplatin. The toxicity observed in these trials was mild and generally well tolerated. Mild sedation occured in 71 per cent, more marked sediation in 5 per cent and only one patient had a dystonic reaction. Forty-four per cent of patients had diarrhoea but it was not clear whether this was due to metoclopramide or cisplatin.

Unfortunately, children appear to be more susceptible to the extrapyramidal effects of metoclopramide than adults. In the early 1970s reports began to emerge of alarming dystonic reactions occurring in children receiving metoclopramide in conventional doses.[12] Terrin et al.[13] reported their experience with intravenous metoclopramide ($0 \cdot 5$ to $2 \cdot 0$mg/kg, 4–8 hourly for 48 h concomitantly with cytotoxic chemotherapy) in 8 children and teenagers aged 6–19 years. Seven of the 8 patients experienced a total of 13 adverse reactions:

extrapyramidal reactions 10
severe agitation 1
severe agitation, plus extrapyramidal reactions 2

Only the oldest patient, aged 19, did not have an adverse reaction. In 7 of the 13 reactions the patients had received 1mg/kg or less of metoclopramide. Diphenhydramine reversed all of the extrapyramidal reactions within minutes. In view of this the authors tried administering intravenous diphenhydramine $0 \cdot 5$mg/kg prophylactically before the first dose of metoclopramide and 12-hourly afterwards. Only one of the 5 patients given the diphenhydramine-metoclopramide combination had further dystonic reactions. Control of emesis was said to be good, with fewer than 3 episodes of vomiting. The reason why children are more susceptible than adults to metoclopramide-induced dystonic reactions is not clear but the explanation does not appear to lie in differences in the pharmacokinetics.[14]

Metoclopramide appears to be a useful drug for the control of nausea and vomiting induced by cisplatin. Its usefulness with other cytotoxic drugs is less clearly defined and more work is required. Care must be taken with children to avoid extrapyramidal reactions and consideration might be given to using concomitant prophylactic diphenhydramine. High-dose metoclopramide is supplied in 20ml ampoules containing 5mg/ml. The manufacturers recommend that it be diluted in at least 50ml of an appropriate infusion fluid and be infused over at least 15 min. The dose may be repeated 2-hourly. Metoclopramide is also available as tablets (10mg), elixir (5mg/ml) and paediatric liquid (1mg/ml using a 1ml pipette).

Domperidone

Domperidone is a unique benzimidazole derivative which acts as a peripheral dopamine antagonist at the CTZ in the brain stem and probably also in the stomach where it promotes gastric emptying and stimulates gastrointestinal motility. It differs from other neuroleptic antiemetics in that it does not readily cross the blood-brain barrier. It is therefore able to act at the CTZ but does not penetrate to the basal ganglia and is consequently only rarely associated with extra-pyramidal or other central side-effects. Dystonic reactions may, however, still occur occasionally and we have witnessed occulogyric crises in 2 children receiving domperidone in conventional doses. On both occasions, the attacks ceased within a few minutes of administering intravenous benztropine.

Domperidone has shown promise in clinical trials in adults receiving cytotoxic chemotherapy and has been the subject of a number of trials in children. In an open study in 12 children who received 8–16mg of intravenous domperidone per day, antiemetic activity was estimated to be excellent or good in 71·5 per cent of 77 courses of treatment. Vomiting was completely absent on more than 75 per cent of the total days of treatment.[15] The children studied received a variety of different chemotherapy regimes of varying emetic potential; none of the patients received cisplatin. Swann et al.[16] compared intra-venous metoclopramide (0·5mg/kg) with domperidone (up to 1·0mg/kg) in a randomized crossover study in 18 children who together received 20 cycles of chemotherapy. Thirteen patients vomited less after domperidone, 2 vomited more and 3 as often as after metoclo-pramide. The duration of effect of domperidone appeared to be about 4 h. No adverse reactions were recorded either with domperidone or metoclopramide. O'Meara and Mott[17] investigated domperidone as a single agent in escalating doses determined by efficacy and side-effects in 27 children aged 1 year 10 months to 13 years. Domperidone was given intravenously prior to chemotherapy and 4-hourly afterwards for up to 2 further doses. Domperidone suppositories were provided for use if required 4-hourly for up to 24 h after chemotherapy. They concluded that domperidone was an effective agent, achieving reasonable or good control in 47 of 58 drug trials. The optimum dose appeared to be 0·7mg/kg per dose and the duration of action was 3–4 h. The only toxicity observed was pain at the site of intravenous injection if domperidone was not sufficiently diluted. Fifteen of 17 patients who had previously experienced control of emesis with other antiemetics chose domperidone when given the option to choose.

Higher doses of domperidone have been used by some investigators. Craft anecdotally reported the use of doses of 1·1 to 2·0mg/kg with the clinical impression of greater efficacy at higher doses with no increase in side-effects.[18] Ward,[19] reporting his rather disappointing experience with intravenous domperidone, advocated the investigation of higher dose regimes analogous to high-dose metoclopramide. Unfortunately, plans to conduct such a study were thwarted by the report of the sudden death of an adult with oesophageal carcinoma whilst receiving high-dose domperidone.[20] Following this and other reports of possible cardiac toxicity, the manufacturers decided against further high-dose studies and subsequently withdrew the intravenous preparation other than for named patients.

Domperidone is currently available as tablets (10mg), suspension (5mg/5ml), suppositories (30mg) and, for named patients only, injection (5mg/ml). The manufacturer's recommended intravenous dose for children is 0·1mg/kg, diluted 1 in 10 with normal saline and infused over 10–30 min; a maximum of 2mg/kg in any one day is suggested. The suppositories may be particularly useful for outpatients; the dose is 30–120mg daily.

Cannabinoids

Cannabis has been used therapeutically since 2737 BC and was described by a Chinese emperor as a 'liberator of sin' and a 'delight giver'. It was introduced to the West by Napoleon's armies in the early 19th century. Interest in the antiemetic activity of cannabinoids originated in the anecdotal reports by adult patients who smoked marijuana that smoking before chemotherapy diminished the severity of post-chemotherapy nausea and vomiting. Subsequent experience of the use of delta-9-tetrahydrocannabinol (THC), the major psychoactive ingredient of marijuana, and the synthetic cannabinoids nabilone and levonantradol has been reviewed by Vincent et al.[21]

The mechanism by which cannabinoids exert their antiemetic effect is not really known but they are believed to act on the cerebral cortex and, via descending pathways, the vomiting centre. Their predominant side-effects involve the central nervous system. THC has been reported to produce changes in mood, memory, concentration, cognitive and motor abilities and distortions of spatial and self-awareness. Subjective feelings of hunger, increased auditory acuity, confusion, temporal disintegration, vivid visual imagery and depersonalization have been described. In trials in adults, younger patients seem to be less severely affected than older ones. The antiemetic action of THC may sometimes be associated with a psychological 'high'. Nabilone seems to have fewer psychological side-effects. Levonantradol is the only cannabinoid which can be given parenterally.

The antiemetic effect of THC in children receiving chemotherapy was compared by Eckert et al.[22] with oral metoclopramide syrup and prochlorperazine tablets in 2 small, double-blind, controlled trials. THC appeared to be more effective than either of the other antiemetics. The numbers involved in the trials were small and the control antiemetics may have been given in too small doses with too long intervals between them; however, these studies confirmed that THC has an antiemetic effect in children. The predominant side-effect was sedation. Two patients reported a psychological 'high' whilst receiving THC. One had an episode of agitation, anxiety and bad dreams, the other reported feelings of euphoria, lightness and increased appetite.

Dalzell et al.[23] compared nabilone with oral domperidone in a double-blind crossover trial involving 25 children aged 10 months–17 years. Children weighing less than 18kg received either nabilone 0·5mg twice daily or domperidone 5mg twice daily. Those weighing between 18 and 36kg received nabilone 1mg twice daily or domperidone 10mg 3 times daily and those weighing more than 36kg received either nabilone 1 mg or domperidone 15mg both 3 times daily. In all cases, the first dose was given the evening before starting chemotherapy and the last dose 24 h after finishing it. All of the patients received combination chemotherapy likely to cause nausea and vomiting. A few of the regimes included cisplatin. The mean number of vomits and the severity of nausea were significantly less in the nabilone group. Twelve of 18 patients or parents expressed a preference for nabilone. Twelve of 22 patients became drowsy, 8 felt dizzy and 3 experienced adverse mood changes. One child had hallucinations of body size and shape and was withdrawn from the trial. A number of other, minor, and well tolerated, side-effects were also listed. Three of the children included in this trial were less than 2 years old. All 3 responded favourably to nabilone and afterwards their parents preferred nabilone to domperidone.

It has been suggested that the concomitant administration of a phenothiazine with nabilone might reduce the incidence and severity of psychological side-effects. Nabilone and prochlorperazine were given to a group of 34 adults by Cunningham et al.[24] Adverse effects were significantly less common with the combination without impairing the antiemetic effect. There are no reports of similar trials in children.

Levonantradol is the only available cannabinoid which can be given parenterally. There is little information about its use in children. Cronin et al.[25] described its use in 31 patients, the youngest of whom was 11 years old. In an open, dose-finding study, levonantradol was administered 4-hourly by intramuscular injection; a route which most paediatricians would consider unacceptable for their patients. The effective dose varied between 0·5 and 1·5mg. Dysphoric reactions were more common with the higher dose. The commonest side-effects were somnolence and a dry mouth.

Other agents

Corticosteroids were investigated as antiemetics after it was noticed that post-chemotherapy nausea and vomiting occurred less frequently following chemotherapy regimes which included a corticosteroid as one of the components. The site of their antiemetic action is not known. Experience with adults suggests that high-dose dexamethasone (10mg i.v.) is superior to placebo, prochlorperazine and high-dose metoclopramide.[26] The addition of dexamethasone to high-dose metoclopramide sometimes achieves control in patients resistant to high-dose metoclopramide alone. Unwanted effects include euphoria, insomnia, itching and swelling of the throat, and perianal discomfort. Our own anecdotal experience with children suggests that high-dose dexamethasone may be useful and that toxicity is usually minimal.

In a randomized double-blind trial, Mehta et al.[27] compared methylprednisolone (4mg/kg) with chlorpromazine (0·5mg/kg) in 20 consecutive patients aged between 2 and 22 years of age. The antiemetics were administered by rapid intravenous injection 30 min before chemotherapy and were repeated after 6 hours if necessary. They found methylprednisolone to be as effective as chlorpromazine in controlling nausea and vomiting but the incidence of sedation was less in the group receiving the steroid. No adverse side-effects were reported.

Lorazepam is a benzodiazepine with antiemetic, sedative and amnesic effects. In addition to reducing the severity of nausea and vomiting, it may actually abolish the patient's memory of having received chemotherapy.[26] Adverse effects have included perceptual disturbances, hypotension and urinary incontinence.

Antiemetic combinations

Since cytotoxic drugs are usually used in combination and each drug may exert its emetic effect at different sites, a logical approach would be to use antiemetic drugs in combinations chosen to obtain maximum benefit with minimum toxicity. The drugs chosen for such regimes should be believed to act at different sites and should not have over-lapping adverse effects. There is a growing literature concerning the use of this approach in adults but, as yet, little has been published about children. For several years, our standard antiemetic regime for inpatients has used chlorpromazine and promethazine (0·5mg/kg, max 25mg), intravenously, 2-hourly, alternately. Adverse effects include sedation and, occasionally, hypotension.

TREATMENT OF ANTICIPATORY NAUSEA AND VOMITING

Anticipatory nausea and vomiting are notoriously difficult to treat and do not usually respond to antiemetic medication. The inclusion of patients with anticipatory symptoms in antiemetic trials may result in the efficacy of antiemetics being underestimated. O'Meara and Mott[17] demonstrated that children with anticipatory nausea and vomiting responded poorly to domperidone when compared with children without anticipatory symptoms.

The failure of drugs to control anticipatory nausea and vomiting has stimulated the search for alternative treatments. Interest has concentrated on the development of psychological and behavioural methods to encourage patients to re-learn more appropriate responses to the stimuli to which they have become adversely conditioned. Since anxiety appears to constitute the predominant emotional component of anticipation, psychological methods frequently seek to decrease its intensity. As with drugs, studies published so far have predominantly concerned adults but there is a growing interest in the problem in children and some paediatric oncology units now include a clinical psychologist amongst their staff. The methods currently being evaluated include hypnosis, systematic desensitization and relaxation therapy in various forms.

LaBaw et al.[28] studied a group of children aged 4–19 years with advanced cancer. Self-hypnosis was taught in group and individual sessions. Whilst in trance, maladapted responses to stress were discouraged and more constructive responses were encouraged. The authors claimed that one of the benefits of treatment was a diminution of anticipatory nausea and vomiting; however, little evidence was offered in support of this claim.

Morrow and Morrell[29] compared 'systematic desensitization' with counselling and no treatment in a group of 60 patients, the youngest of whom was 19 years old. Systematic desensitization involves the teaching of progressive muscle relaxation followed by the presentation of a hierarchy of imagined stimuli associated with the administration of chemotherapy. The patient is encouraged to maintain his state of relaxation as each stimulus is presented. When he is able to remain relaxed whilst contemplating the stimulus, he is taken on to the next, more intense, stimulus. Anticipatory symptoms occurred less frequently and were less severe in patients who had received systematic desensitization.

Relaxation training with guided imagery or electromyographic biofeedback are amongst other methods which have been tried in adults and have been reviewed by Moher.[30]

Although drugs are usually ineffective in alleviating anticipatory emesis, it has been suggested that lorazepam may be useful in preventing and possibly treating anticipatory symptoms because of its amnesic and anxiolytic effects.

CONCLUSION

Following the introduction of intensive combination chemotherapy regimes which include potent cytotoxic drugs of great emetic potential, the need for effective antiemetics has become all too apparent. Recent research has begun to elucidate the mechanisms by which cytotoxic drugs cause post-chemotherapy nausea and vomiting and, at the same time, the importance of anticipatory vomiting has become clear. A number of new, effective, antiemetics has been introduced but still the prevention of chemotherapy-induced nausea and vomiting remains imperfect. An aggressive approach needs to be adopted, attempting to control emesis right from the start of treatment. More research is needed in children receiving cancer chemotherapy to ensure that currently available antiemetics are being used to maximum effect. The quest for new, more effective agents needs to continue and trials of antiemetic combinations in children are needed. At present, anticipatory nausea and vomiting remain a major problem and further studies of behavioural therapy are required.

With currently available drugs and techniques, it is usually possible to reduce the frequency and severity of cytotoxic-induced emesis. It is not yet possible to prevent it completely. There is still room for improvement.

REFERENCES

1. Coates A., Abraham S., Kaye S. B. et al. (1982) On the receiving end—patient perception of the side-effects of cancer chemotherapy. *Eur. J. Cancer Clin. Oncol.* **19**, 203–8.
2. Borison H. L. and Wang S. C. (1953) Physiology and pharmacology of vomiting. *Pharmacol. Rev.* **5**, 193–230.
3. Lindstrom P. A. and Brizzee K. R. (1962) Relief of intractable vomiting from surgical lesions in the area postrema. *J. Neurosurg.* **19**, 228–36.
4. Borison H. L. and McCarthy L. E. (1983) Neuropharmacology of chemotherapy-induced emesis. *Drugs* **52** (Suppl. 1), 8–17.
5. Dolgin M. J., Katz E. R., McGinty K. et al. (1985) Anticipatory nausea and vomiting in paediatric cancer patients. *Paediatrics* **75**, 547–52.
6. Bernstein I. L. (1978) Learned taste aversions in children receiving chemotherapy. *Science* **200**, 1302–3.
7. Bernstein I. L., Webster M. M. and Bernstein I. D. (1982) Food aversions in children receiving chemotherapy for cancer. *Cancer* **50**, 2961–3.
8. Stockwell M., Adams M., Andrew M. et al. (1983) Central venous catheters for out-patient management of malignant disorders. *Arch. Dis. Child.* **58**, 633–5.
9. Kearsley J. H. and Tattersall H. N. (1985) Recent advances in the prevention or reduction of cytotoxic-induced emesis. *Med. J. Aust.* **143**, 341–6.
10. Wempler P. (1983) The pharmacology and clinical effectiveness of phenothiazines and related drugs for managing chemotherapy-induced emesis. *Drugs* **25** (Suppl. 1), 35–51.
11. Gralla R. J. (1983) Metoclopramide: a review of antiemetic trials. *Drugs* **25** (Suppl. 1), 63–73.
12. Casteels-Van Daele M., Jaeken J., Van der Schueren P. et al. (1970) Dystonic reactions in children caused by metoclopramide. *Arch. Dis. Child.* **45**, 130–3.
13. Terrin B. N., McWilliams N. B. and Maurer H. M. (1984) Side-effects of metoclopramide as an antiemetic in childhood cancer. *J. Pediatr.* **104**, 138–40.
14. Bateman D. N., Craft A. W., Nicholson E. et al. (1983) Dystonic reactions and the pharmacokinetics of metoclopramide in children. *Br. J. Clin. Pharmacol.* **15**, 557–9.
15. Chantraine J. M. and Reginster-Bous M. (1979) The antiemetic action of domperidone (R33812) in children undergoing a course of cytotoxic treatment. *Rev. Méd. Liège* **34**, 199–202.
16. Swann I. L., Thompson E. N. and Qureshi K. (1979) Domperidone or metoclopramide in preventing chemotherapeutically induced nausea and vomiting. *Br. Med. J.* **2**, 1188.
17. O'Meara A. and Mott M. G. (1981) Domperidone as an antiemetic in paediatric oncology. *Cancer Chemother. Pharmacol.* **6**, 147–9.
18. Craft A. W. (1983) Clinical experience with domperidone in paediatric oncology patients. *Clin. Res. Rev.* **3**, 45–8.
19. Ward P. S. (1983) Recent clinical experience with domperidone in the treatment of cytotoxic induced nausea and vomiting in paediatrics. *Clin. Res. Rev.* **3**, 35–9.
20. Joss R. A., Goldhirsch A., Brunner K. W. et al. (1982) Sudden death in cancer patient on high-dose domperidone. *Lancet* **i**, 1019.
21. Vincent B. J., McQuiston D. J., Einhorn L. H. et al. (1983) Review of cannabinoids and their antiemetic effectiveness. *Drugs* **25** (Suppl. 1), 52–62.
22. Eckert H., Waters K. D., Jurk I. H. et al. (1979) Amelioration of cancer chemotherapy-induced nausea and vomiting by delta-9-tetrahydrocannabinol. *Med. J. Aust.* **2**, 657–9.
23. Dalzell A. M., Bartlett H. and Lilleyman J. S. (1986) Nabilone: an alternative antiemetic for cancer chemotherapy. *Arch. Dis. Child.* **61**, 502–5.

24. Cunningham D., Forrest G. J., Soulkop M. et al. (1985) Nabilone and prochlorperazine: a useful combination for emesis induced by cytotoxic drugs. *Br. Med. J.* **291**, 864–5.

25. Cronin C. M., Sallan S. E., Gelber R. et al. (1981) Antiemetic effect of intramuscular levonantradol in patients receiving anti-cancer chemotherapy. *J. Clin. Pharmacol.* **21**, 43–50.

26. Anonymous (1986) Corticosteroids and lorazepam as antiemetics in cancer chemotherapy. *Drug Ther. Bull.* **24**, 46–8.

27. Mehta P., Gross S., Graham-Pole J. et al. (1986) Methylprednisolone for chemotherapy-induced emesis: a double-blind randomized trial in children. *J. Pediatrics* **108**, 774–6.

28. LaBaw W., Holton C., Tewell K. et al. (1975) The use of self-hypnosis by children with cancer. *Am. J. Clin. Hyp.* **17**, 233–8.

29. Morrow G. R. and Morrell C. (1982) Behavioural treatment for the anticipatory nausea and vomiting induced by cancer chemotherapy. *N. Engl. J. Med.* **307**, 1476–80.

30. Moher D., Arthur A. Z. and Pater J. L. (1984) Anticipatory nausea and/or vomiting. *Cancer Treat. Rev.* **11**, 257–64.

9. Nutrition

J. Drakeford

INTRODUCTION

Improved treatment and survival of children with cancer has encouraged those involved with their care towards more aggressive forms of nutritional support.[1]

Poor nutrition is mainly seen in children with active disease, particularly in relapse.[2,3,4] Surgery or the development of severe infection exacerbates the problem.[5]

Protein-energy malnutrition is likely at diagnosis and during treatment although the incidence varies according to the tumour type and the stage of the disease (*Table* 9.1).[3] Vitamin deficiencies may occur, especially vitamins A, C and thiamin,[6] whilst taste abnormalities may be due to trace element deficiencies such as zinc, as well as cancer therapy. The biggest problem is ensuring adequate energy intake.[7]

The result is cancer cachexia, the term describing a combination of weight loss, muscle wasting, reduced skin fold fat and increased basal metabolic rate, along with progressive weakness and apathy.[8]

The causes of cachexia are many, not least of which is anorexia, leading to decreased nutrient intake. This may be due to the disease itself or the side-effects of therapy.[9] Other problems include

Table 9.1. Common risk factors for development of protein energy malnutrition (Reproduced from Rickard et al.)[3]

Advanced disease at diagnosis or during treatment
Lack of tumour response
Abdominal or pelvic irradiation
Intensive and frequent course of chemotherapy
Surgery to the abdomen or other abdominal complications such as ileus
Psychological depression

malabsorption, diversion of nutrients to the tumour and production of tumour factors which affect host metabolism.[8, 10, 11]

Treatment designed to destroy cancer cells can also damage normal cells. This lack of selectivity particularly affects rapidly dividing cells, such as bone marrow, intestinal mucosa and hair follicles. Chemotherapeutic agents may also have a toxic effect on the liver, pancreas, kidney and cardiovascular system.[12, 13, 14].

The multimodal approach to therapy, involving surgery, chemotherapy and radiotherapy has a wide range of potential nutritional side-effects (*Table* 9.2). All methods have an adverse effect on food intake and utilization, although it has been argued that successful therapy will result in a better appetite and weight gain.[2, 15] A malnourished child is a listless and unwell child with an increased risk of infection, provoking further anxiety in already overwrought parents. Well-nourished patients tolerate anti-tumour therapy better,[16, 17] have enhanced immunological status,[5, 17] are better tempered and are easier to manage, so improving family morale.

Surgery. Head and neck surgery can lead to serious malnutrition by affecting normal nutritional processes such as chewing and swallowing. Bowel resections, stomach and pancreatic surgery may cause different degrees of malabsorption, whilst all surgery poses the usual risk of infection and increased catabolism. There may be considerable time before a child can eat postoperatively.

Radiation. Sensitivity of mucosal epithelia to radiation can lead to alterations in taste and smell, dysphagia and reduced saliva production. All combine to reduce appetite.[3] Head and neck irradiation may cause mucositis, stomatitis and gingivitis, whilst abdominal

Table 9.2. Nutritional side-effects of cancer treatment[12]

Weight loss
Nausea
Vomiting
Anorexia
Diarrhoea
Stomatitis
Malabsorption
Reduced saliva production
Altered taste sensation
Early satiety
Learned food aversion
Steroid-induced diabetes
Renal protein loss
Constipation
Diversion of nutrients to tumour

treatment can lead to nausea and vomiting and pelvic irradiation to diarrhoea.

Chemotherapy. Cytotoxic agents, used in combination or alone, have the advantage of destroying malignant cells throughout the body and not just locally. However, induction of symptoms similar to those seen after radiation is likely. These include mucosal ulceration, taste changes, nausea, vomiting and diarrhoea. Electrolyte disturbances and fluid imbalance resulting from the latter need to be treated.

It is important to help parents with simple, practical advice that is consistent and reassuring when, and if, such problems occur.[18] (*See* Appendix 1.)

ASSESSMENT OF NUTRITIONAL STATUS

Adequate nutrition in childhood is achieved when there are sufficient nutrients for growth and development.[1] Frequent assessment will prevent malnutrition from going undetected or progressing to a more severe state. It should include clinical examination, medical history (type of treatment, drugs used, etc.) and also a psychosocial review of the child and his family.[5]

Table 9.3. Investigations of nutritional status[3]

Dietary history
Weight as % ideal body weight for height
Skin fold thickness
Monitoring of growth
Nitrogen balance
Biochemical parameters, e.g. serum albumin, transferrin, haemoglobin

Overt malnutrition may not be present but the degree of depletion needs to be measured in order to decide on the intervention required. Although there are no standard, validated procedures which exist for nutritional assessment of children, a number of investigations are recommended.[5] (*See Table* 9.3.) A child with a weight:height ratio of less than 80 per cent that of the 50th centile, should receive some form of nutritional supplementation.[4, 19] Although treatment of the cancer primarily affects ultimate survival, a lack of weight gain in a child represents deterioration of nutritional status.[17]

METHODS OF NUTRITIONAL SUPPORT (*Fig.* 9.1)

The term nutritional support describes the provision of adequate nutrients, regardless of the route of administration. It is an integral

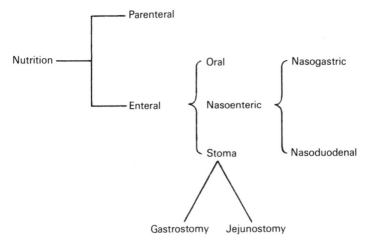

Fig. 9.1. Nutritional support—possible feeding routes.

part of total patient management and should be considered alongside the anti-tumour therapy. Although, as yet, it is unclear whether response to treatment is increased by improving nutritional status,[13] other advantages are well known (*Table* 9.4).

Table 9.4. Advantages of improved nutritional status

Improved wellbeing
Reduction of cachectic symptoms
Reduced wound dehiscence
Lower surgical mortality
Fewer postoperative wound infections
Better tolerance of anti-tumour therapy
Improved drug metabolism
Enhanced immunological status

ORAL ROUTE

To feed a child is a basic instinct and food is normally taken by mouth. However, many children find hospital food unfamiliar and unacceptable, or the timing of meals inappropriate for their therapeutic regime. Favourite foods often become overused or associated with unpleasant procedures by the child and specific food avoidance may continue long after symptoms of discomfort have subsided.[9, 20] This may result in a complete change of food preferences during a hospital admission. Although adults may be persuaded to eat when taste perceptions are altered, children usually refuse to do so until they normalize. Force feeding is never indicated when children become difficult and manipulative at mealtimes, but it is necessary to be calm and firm. It is not uncommon for most of the day's food to be consumed after 5 p.m., due to the many activities of the hospital day. Although hospital catering departments are generally willing to adjust the provision of food, it is worth obtaining the support of the child's family and friends in the preparation of tempting and enjoyable meals.[1,21] Ward level stock of convenience foods such as canned soups, baked beans and milk puddings can be very useful, whilst equipment such as a deep freeze and microwave are great assets. The presentation of food is crucial to its acceptability and care needs to be taken with colour, textures, temperature and portion size.

An anorectic child is unlikely to consume adequate food to meet his requirements. To improve nutrition, simple advice to nursing staff and the family may be adequate. This should be based on the best food choices, supplementation of familiar foods to increase protein and energy intake and the provision of a vitamin and mineral supplement as an insurance against deficiency. Discussion between all support staff will indicate when changes to management are needed, according to the progression of the disease.

LIQUID SUPPLEMENTS

It may be necessary to provide nourishing drinks before, during or after therapy. A variety of commercially produced drinks are available, some of which are prescribable as Borderline Substances (Appendix 2). They range from simple energy sources to those containing balanced amounts of protein, energy, vitamins and minerals. If taken regularly as a supplement between meals, marked improvement in nutrient intake will be achieved. However, acceptance of such drinks is usually shortlived and home-made mixtures with a variety of flavourings can be more effective (Appendix 3). There is little advantage to a theoretical calculation of requirement and making products available, if the drinks remain in the ward fridge. Dietitians and support staff must learn to listen to the views of the parents in order to provide practical help for each individual child.

It has been reported that adults with cancer prefer milk-based drinks to savoury or fruit flavours[22] and this often applies to children. However, the development of bitter and metallic tastes or enhanced sensations of flavour, may make supplements of all types unacceptable.[3] Similarly, symptoms such as nausea and vomiting will frustrate all efforts.

In view of the fact that patients are known to develop aversions to new or unusual foods offered prior to therapy,[10,22] simple glucose polymers remain the most useful way of supplementing familiar drinks and puddings. By providing a relatively tasteless source of energy, they are also helpful when early satiety necessitates the use of energy dense items rather than bulky, low calorie foods.

Early introduction of oral supplements is recommended, preferably before treatment commences, in order both to improve and maintain nutrition throughout the subsequent anti-tumour therapy.

NASOENTERIC FEEDING

When oral intake ceases to be adequate for the child's needs, or when the predictors of malnutrition are present, it is necessary to consider additional methods of nutritional support.

Nutrients can be administered directly into the gastrointestinal tract by nasogastric or nasoduodenal tube.[23] Such regimes may provide total nutrition with feeds given regularly over a 24-h period, or be supplementary to oral food intake and given over reduced time spans, such as overnight. The latter allows the child to eat and drink according to appetite by day, to play and make trips outside the hospital, whilst maintaining acceptable nutrition.

The availability of flexible fine bore tubes and enteral feeding pumps ensures it is a simple and effective procedure, although decisions need to be made on the mode of administration, choice of feed and rate of infusion.

In children, large volume bolus feeds have been replaced by small, frequent feeds, 2–3 hourly. The latter allows better absorption and yet still allows the child a respite between feeds. It also mimics normal feeding patterns more closely than continuous drip feeding which carries the risk of tube displacement and feed inhalation. Overnight drip feeding may be used as a way of maximizing feed intake,[3] but should always be controlled by a feeding pump and not gravity flow methods.

CHOICE OF FEED

Immunosuppressed patients are at particular risk of infection and there has been considerable discussion on the contamination of enteral feeds, resulting in rapid bacterial growth.[24] Commercially produced, sterile feeds are therefore preferred to hospital prepared 'home brews'.[25] Blenderized food is not recommended due to the high bacterial hazard and the blockage of fine bore tubes with food particles. Dilution of blenderized food produces a nutritionally

Table 9.5. Complications of nasoenteric feeding

Nausea
Vomiting
Abdominal cramps
Diarrhoea
Metabolic complications, e.g. hyperglycaemia
Oesophageal reflux
Vitamin/mineral/trace element deficiencies
Tube displacement

---

inadequate feed of uncertain composition, particularly electrolytes. An agreed protocol on the safe preparation and administration of enteral feeds is vital.[26]

Most commercially available feeds are nutritionally complete when given in adequate volume for adults, but are not designed for children. Nutritional adequacy, therefore, needs to be established by appropriate supplementation, if they are to be used as a sole source of nutrition. It is wise to check the provision of calcium, vitamin D, iron, zinc and folic acid if long-term feeding is envisaged.

Gradual introduction of the feed, considering both strength and volume, should avoid the reported complications of feeding (*Table* 9.5). Full strength, full volume feeding may be achieved within 4 days of commencing the regime, depending on the child's condition. Changes should be agreed by all support staff as it is important not to increase the feed volume and strength at the same time, if diarrhoea is to be prevented.

CHEMICALLY DEFINED FORMULAE

Provided gastrointestinal function is adequate, a standard formula based on whole protein, fat and carbohydrate, fortified with vitamins and minerals, should be used. These are well tolerated, inexpensive and often palatable enough to be taken orally. However, if digestion and/or absorption are limited, nutrients need to be presented to the intestinal mucosa in a readily absorbable form. Feeds based on

Table 9.6. Indications for chemically defined formulae

Short bowel syndrome
Gastrointestinal fistulae
Malabsorption
Preoperative bowel preparation

---

peptides and amino acids, simple carbohydrates such as glucose and medium chain triglycerides are occasionally indicated (*Table* 9.6). These products (*see* Appendix 2) are expensive, very unpalatable and may be hyperosmolar, although the greater reliance on small peptides rather than amino acids as a protein source has improved them considerably. Nitrogen absorption appears to be more efficient from peptides than free amino acids[27,28] and therefore partial protein hydrolysates are now employed.

GASTROSTOMY/JEJUNOSTOMY FEEDING

Feeding via a stoma may be required when there is intractable vomiting or oesophageal involvement in the disease. Such invasive procedures are not widely used but may provide a simpler, safer and cheaper alternative to parenteral nutrition, whilst avoiding frequent repassing of nasoenteric tubes,[29] which may damage the oesophageal mucosa leading to stricture formation. This is particularly so in children on chemotherapy who have oral candida. Standard, whole protein feeds are tolerated, provided the rate of infusion is carefully controlled in patients with a jejunostomy.[30] Continuous or frequent, small volume feeding is essential in the latter, if osmotic effects are to be avoided. Bolus feeding can be used when feeding is directly into the stomach.

PARENTERAL NUTRITION

The intravenous administration of nutrition is expensive compared with enteral feeding and is likely to cause more complications. The more physiological method of enteral feeding, which is also easier to administer, is therefore preferred where gastrointestinal function is adequate.[31]

Parenteral feeding is often necessary, however, during periods of intensive treatment and may provide partial or total nutrition (*Table* 9.7). Complete parenteral nutrition has been shown to reverse weight loss and improve biochemical parameters, even in the presence of intensive chemotherapy.[2,19] Although it may not significantly improve survival, it can decrease treatment side-effects and improve nutritional status.[32]

Access to the circulation may be via a peripheral vein but nutrition is limited to short periods, due to vein thrombosis with hypertonic solutions. Long-term feeding through a central venous catheter, introduced into a major vein, such as the subclavian, allows more concentrated solutions to be given. Precise infusion control is ensured

Table 9.7. Indications for total parenteral nutrition

Intestinal obstruction
Paralytic ileus
Coma
Fistulae
Severe malabsorption
Intractable vomiting

by sophisticated pumps which incorporate alarms to warn of deviation from the set flow rate or of air in the system.

COMPLETE PARENTERAL NUTRITION

The regime should provide adequate fluid, energy and nitrogen, together with electrolytes, minerals, vitamins and trace elements.[33]

Fluid

Fluid requirements should be calculated for each child, preferably according to their expected weight, so that weight gain may be achieved. Expected weight may be estimated in a number of ways:

a. Take the same centile as birthweight (for infants).
b. Take the centile the child was at when he stopped gaining weight or started to lose.
c. Use a previous known centile.
d. If malnutrition is of recent, acute onset, use the length centile as a guide.

Calculation of requirement in this way may mean a relatively high energy and protein intake when compared with actual weight. At least 1ml of fluid is recommended for every kilocalorie (4·184kJ) in the infusate. Additional fluid may be needed to compensate for abnormal losses such as diarrhoea.

Protein

The usual protein source is a balanced mixture of crystalline L-amino acids, necessary for tissue synthesis and maintenance. In order to ensure full utilization of the nitrogen, adequate energy must be provided in the form of carbohydrate and fat. At least 126 non-protein kilojoules (30 non-protein kcal) are needed for each gram of protein (equivalent to 628–837kJ/g or 150–200kcal nitrogen).

Carbohydrate

Glucose is the carbohydrate of choice[35] and should provide 50–60 per cent energy. Peripheral vein feeding is limited by osmolarity to the use of 10 per cent glucose solutions or less, while central venous access allows higher concentrations to be tolerated.

Fat

This is an excellent source of energy, provides essential fatty acids and is used as a carrier for fat-soluble vitamins. An isotonic lipid emulsion is used, based on soya bean oil, stabilized with egg yolk phospholipid and with added glycerol. When given as part of a total nutrition regime, normal caloric balance is maintained with 35–40 per cent energy as fat. It should be used with caution, however, in children with cancer and is contraindicated if the drugs given affect liver function or where there is septicaemia or disturbances of fat metabolism.[34]

Minerals and vitamins

Commercial preparations of essential trace elements and vitamins (water- and fat-soluble) are available for supplementing solutions. Additional phosphate, calcium, magnezium and zinc are added when indicated. Parenteral nutrition should be increased gradually over 4–6 d and similarly decreased at the end of the feeding period. This should minimize the risk of hyperglycaemia, fat and fluid overload. If feeding is interrupted, a 10–15 per cent glucose infusion will prevent hypoglycaemia.

Table 9.8. Complications of total parenteral nutrition (Reproduced from Phillips, 1982)[37]

Metabolic:	Hyper/hypoglycaemia
	Hyper/hypo-
	magnesaemia
	natraemia
	chloraemia
	calcaemia
	phosphataemia
	Acidosis/alkalosis
	Trace element, vitamin, fatty acid deficiencies
	Over- and under-hydration
	Hyperosmolality
Infective:	Bacterial
	Fungus
Psychological:	Anxiety neurosis

The preparation of feeding solutions should be in specialized units by pharmacy staff but may be by nursing staff at ward level. The former generally provide single containers with mixed solutions and additives ready for use. This system is more economic of time and money and reduces infection risk, compared to multiple bottle systems.[35,36]

Despite the many potential complications of parenteral nutrition,[37] (*Table* 9.8), long-term or intermittent feeding can be very successful. Careful attention to the feeding line by experienced staff is the key to this success.[38]

THERAPEUTIC DIETS

In addition to the nutritional support so far discussed, dietary modification may also be necessary at intervals throughout the course of the disease.

Low lactose diets, following episodes of diarrhoea, may be required. Consumption of 'live' yoghurt can prove beneficial by reducing flatulence and diarrhoea due to its high lactase activity and autodigestion of lactose.[39] A low residue diet may also be helpful. In contrast, high fibre diets may be required as an adjunct to the use of stool softeners and laxatives in chronic constipation. All such modifications should be organized in co-operation with the hospital dietitian.

The use of special diets in the treatment of cancer remains controversial. Vegetarian diets based on predominantly raw food have been advocated for adults[40] and high dose vitamin A and C supplementation has also been recommended.[6,8] At present, a healthy scepticism remains, particularly in view of the problems encountered in ensuring adequate energy intake amongst children with cancer.[41]

CONCLUSION

Good nutritional support depends upon assessment, planning, monitoring and control of the system. It involves co-operation between medical, nursing, technical, biochemical, dietetic and pharmacy staff, not forgetting, of course, the child and his family. Liaison with community staff will ensure that parents receive consistent and reassuring advice.

Although all efforts may not be wholly successful in preventing nutritional depletion during intensive therapy, considerable emotional support will be gained by the family, together with a sound nutritional philosophy that will be continued once the intensive phase is over.

Appendix 1

Practical Advice for Parents

Eating well means having a variety of foods on a regular basis, in order to provide all the essential energy (kilojoules), protein, vitamins, minerals, fluid and roughage.

Problems which arise need simple and practical advice.

'But I don't want to eat'

Children always have good days and bad days, but the bad days become more frequent when they are unwell, or having treatment. They become moody and irritable and may refuse to eat altogether.

Keep snacks handy and tempt him with small amounts of his favourite foods. Don't be surprised if he turns against these—this is not unusual as his sense of taste may change.

Food often tastes better if cold or at room temperature, rather than hot.

Use a high protein drink (*see* p. 159) as an occasional meal substitute.

Accept that he will eat slowly—at least this allows him to chew his food well and gives you all time to relax.

Accept offers from friends and family who want to help prepare food in advance. It can be frustrating to spend hours in the kitchen only to find the food is refused.

Have you a freezer or microwave oven? Use it. If not, keep individual portions of foods which can be quickly prepared. For example:

Sausages, beefburgers, fish fingers, boil-in-the-bag fish
Tins of spaghetti, baked beans, macaroni cheese
Soup, sandwich fillings
Packets of savoury rice
Tinned sponge puddings and custard or yoghurts

Remember that fluid is very important, so encourage frequent drinks throughout the day.

If the problem persists, seek help from your doctor or dietitian.

'I'm full up'

A feeling of being very full is aggravated by fried, greasy and spicy foods.

Five or six snacks will be better than three meals.

Offer drinks half an hour before or after food, instead of with meals.

'Everything tastes funny'

Children often find their sense of taste changes.

Avoid foods which are very hot—they will taste better cold or at room temperature.

Chicken, fish and cheese are usually better than red meats.

If food tastes bitter, add a little sugar or fruit juice or try mayonnaise and bottled sauces.

Sweet, milky drinks may not be acceptable—try fruit drinks instead.

'I feel sick'

Hopefully, this will only be temporary, but ask the doctor to prescribe something to help.

Keep the child away from the kitchen while preparing food, to avoid the smell of cooking.

A well ventilated room will help to get rid of the cooking smells.

Dry biscuits, crackers or toast may help.

Avoid rich foods with sauces and greasy foods.

Encourage the child to eat slowly—sipping drinks through a straw may help.

Avoid tight-fitting clothes and sudden movements.

Constipation?

Encourage plenty of fluids, especially fruit juices and water. Aim for 6–8 cups daily. An early morning hot drink may help.

Try more roughage. The following foods all contain roughage (or fibre):

Wholegrain breakfast cereals
Wholemeal bread (not just brown)
Digestive biscuits, oatcakes, fruit cakes
Fresh and dried fruit of all types
All kinds of vegetables, including baked beans, potatoes
A suitable laxative may be necessary.

Diarrhoea?

Fluid is particularly important—all types may be given but avoid fizzy drinks.

Avoid highly spiced or sweetened foods.

Choose more white bread and low fibre cereals, like Cornflakes or Rice Krispies, rather than the foods listed for constipation.

Some foods tend to make diarrhoea worse—such as baked beans, cabbage, peas and sweetcorn.

Natural yoghurt may help, especially the 'live' varieties from health food shops.

'My mouth is dry and/or sore'

Prepare soft, moist food with sauces, or gravy. Use custard, ice cream, yoghurt or mix up milky drinks.

Avoid very acid foods like citrus fruits or add a little sugar to them.

Avoid rough foods like toast and hot foods which may irritate the mouth.

Use a straw for drinks.

Sucking ice cubes, ice lollies or fruit sweets may freshen a dry mouth.

Ask for advice on the use of mouthwashes or artificial saliva.

Encourage good oral hygiene and frequent mouthwashes.

Appendix 2

Prescribable Nutritional Supplements

The following are prescribable as Borderline Substances for specific conditions:

Brand name	Presentation	Comments
Glucose polymers		
Polycal (Cow & Gate)	Powder	Useful as a relatively
Caloreen (Cassene)	Powder	tasteless source of energy,
Maxijul (SHS)	Powder	particularly in drinks.
Polycose (Abbott)	Powder or liquid	
Calonutrin (Geistlich)	Powder	
High energy drinks		
Fortical (Cow & Gate)	Liquid	Available in apple, apricot, neutral, lemon, blackcurrant and orange flavours.
Hycal (Beecham Products)	Liquid	Available in raspberry, lemon, orange and blackcurrant flavours.
Maxijul (SHS)	Liquid	Available in natural, blackcurrant, lemon and lime flavours.
Protein supplements		
Casilan (Glaxo-Farley)	Powder	
Maxipro (SHS)	Powder	
Sip feeds		
Fortisip (Cow & Gate)	Liquid	Available as strawberry, chocolate and vanilla milk-based drinks.
Fresubin (Fresenius-Dylade)	Liquid	Available as vanilla, peach, nut and chocolate milk-based drinks.

Brand name	Presentation	Comments
Whole protein tube feeds		
Clinifeed range (Cassene)	Liquid—ready to feed	Clinifeed Favour is lactose free.
Ensure range (Abbott)	Liquid or powder	All varieties are lactose free.
Fortison range (Cow & Gate)	Liquid—ready to feed	Very low lactose. Soya-based feed available.
Isocal (Bristol-Myers)	Liquid—ready to feed	Lactose free. Contains medium chain triglycerides.
Nutrauxil (Kabivitrum)	Liquid—ready to feed	Very low lactose.
Triosorbon (E. Merck)	Powder	Contains minimal lactose.
Wyeth Standard Enteral Feed (Wyeth Laboratories)	Liquid—ready to feed	Low lactose.

These enteral feeds contain balanced amounts of protein, energy, vitamins and minerals. They should not be used for infants and may require modification when used as a sole source of nutrition for children.

Brand name	Presentation	Comments
Chemically defined formulae		
Elemental 028 (SHS)	Powder	Protein as amino acids.
Flexical (Bristol-Myers)	Powder	Protein as peptides and amino acids.
Nutranel (Cassene)	Powder	Protein as peptides, amino acids.
Peptisorbon (E. Merck)	Powder	Protein as peptides, amino acids.
Pepdite 0–2/2 + (SHS)	Powder	Protein as peptides—suitable for infants and young children.
MCT Pepdite 0–2/2 + (SHS)	Powder	As above but contains medium chain triglycerides.
Vivonex (Norwich Eaton)	Powder	Protein as amino acids. Very high osmolality—*not suitable for children.*

The above formulae are unpalatable and generally need to be given via nasoenteric tube. Modification and/or supplementation may be necessary when used as a sole source of nutrition for children. Gradual introduction of the feeds is necessary due to their relatively high osmolality.

Appendix 3

High Protein Hints

Fortified milk

60g dried skimmed milk powder
600ml fresh cow's milk

Whisk the milk powder into the fresh milk for a high protein milk which can be used in drinks, on cereals and in cooking.

High protein drinks

Nourishing drinks such as Build Up, Complete, Vitafood and Complan can be bought from chemist shops and used as a 'meal in a glass'.

A cheaper, home-made milk shake is:

300ml fresh cow's milk $\qquad\rangle$ 1424kJ
30g (2 tablespoons) dried skimmed milk powder $\Big\}$ (340kcal)
30ml (2 tablespoons) milk shake syrup $\qquad$ 20g protein

Ice cream may be added for extra taste or use cocoa, coffee and malted milk powders for a hot drink.

Other recipe ideas

Breakfast in a Glass

150ml chilled natural orange juice
1 egg
1 tablespoon glucose polymer $\qquad$ 1130kJ (270kcal)
150ml plain yoghurt $\qquad$ 15g protein
1 tablespoon sugar or honey

Place all ingredients into a liquidizer and blend for 5–10 sec. Serve immediately.

Banana Egg Nog

1 egg
200ml milk $\qquad$ 1215kJ (290kcal)
1/2 banana—chopped $\qquad$ 13g protein
1–2 teaspoons sugar

Place all ingredients in a liquidizer and blend for 10–15 sec.

Honey and Egg Flip

1 egg
200ml milk
1 teaspoon honey   1020kJ (244kcal)
1 teaspoon sugar or 1 tablespoon glucose 13g protein
  polymer

Place all the ingredients into a liquidizer and blend for 10–15 sec.

Orange Drink

200ml natural orange juice
1 egg   710kJ (170kcal)
1 teaspoon sugar or 1 tablespoon glucose 7g protein
  polymer

Place all ingredients into a liquidizer and blend for 10–15 sec.

Banana Yoghurt Shake

300ml milk—chilled
1 tablespoon glucose polymer (optional)   2110kJ (504kcal)
150ml hazelnut yoghurt (or try other   19g protein
  flavouring)
1 tablespoon sugar
1 banana—chopped

Place all ingredients in the liquidizer, blend for 10–15 sec, and serve immediately.

Chocolate Cooler

300ml milk—chilled
4 teaspoons drinking chocolate
1 teaspoon sugar   1730kJ (413kcal)
1 tablespoon glucose polymer (optional)   14g protein
4 tablespoons vanilla ice-cream
A little drinking chocolate—for sprinkling

Place all ingredients in the liquidizer and blend for about 10 sec. Pour into 1–2 glasses and sprinkle a little chocolate powder on top.

REFERENCES

1. Van Eys J. (1977) Nutritional therapy in children with cancer. *Cancer Res.* **37** (Part 2), 2457.
2. Van Eys J. (1979) Malnutrition in children with cancer. *Cancer* **43**, 2030.
3. Rickard K. A., Baehner R. L., Coates T. D. et al. (1982) Effect of nutritional status on responses to therapy. *Cancer Res.* **42** (2 Suppl.), 747.
4. Carter P., Carr D., Van Eys J. et al. (1983) Nutritional parameters in children with cancer. *J. Am. Diet Assoc.* **82** (No. 6), 616.
5. Neuman C. G., Jelliffe D. B., Zeifas A. J. et al. (1982) Nutritional assessment of the child with cancer. *Cancer Res.* **42** (2 Suppl.), 699.
6. Calman K. C. (1978) Nutritional support in malignant disease. *Proc. Nutr. Soc.* **37**, 87.
7. Carter P., Carr D., Van Eys J. et al. (1983) Energy and nutrient intake in children with cancer. *J. Am. Diet. Assoc.* **82**, 610.
8. Calman K. C. (1984) Diet and cancer. *Appl. Nutr.* **11**, 8.
9. Bernstein I. L. (1982) Physiological and psychological mechanisms of cancer anorexia. *Cancer Res.* **42** (Suppl.), 715.
10. Dickerson J. W. T. (1984) Nutrition in the cancer patient: a review. *J. R. Soc. Med.* **77**, 309.
11. Walsh T. D., Cheater F. M. (letter) (1983) *Lancet* **2**, 288.
12. Donaldson S. S. (1982) Effects of therapy on nutritional status of the paediatric cancer patient. *Cancer Res.* **42** (2 Suppl.), 729.
13. Costa G. and Donaldson S. S. (1979) Current concepts in cancer. *N. Engl. J. Med.* **300**, 1471.
14. Holmes S. (1984) Chemotherapy and the gastrointestinal tract. *Nurs. Times* Feb. 22, 29.
15. Wheeler K. (1986) Caring for children with cancer. *Update* **12**, 21.
16. Van Eys J. (1986) The pathophysiology of undernutrition in the child with cancer. *Cancer* **58** (No. 8), 1874.
17. Rickard K. A., Coates T. D., Grosfeld J. L. et al. (1986) The value of nutrition support in children with cancer. *Cancer* **58** (Suppl.), 1904.
18. Kelly K. (1986) How to nourish the cancer patient by mouth. *Cancer* **58** (Suppl.), 1897.
19. Van Eys J., Cangir A., Carter P. et al. (1982) Effect of nutritional supportive therapy on children with advanced cancer. *Cancer Res.* **42** (2 Suppl.), 713.
20. Bernstein I. L. (1986) Aetiology of anorexia in cancer. *Cancer* **58**, 1881.
21. Corr J. (1984) The role of the dietitian working in an oncology unit. *Appl. Nutr.* **11**, 12.
22. Aker S. N. (1979) Oral feeding in the cancer patient. *Cancer* **43**, 2103.
23. Editorial (1986) Enteral feeds for adults: an update. *Drug. Ther. Bull.* **24** (No. 16), 61.
24. Anderton A. (1983) Microbiological aspects of the preparation and administration of nasogastric and naso-enteric tube feeds in hospital—a review. *Hum. Nutr. App. Nutr.* **37A**, 426.
25. Anderton A., Howard J. P. and Scott D. W. (1983) Microbiological control in enteral feeding. *Hum. Nutr. App. Nutr.* **40A** (No. 3), 163.
26. (1986) *Microbiological Control in Enteral Feeding: A Guidance Document.* The Parenteral and Enteral Nutrition Group of the BDA.
27. Silk D. B. A., Fairclough P. D., Clark M. L. et al. (1980) Use of a peptide rather than free amino acid nitrogen source in chemically defined 'elemental' diets. *J. Parenter. Enter. Nutr.* **4** (No. 6), 548.
28. Adibi S. A. (1985) Advances in enteral nutrition with emphasis on the source of nitrogen. *Proceedings of the Aspen Conference.*

29. Russell C. A. (1984) Fine needle jejunostomy feeding in patients with oesophageal or gastric carcinoma. *Appl. Nutr.* **11**, 1.
30. Hindmarsh J. T. and Clark R. G. (1973) New jejunostomy feed. *Br. Med. J.* **3**, 609.
31. Irving M. (1985) Enteral and parenteral nutrition. *Br. Med. J.* **291**, 1404.
32. Nixon D. W. (1986) The value of parenteral nutrition support: chemotherapy and radiation treatment. *Cancer* **58** (Suppl.), 1902.
33. Lee H. A. (1980) The development of complete parenteral nutrition from first principles. *Br. J. Pharm. Prac.* **1** (Suppl.), 29.
34. Wheeler N. (1984) Parenteral nutrition. In: Kelts D. G. and Jones E. G. (eds.) *Manual of Paediatric Nutrition*. Boston, Little, Brown.
35. Nunn A. J. (1980) Aspects of pharmacy involvement. *Br. J. Pharm. Prac.* **1** (Suppl.), 42.
36. Forbes D. R., Faulkner S. and Dunn M. (1986) Low-cost aseptic service of TPN and cytotoxic reconstitution. *Pharm. J.* **237**, 620.
37. Phillips C. D. and Odgers C. L. (1982) Parenteral nutrition: current status and concepts. *Drugs* **23**(4), 279.
38. Nugent M. and Park R. (1984) Role of nutrition team—the Victoria Infirmary, Glasgow. *Appl. Nutr.* **11**, 15.
39. Kolars J. C. and Levitt M. D., Aoji M. et al. (1984) Yoghurt—an autodigesting source of lactose. *N. Engl. J. Med.* **310** (No. 1), 1.
40. Forbes A. (1986) *The Bristol Diet*. London, Arrow Books.
41. Herbert V. (1986) Unproven (questionable) dietary and nutritional methods in cancer prevention and treatment. *Cancer* **58** (Suppl.), 1930.
42. *Eating Problems—How to Cope*. CLIC leaflet. Cancer & Leukaemia in Childhood Trust, 12 Fremantle Square, Bristol 6.

ACKNOWLEDGEMENTS

Acknowledgements to Anita MacDonald for help with the recipes, and the pharmacy staff of the Bristol Royal Hospital for Sick Children.

10. Central Venous Catheters

E. Kiely

INTRODUCTION

The wide variety of available central venous catheters suggests that no single catheter is suitable for all patients. It also means that individual requirements can be met. With a personal experience of almost 400 central venous catheters in children, the author has acquired some views on catheters and techniques and these are expressed in this chapter.

There are many valid opinions on the question of which catheter to use and by which approach. As with other surgical problems, efforts should be directed towards mastery of a limited number of techniques.

The availability of a wide bore catheter greatly reduces the need for venepuncture in childhood cancer. The anxiety and upset associated with needles can be abolished and a needless cause of suffering removed. Consequently, a catheter should be inserted early in the course of the illness, particularly if the chemotherapy is very toxic or prolonged.

TYPES OF CATHETER

A wide range of catheters is available. Catheters used in childhood malignancies are likely to remain in place for many months. They should, therefore, be constructed of non-irritant and non-thrombogenic material and should be pliable. Silicon rubber (silastic) fulfils these criteria and catheters constructed of this material have been available for many years.

There are two basic types which are suitable for use—cuffed and uncuffed catheters. Cuffed catheters have a collar of synthetic felt glued to the subcutaneous part of the catheter. Tissue ingrowth into this collar fixes the catheter in position and prevents catheter movement. It also prevents accidental removal and may prevent

163

bacterial migration along the catheter from the skin entry site. Broviac and Hickman catheters* are the most commonly used cuffed catheters and come in various sizes from 1·3 to 3·2mm outside diameter. Other manufacturers make similar catheters.

Multilumen catheters are useful in certain circumstances, but have been rarely used in the author's experience. The other variety of cuffed catheter in use is the totally implantable device which includes a catheter and injection port. These are much more expensive but have a well defined, though limited, role. It is too early to say whether or not these devices are at less risk of infection.

A large range of uncuffed catheters is available. The smaller catheters can be introduced from peripheral veins and can also be used if caval stenosis has occurred. Uncuffed catheters are unsafe for home use because of their tendency to dislodgement and are not recommended for routine use in these circumstances.

Author's preference

A cuffed catheter of 2–3mm outside diameter is suitable for most uses and is unlikely to block.

ACCESS SITES

Any vein may be used. However, large catheters are most easily inserted into large veins. Internal and external jugular, axillary, long saphenous and femoral veins are the most easily accessible by cut down. The cephalic vein in the deltopectoral groove is variable in size and frequently absent and is not recommended for routine use.

The subclavian veins are most commonly used for percutaneous insertions. The internal jugular veins are also suitable, but much less frequently used under these circumstances.

ANAESTHESIA

Either local or general anaesthesia is necessary in all cases. A general anaesthetic usually means the use of an operating theatre or an intensive care unit. With local anaesthetic, the procedure can be performed at the bedside, although it is hard to see why this should be an advantage.

---

* Evermed, PO Box 296, Medina, Washington 98039, USA.

Author's preference

Intubated general anaesthesia in the operating theatre provides optimal conditions as regards lighting and sterility. In addition, the absence of patient anxiety, discomfort and movement allows for a precise and unhurried procedure. Difficulties with catheter positioning are not rare and if the patient is awake, the difficulties are compounded.

TECHNIQUES OF INSERTION

Under all circumstances a subcutaneous tunnel is constructed so that the entry site into the vein and exit site from the skin are several inches apart.

Open operation

If the jugular vein is being used, the entire neck and anterior chest are prepared and included in the operation field. A radiolucent roll beneath the shoulders and slight head down position may be helpful. The operation field is covered with an adherent plastic drape so that the catheter cannot come into contact with the skin. A 1–2cm incision is made over the middle of the sternomastoid muscle. It is essential to allow enough space below the incision for finger pressure to occlude the internal jugular vein should bleeding occur during the procedure. The platysma is divided and this is sufficient to expose the external jugular vein. The internal jugular is most easily approached through the belly of the sternomastoid muscle by splitting its fibres longitudinally. The internal jugular is mobilized by incising the carotid sheath over it and lifting the vein out. The posterior attachments are freed using a combination of sharp and blunt dissection. The vagus nerve which is nearby is not usually encountered.

About 1·5cm of vein is mobilized and slings are passed around the vein proximally and distally. The catheter is then filled with 0·9 per cent saline and the cap is fitted to the hub. An exit site on the chest wall is chosen, usually above and lateral to the nipple. Through a short incision here, a subcutaneous tunnel is developed up to the cervical incision. The lower part of the tunnel must be wide enough to accommodate the cuff on the catheter. Using an artery forceps, a strong thread is drawn down through the tunnel and tied to the distal end of the catheter. The catheter is then drawn up to the neck incision and the cuff positioned in the lower half of the tunnel. The catheter is laid down over the chest wall and transected with a bevel just above the level of the nipple. This ensures that the tip will be in the middle of the right atrium. Using sharp, fine pointed scissors, a small venotomy is made between the slings. The catheter is inserted fully into the vein and care taken that the bend on the catheter is not too acute. The venotomy is tightened around the catheter if necessary by using a 6/0 prolene suture. Purse string sutures should not be used as they may transect the catheter during removal.

A chest X-ray is taken to ensure that the tip is in the correct position. Screening allows for precise positioning and is particularly useful when the external jugular vein is used. The wound should not be closed until the X-ray has been seen.

Wound closure is obtained using a 5/0 or 6/0 absorbable suture to platysma with a subcuticular suture to the skin. No dressing is required.

The same procedure is used for groin or axillary vein insertions. In the former, the catheter exits above the knee and in the latter on the arm or chest wall.

Percutaneous insertion

The patient is positioned in a similar manner, with a roll beneath the shoulders and slightly head down. The infraclavicular route is most commonly used and the operation field is prepared as for an open procedure.

The junction of the internal jugular and subclavian veins lies behind the sternoclavicular joint. The sharp anterior edge of the first rib can be felt beneath the medial one-third of the clavicle and the vein of course crosses the rib behind this part of the clavicle.

Many different kits are available for percutaneous central vein cannulation. All involve insertion of the catheter through a cannula. In the case of the cuffed catheters which have an attached hub, the insertion cannula peels into two halves. The initial step is needle puncture of the subclavian vein. Through a short incision below the mid-point of the clavicle, the needle is advanced medially at an angle of about 45° to the chest wall and in a slightly cranial direction. The needle can be felt to pass over the rib and into the vein lateral to the sternoclavicular joint.

Entry into the vein may be felt as a distinct click, but more usually is recognized by the aspiration of blood.

Depending on which device is used, a cannula may be advanced over the needle, or a guide wire through it. In the latter case, a dilator–cannula combination is advanced over the guide wire into the vein. In either case, a subcutaneous tunnel is fashioned to move the catheter exit site further away from the vein. The catheter is trimmed as for the open procedure and then inserted through the cannula. The position is checked on X-ray before completion of the procedure.

IMPLANTABLE DEVICES

General anaesthesia is virtually always required for this procedure. Either insertion technique may be used for the catheter. A further incision is then necessary, below the costal margin. Through this incision a pocket is developed for the injection chamber which will lie superficial to the ribs. Meticulous haemostasis is necessary before implanting the chamber. When the vein has been isolated (open) or cannulated percutaneously, then the chamber and catheter are joined together and flushed with heparinized saline. The catheter is then drawn up to the upper incision and the chamber is sutured in place. The catheter is trimmed as before and inserted. The wounds are closed as usual with an absorbable suture for fat and a subcuticular suture for skin. No dressings are required. An X-ray is taken prior to wound closure.

TECHNICAL PROBLEMS

Always check to see if any of the veins have previously been used and avoid these if possible. When performing open procedures, proximal and distal control of the vein should always be obtained prior to venotomy.

Significant venous malformations are unusual and are nearly always acquired. The main problems are related to venous occlusion or stenosis—the result of incorrect positioning of a previous catheter. If the catheter tip is positioned in the inferior or superior vena cava then an infusion of irritant solutions may thrombose the vein.

The only significant congenital venous malformation is a persistent left superior vena cava. This usually drains into the coronary sinus. The problem is recognized by the position of the catheter on X-ray. The catheter cannot be allowed to perfuse the coronary sinus and it should be removed. On the rare occasion where no alternative is available, then a very narrow bore catheter can be advanced into the right atrium through the coronary sinus, but this is a measure of last resort.

Occasionally the catheter will not advance or it persistently takes the wrong course. Twisting the catheter as it is advanced often solves this problem. X-ray screening with or without contrast may reveal the source of the trouble and gives valuable information when problems persist. If this facility is unavailable and several attempts are unsuccessful, then recourse is made to another site of insertion. It is unwise to persist for prolonged periods if other unused veins are available.

Although the veins are not usually ligated during open procedures, it is unusual to be able to use the same vein twice. For this reason, other veins are explored if a second or third catheter becomes necessary.

The same problems with insertion and positioning occur with percutaneous catheterization. They are managed in a similar fashion. For subclavian catheterization, the head should be turned towards the operator to avoid misdirecting the catheter in the neck. The left subclavian vein is used preferentially as the course of the catheter is smoother than when it is inserted from the right side. Once again, persistent problems should encourage the operator to change veins and/or technique. Inadvertent arterial puncture is not usually a problem and does not need exploration. Arterial laceration—manifested by signs of blood loss and a rapidly enlarging haematoma—may rarely necessitate exploration. One advantage of percutaneous puncture is that the same vein may be repeatedly used.

Finally, open procedures are preferable if a bleeding disorder is present.

Author's preference

Open operation using the right internal jugular vein is the safest and swiftest method of central venous catheterization in the author's experience. The external jugular veins are often of adequate size but the catheter is frequently misdirected on entry into the subclavian. The veins in the groin are very readily accessible also but will not take the larger catheters.

CATHETER POSITION

The optimal position for the catheter tip is in the middle of the right atrium. The author has not seen a single case of caval thrombosis in catheters so positioned. One case of atrial thrombosis with pulmonary embolism was seen, however. Neither has the author encountered atrial perforation and cardiac tamponade, although this is a complication which is well described. Cardiac tamponade can, of course, occur if the catheter tip is left in the lower SVC due to high investment of the pericardium. The generally favourable experience with ventriculo-atrial CSF shunts confirms that atrial placement is safe. Complete freedom from risk is impossible.

FIXING THE CATHETER

The catheter is fixed at its exit site with one or two fine prolene sutures. An adhesive is used which will stick silastic to skin. We have used Dow Corning medical adhesive B* for many years and it works very well. A small gauze square is applied to the exit site and further adhesive applied. The dressing and catheter are then taped to the skin. This form of dressing abolishes all movement between catheter and skin and should be left untouched for at least 2 weeks. At this time, the cuffed catheters are fixed in position and only light dressings are needed subsequently. The same type of dressing is carefully re-applied every 2–3 weeks when uncuffed catheters are used.

Occlusive dressings are not needed and adherent plastic films are sometimes associated with excoriation of the skin.

CATHETER REMOVAL

Uncuffed catheters are easily removed—this is their main disadvantage. Cuffed catheters are removed in one of two ways. Steady traction on the catheter will detach the cuff, allowing the catheter to be removed. The cuff remains attached to the subcutaneous fat and is felt as a lump under the skin. This is rarely troublesome. If the cuff is within a centimetre or two of the exit site, it can be dissected free. If not, a further incision is necessary to remove the cuff.

Occasionally, these catheters remain in place for so long that a tight fibrous sheath forms around the intravascular part of the catheter. This may prevent catheter removal—a situation well known to those who insert CSF shunts. Under these circumstances, the catheter is tied off close to the vein and left in place.

CATHETER USAGE

Strict asepsis is the rule when using the catheter. This entails, at the very least, the use of sterile gloves and dressing packs. The junction between the giving set or syringe and the catheter is liberally swabbed with antiseptic before and after the circuit is broken. Sterile caps for the catheters are available when they are not in use and the catheter can be filled with a heparinized saline lock. A concentration of 1 unit of heparin to 1ml 0·9 per cent saline works well in practice.

* Dow Corning Europe Medical Products, Brussels, Belgium, pa.

The child's parents can also be taught to use the catheter. Catheter sepsis rates for home use are certainly no higher and often lower than rates for hospital use. There may be other reasons for this than the obvious care that parents will take with their children.

The catheter should not restrict activities unduly. Swimming is allowed in the sea and well maintained swimming baths. Most sports should be possible, although heavy contact sports should probably be avoided.

CATHETER BREAKS AND BLOCKAGES

Catheter breaks are relatively easily managed. All manufacturers supply repair kits for their catheters and sepsis is not a frequent complication of catheter repair. The life of a catheter may be considerably lengthened by the use of a repair kit.

Blockage is uncommon with the larger bore catheters. It is a problem, however, with those less than 2mm outside diameter. Prolonged intravenous feeding is the main offender and results in the build-up of a chalky deposit in the lumen. Blockage by blood clot also occurs and may be cleared by the use of heparin or streptokinase. Either way, as the catheter gradually silts up, it becomes less suitable for blood withdrawal but may be used for quite a time for infusion.

SUMMARY

Early recourse to a central venous catheter is justified in these children. Complications related to insertion at open operation are extremely rare. The great majority of children undergoing chemotherapy need only one catheter during the course of their illness and it is unusual to remove the catheter for infection or blockage within 4 months.

At the present time, cuffed catheters are vastly superior in performance to all other designs. There is a limited role for multilumen catheters or totally implantable devices.

FURTHER READING

Broviac J. W., Cole J. J. and Scribner B. H. (1973) A silicone rubber atrial catheter for prolonged parenteral alimentation. *Surg. Gynecol. Obstet.* **136**, 602–6.

Editorial (1985) Indwelling venous catheters. *Lancet* i, 499.

Fonkalsrud E. W., Ament M. E., Berquist W. E. et al. (1982) Occlusion of the vena cava in infants receiving central venous hyperalimentation. *Surg. Gynecol. Obstet.* **154**, 189–92.

Groff D. B. and Ahmed N. (1974) Subclavian vein catheterization in the infant. *J. Pediatr. Surg.* **9**, 171–4.

Hickman R. O., Buckner C. D., Clift R. A. et al. (1979) A modified right atrial catheter for access to the venous system in marrow transplant patients. *Surg. Gynecol. Obstet.* **148**, 871–5.

Pessa M. E., Howard R. J. (1985) Complications of Hickman-Brovia catheters. *Surg. Gynecol. Obstet.* **161**, 257–60.

Reed W. P., Newman K. A., Tenney J. H. et al. (1985) Autopsy findings after prolonged catheterization of the right atrium for chemotherapy in acute leukaemia. *Surg. Gynecol. Obstet.* **160**, 417–20.

11. Play Therapy

J. Kuykendall

In the past, children's play was considered by some a 'superfluous activity', an activity only important as it allowed the child a release of excess energy. Other theorists' research reflected this and recognized that play offered and effected much more. Their work stated that play was essential as a problem-solving approach into adulthood, that play was fun, exploratory and relieved boredom; that play maintained and promoted normal development, that there was no difference between play and the work of the child. Play was the *best* use of the child's time.

Many organizations (nursery school, day nursery and hospital play schemes) have already embraced this important message with more and more hospitals responding to it. Play has been elevated from its 'excess energy' status to become a vital learning method in the social, intellectual and emotional development of the sick as well as the healthy child.

The sick child, however, is certainly at a disadvantage for maintaining play.[1] It has been documented that immobilization[2] in bed, traction, plaster casts, transfusions, eye patches and catheters may greatly diminish the child's mobility and desire to involve himself in play. This, in turn, can threaten a child's sense of worth and self-confidence, diminishing further his ability to seek out the natural need to play.

A sterile environment, an environment with inappropriate materials and, sadly, staff too, can discourage children from play. Even in optimal surroundings, children may be so overwhelmed by separation from parents, by the hospital size and structure, by its unfamiliar sounds and unpleasant odours as well as by those nasty medicosurgical procedures, that they have withdrawn from this very threatening environment. Other children with chronic illness, multiple re-admission and handicap are already at high emotional and social risk.[3,4] Overwhelmed children and very unhappy ones cannot play.

The Expert Group on Play recognized that, unlike well children, sick children required a special person trained in child development and play, a person who would not lead the play but act as a catalyst for it.[3] This hospital play worker, an integral member of the paediatric team, implements all types of play so as to address the child's total needs.[1] This includes looking specifically at the appropriate play materials to foster the emotional welfare of the child so that emotional problems do not outweigh the health care benefits.[5] The play specialist looks at how the hospital, along with its procedures, threatens emotional and overall development. The challenge is to create a play system that, at the least, makes hospital stress manageable and then allows the child to assimilate the new reality into his life. Play in hospital constitutes a scheme for the child to experiment with the external threatening hospital world and himself. Through this play, he can gain a sense of mastery while being prepared for the events of hospitalization.

The Platt report notes that children should be prepared for procedures[3] with many studies suggesting that preparation results in less anxious mothers,[6] with children whose recovery and discharge is less complicated and traumatic.[7,8] Yet preparation is a complex issue—how does one prepare? And with what materials? And for what procedure(s) and to what extent? How does one find out what the child perceives as the problem? How does the preparation gear itself to children of different ages, with different experiences, with different medical, surgical, social and cultural presentations? Klinging and Klinging state that the child does not even perceive 'routine' medicosurgical procedures as routine.[9] How difficult it is to establish what is going to be threatening to *any* individual child.

Research has shown significant stress reduction in play preparation programmes that combine giving information, demonstrating it and having the child play with the equipment,[10] for the medicosurgical procedure that he is to undergo.[11] This cognitive/psychological approach helps the child acknowledge and play through fantasies, false perceptions and misconceptions as well as reality problems surrounding the impending event. This approach should begin with the pre-admission visit to hospital. Melamed et al.[12] reported lower self-reported anxiety and lower observed behavioural anxiety in children prepared for hospital one week in advance.

The one-hour programme devised by the author and colleagues invited patient, siblings and parents 1–2 weeks prior to admission. It consisted of a 20-min slide presentation with tape entitled 'Charlie comes to hospital' (Charlie is a doll). This overview was intended to show many places, people and the admitting process that the younger child would encounter in hospital. Older children were shown the programme with the tape 'David comes to hospital' narrated by a

9-year-old multiple re-admission patient. The scenes depicted the hospital admitting process but, additionally, how David felt about his various experiences.[13] The slide shows were followed by a question and answer period led by one of the ward sisters; afterwards, Sister took the participants on a controlled ward visit where they found that each child had his own bed with overhead light, locker and corkboard to display his 'get well' cards (a psychologically important point to reinforce). The third part was playing with real hospital equipment. Children were divided into small groups so that the hospital play specialists could demonstrate and then record the child's reactions to both the demonstration and the use of materials presented (family of dressed dolls, admission bracelet, medicine cup, BP cuff and sphygomomanometer, auroscope, patellar hammer, tongue depressors, stethoscope, thermometer, gowns, etc.). Finally, each participant, over biscuits and drinks, received his own certificate of attendance. Observation suggested that families who attended settled in more rapidly and were more relaxed and more co-operative throughout their stay. This supports the idea that a positive initial interaction with an unfamiliar situation is enhanced when the situation becomes familiar.

Once in hospital, the patient's anxiety may involve intrusive procedures (injections, blood tests, lumbar punctures, catheterization) as well as all the 'routine' ones.

Martin, a 6-year-old with ALL, would scream whenever the doctor appeared wearing a red stethoscope around his neck. Following the doctor's departure, staff observed how solemnly Martin placed the red stethoscope on Action Man's chest and told him 'that he wouldn't have any blood left soon'.

How difficult it is to establish what is threatening to any individual child. While our observations have shown that most children, especially the chronically or terminally ill, demonstrate a high amount of play involving injections and blood tests, there are other issues equally important to be played through.

Lucy, a 4-year-old with a medulloblastoma, already in hospital 1 month, walked up to the Wendy house and slammed the door saying, 'Lucy doesn't live here anymore'. The hospital play specialist went into the Wendy house and asked Lucy to knock again. This time she was told how much she was missed at home and how quickly everyone wanted her to get better and return home. Afterwards, Lucy appeared happier and joined in the group cooking activity.

There are so many ways that allow a child to express worrying and negative feelings in an acceptable, safe and indirect manner.

Gregory, a 6-year-old sibling, released considerable aggression through the use of his animal puppet. The puppet yelled at a doll 'who didn't care about him anymore and who spent all her time with

Michael' (his 17-year-old brother dying from chronic myelogeneous leukaemia). Through several therapeutic play puppet sessions, he became able to realize some of his negative feelings directed at Michael and his mother.

Such play not only gives vital clues to what a child is experiencing but enables the caregiver to intervene adaptively and support the family unit.

Gregory, who had always received his mother's preferential attention, was forced into a different role that he was frightened by and deeply resented. After Michael's death, his mother informed us that Gregory was unusually aggressive towards his playmates at school and was doing poorly in both attendance and in schoolwork. It was decided that the hospital play specialist, together with the psychologist, would intervene. Gregory presented as a withdrawn and depressed 6-year-old. Through several sessions with puppet and messy play, he voiced that 'if Michael went away, then Mummy could take care of the other children' and 'Gregory killed Michael. Bad, naughty Gregory'. Through the play, he was able to acknowledge and, with support, let go of the thoughts and negative feelings associated with his brother's death.

As he had not wanted to attend the funeral, it was queried whether he would somehow like to say goodbye to Michael. Gregory created with the vicar a short memorial service and invited his mother, older sister, who had already left home, and the family cat. This was a positive step for him. In a final session with him, Gregory was able to talk openly about Michael and he asked what it felt like to be dead. He also wondered if Michael would come back to visit. These queries dramatically illustrated his normal way of thinking about death as a reversible temporary condition. Simple, truthful and maturationally appropriate answers given at that time will allow Gregory to continue his discussions when his need to understand death expands. Clearly, therapeutic play acted as a catalyst for this sibling prior to and during the intervention period.

It is essential to note the entire family as the 'patient', as the needs of all within the family unit are compromised. This is especially true in the case of the siblings. The siblings are often not presented with play opportunities to address their feelings and knowledge regarding the hospitalized child even if that child is chronically or terminally ill. It is reported in work by Spinetta and Spinetta[14] that siblings fared worse in overall emotional adjustment and worse than both parents and patient during times of crisis. Our visitors' playroom, staffed by two full-time hospital play specialists, provided opportunities for these siblings to discuss the many misconceptions as well as feelings of guilt, resentment and anger towards the specially-treated child patient. Their drawings, Wendy house, play and conversations are carefully reported to the ward staff for appropriate support interventions.

Sometimes drawing and painting provide the child with a medium for expression. Sean, an 8-year-old with osteogenic sarcoma who had already had his right leg amputated and developed metastases to his lungs, produced a picture of an empty house surrounded by a fence without a gate. This picture also had a huge black cloud suspended above the entire house. It reflected his feelings of depression, impotency and isolation at not being able to get away from this ever-present and invasive cancer. Drawings can inform us of the child's overall feelings concerning the external threats as well as how he perceives himself in relation to them.[15,16] Staff drawings can complement a child's presentation to keep the 'dialogue' flowing. Staff must be very sensitive in eliciting a child's response to his drawing as the content may be too threatening to verbalize.

Play preparation is another approach for the family-patient. The child together with Mum/Dad is admitted directly into the play-room. This allows the play worker the opportunity to introduce herself and present materials to help the family to settle in. It enables her to observe the initial anxieties and begin the trust relationship with this family. Knowledgeable of the child's vocabulary and aware of the day's observations, the caregiver presents the play prep. box. The surgical play prep. box contains only the materials that the child will see, hear and feel and includes the 'Do Not Feed Me' sign and badge, gowns, medi-wipes, syringes, plasters, surgical tape, medicine cup, theatre slippers-hats-masks-gown-overalls-anaesthetic masks, pictures of the porter, anaesthetists, recovery room and how the doctors and nurses dress within the operating and recovery rooms; also, relevant books made for each specific operation are included. Play prep. is always done with the parent present and usually in a group setting. Through a series of alternating, threatening and non-threatening statements, a linear story unfolds as to why children come into hospital.

Explanations are always brief, simple and honest . . . older children tend to tell us directly why they think they have come in. This gives us the first opportunity to rectify the many false perceptions and fantasies they have as well as reassure all the children that only that specific part of their body will be mended.

The play prep. concepts include:

1. Making sure that the child eats enough before going to sleep when the 'Do Not Feed Me Badge' is attached to the child and the 'Nil by Mouth' sign hung above the bed.
2. The wearing of the hospital gown with the child's choice of favourite colour recorded. (It is extremely important to give as

much realistic choice in such a non-negotiable place as a hospital.)

3. Receiving the pre-med. in the medicine cup and/or syringe. Plenty of time is allowed for the child to hear that injections hurt, to acknowledge the fact and to create some coping strategy. For Sean, an 8-year-old with osteogenic sarcoma, it was taking 3 deep breaths before he allowed the staff to take blood or give an injection. Other children give realistic commands to staff, e.g. 'Be quick', while others decide to hold their mother's hand and look away. Children are always praised to the degree that they have been able to assist in the procedure.

4. Explanations that this pre-med. dries the mouth and that, although it might feel odd, it is exactly what the doctor needs before he can mend the child.

5. Also, the fact that some children feel drowsy, others may want to go to sleep, while still others may stay wide awake. These are all normal for any individual child but that no-one has to worry as all children will receive their special sleep in the operating room before the doctors remove or repair the designated area only. Even with this additional reassurance, some children fear the loss of any part of their body saying that they need all their parts to live.[17] Throughout the play preparation, children are encouraged to handle all the materials as the story unfolds.

6. Children being asked what they imagine the doctors and nurses wear in the operating room/recovery room. As they shout out their answers the play specialist puts on the corresponding article. This dress-up presentation relieves them as they now know that Martians or ET are not employed within the health service.

7. Being told that a porter will take them with their favourite nurse to the operating room and that Mum/Dad will be with them as soon as they return (if that is the case). Since masks are very threatening to a child, we ask the parents to demonstrate how to breathe through them. This role modelling then enables many of the children to ask for their turn. It is explained that the special sleep comes from the medicine in the mask (or through the butterfly needle which feels like a cat scratching the back of their hand). This sleep is special because the child always wakes up from it *only* when the doctor has finished the procedure. After sleeping a while in the recovery room the doctor and nurses will say that it is all right to return to the children's ward.

Children are told that they may sleep for a while and that the area that was mended may hurt but that the doctor has already written out medicines to help that hurt go away. Each day they will feel better and some children may even want to go into the playroom the next day.

It is explained that since the medicine that gave them the special sleep is still in their tummy nurses will give them water first and later on they can have their favourite drink. Again this is recorded so that the child feels that he is actively included within his stay in hospital. Later on he will be able to eat some food.

This basic format is modified according to need. Some children may require 2 or more sessions, especially if they will wake up in a place (ITU, CCU) other than their own bed. Postoperative play prep. for emergency procedures affords children the same opportunity to acknowledge and deal with misconceptions while gaining some mastery over events that happened too quickly to prepare for.

Highly specialized preparation for CAT scan, masks, radiotherapy department, Hickman catheters, can be achieved using hospital books for individual procedures, models or visits. No matter what method is used, play not only gives some normality to the child but remains a fundamental language of the child whether in hospital or in the community.

Let's not be afraid to *play*.

REFERENCES

1. Noble E. (1967) *Play and the Sick Child*. London, Faber and Faber, p. 92–3.
2. Blom G. E. (1958) The reactions of hospitalized children to illness. *Paediatrics* **22**, 590.
3. DHSS (1959) *The Welfare of Children in Hospital. Report of the Committee*. The Platt Report, HMSO.
4. Walker, Gortmaker and Weitman (in Pless IB, 1984) 'Clinical assessment' physical and psychological functioning: *Pediatr. Clin. North Am.* **31**, 33–45.
5. Droske S. C. and Francis S. A. (1981) *Paediatric Diagnostic Procedures, With Guidelines for Preparing Children for Clinical Tests*. Chichester, Wiley.
6. Skipper J. K. (1966) Mothers' distress over their children's hospitalization for tonsillectomy. *J. Marr. Fam.* **28**, 145.
7. Mellish R. (1969) Preparation of a child for hospitalization and surgery. *Paediatr. Clin. North Am.* **16**, 3.
8. Visintainer M. A. and Wolfer J. A. (1975) Psychological preparation for surgical paediatric patients: the effect on children's and patients' responses and adjustment. *Paediatrics* **56**, 187–202.
9. Klinging D. R. and Klinging D. G. (1977) *The Hospitalized Child. Communication Techniques for Health Personnel*. New Jersey, Prentice-Hall.
10. Plank E. (1971) *Working with Children in Hospital*. Cleveland, Case-Western Reserve University Press.
11. Ferguson B. F. (1979) Preparing young children for hospitalization: a comparison of two methods. *Paediatrics* **64**, 656–64.
12. Melamed B. C., Meyer R., Gee C. et al. (1976) The influence of time and type of presentation on children's adjustment to hospitalization. *J. Pediatr. Psychol.* **5**, 31.
13. Melamed B. C. and Siegal L. T. (1975) Reduction of anxiety in children facing

hospitalization and surgery by use of filmed modelling. *J. Consult. Clin. Psychol.* **43**, 511.

14. Spinetta J. and Deasy-Spinetta P. (1981) *Living with Childhood Cancer.* St. Louis, Mosby.
15. Dileo J. M. (1973) *Children's Drawings as Diagnostic Aids.* New York, Brunner/Mazel.
16. Swanwick M. (1985) Play as a coping mechanism. *Nursing,* 39, Baillière Tindall, 1154–6.
17. Gellert E. (1978) What do I have inside me? How children view their bodies. In: Gellert E. (ed.) *Psychosocial Aspects of Paediatric Care.* London, Grune & Stratton.

12. Oncology Social Work

D. Donnelly-Wood

INTRODUCTION

This chapter is essentially a practical one. Although total care of patient and family is shared by all the paediatric oncology team, major responsibility for the psychosocial side of that care is carried by the team's social worker(s), joined where available by specialist colleagues from community nursing or health visiting. By describing the social worker's involvement through the course of the child's disease, this chapter will demonstrate what is available to most families of children with cancer. It is important to remember, however, that what is described reflects the practice of one particular unit. Practice does vary in detail from centre to centre according to local conditions, resources and workloads. Nevertheless, the broad picture remains fairly constant. The intention is not to review the theory of, and research into, the psychosocial problems affecting the families of children with cancer. That is already well done elsewhere in this book and in many other publications. These reflect both the growth of the problems, paradoxically caused largely by the improvement in treatments and survival rates, and the growing awareness of the need to help prevent, minimize or solve them among the professionals in this field.[1,2,3] One of the responses has been the development of specialist paediatric oncology social workers.

PAEDIATRIC ONCOLOGY SOCIAL WORKER

The specialist social worker has become an important member of the paediatric oncology team with the introduction of the multi-disciplinary teamwork approach (*see* Appendix 4). The social worker brings specialist skills in establishing therapeutic relationships quickly and sensitively: in assessment; in counselling and communication; in groupwork; and in organization and liaison. His/her specialist knowledge includes that of social systems; of groups and family dynamics, particularly in stress situations; of interpersonal relationships and of statutory, voluntary and community resources. He/she also brings the freedom of being able to leave the hospital setting to visit patients and families at home; and brings the time to sit with patients and parents, for hours on end, if and when that is needed, and listen. Equally importantly, the social worker can be perceived by parents and children as someone who is not medical or nursing staff and, though a member of the unit team, is not part of all the 'medical' things that are happening.

The social work involvement with patient and family has 3 main aims—support in crisis, assessment, and the prevention of identified problems or the minimizing of their effects. Involvement is generally concentrated around certain specific times in the course of the child's disease,[4] though some families seek and need fairly continuous help while a few will accept only very limited support. The key times are: initial diagnosis, maintenance, relapse, cessation of active therapy, terminal phase, death, bereavement.

INITIAL DIAGNOSIS

Initial diagnosis is the most important of the key times. It is during the time of diagnosis and initial therapy that the relationship between unit and family is established and the foundation for future work is laid. The social worker becomes involved with all families automatically and should be introduced as an integral and valued member of the team. This is important since many of the families would not normally have contact with social workers and, indeed, some would see such contact as a social stigma. However, as Ross and Klar have described,[4] the involvement of the social worker with all families as a matter of course normalizes the relationship, removes the perceived stigma and makes acceptable the help and support offered.

Usually the social worker first sees parents as soon as possible after they have been given the diagnosis. They are usually in shock and frequently in grief since their first reaction to being told their child has cancer is often to expect imminent death. They are certainly in crisis and need support. They need to be able to express their feelings if they wish to, and they need to be able not to express them if that is what they want. The social worker must bring great sensitivity to discerning the difference and then to creating an atmosphere conducive to meeting their needs.

At this time, assessment of parents' management and coping ability will commence. Overt questioning may be inappropriate at the very beginning, though should not be shirked later, but even during the first interview various clues may reveal a lot. The relationship between mother and father, for instance, so important to coping ability as well as a possible problem area of its own, can be revealed through body language—how they sit together, whether they touch, whether they listen to each other or look at each other, what words they use to each other and to a third person.

Anger is a common reaction now and must be identified and expressed. It can be directed at a whole variety of targets, e.g. environment, another hospital, general practitioner, God. Sometimes parents are ashamed or frightened by the intensity of their anger and need to be reassured that such a feeling is normal and permissible. The social worker may have to encourage, or give them 'permission', to feel as they do. Similarly, the common feeling of personal guilt for their child's disease must be identified, expressed and established as normal, otherwise it, like other feelings, can fester, grow and cause major problems later.

COMMUNICATION

The policy of open communication in paediatric oncology units is now well established. Parents and patients are told the truth—for patients it is consistent with their level of understanding—and nothing is consciously hidden from them. The aim is that the whole relationship between unit, parents and patient is characterized by the trust that can only come from openness and honesty. Part of the social work task is constantly to monitor that this is taking place, liaise between parents and doctors, and feed back to medical and nursing staff what parents and patients know. This task starts with the first interview with parents. The social worker asks them what they have been told and so obtains from them their understanding of the situation. What a doctor believes he has told parents is not always what they think they have heard. Many parents only hear the diagnosis during their first talk with a doctor and do not remember subsequent information. Some simply do not understand all the things that have been said but, for one reason or another, are unable to ask for further explanation. Many parents are more likely to admit a lack of knowledge or understanding to the 'non-medical' social worker who can then feed back to doctors the need for further discussion on particular topics. Knowledge and understanding can be reinforced then by further discussion with the social worker who is usually the one with the time to sit and talk at length. Various publications can also help and many units use a variety of these (*see* Appendix 1).

This is an appropriate place to sound an important note of caution. It applies to the whole of our continuing relationship with families, but nowhere is it more important than in these early stages. It is very easy to make assumptions about how parents—or patients or other family members for that matter—should react or are reacting to the situation. We make judgements about them all the time, that is quite normal and natural. Those assumptions and judgements are usually reasonable and are often correct. However, without first being checked, they should not form the basis for our relationship with the people concerned, nor the basis for action. People can be labelled as 'difficult'; families can be known as 'problem families' because assumptions have been made which have not been checked. Unfortunately, such labels can have profound and far-reaching consequences for our treatment of such families, alienating them— for families can be very sensitive to and perceptive of how they are viewed by doctors, nurses, social workers and other members of the team—and isolating them from the help and support that they need. In fact, it is often the families in greatest need who suffer most. Frequently, it is the social worker who must do the 'checking out' of the team's assumptions. Are the parents indeed difficult or are they awkward at expressing their needs? Some can be aggressive, but maybe aggression is the only language they know in foreign and threatening situations. Maybe they find hospitals—familiar territory, almost 'home', to staff—intimidating. Perhaps their being 'difficult' is their way of holding on to their own identities in a strange and frightening situation where control of their lives has been taken from them and they have become almost totally dependent. What is 'difficult' anyway?

Parents, especially, who are nervous, frightened, insecure and feeling they are being criticized, will usually not be able to talk to doctors and nurses about their feelings. They fear their words may be interpreted as criticism of, and ingratitude to, the very people who are fighting so hard for their child. They may worry that their feelings, if expressed, will earn them an even lower place in the estimation they feel the staff have of them. In these cases the social worker becomes a 'safe' person to whom they can reveal themselves and is therefore the most appropriate person to check out the assumptions made. The social worker almost becomes the 'conscience' of the unit, interpreting the behaviour of the parents to other team members, while helping parents to behave more appropriately; and interpreting the attitude of some staff members while helping those colleagues change negative attitudes that come from unchecked assumptions.

SIBLINGS

Parents need advice on how to handle their other children. At this stage, all their attention and concern is focused on the sick child, but the needs of siblings are important and require attention. The illness of their brother or sister will inevitably have some effect, for good or bad, on siblings and parents need to realize this. Bad effects can be minimized and good effects encouraged. The siblings need to be included in what is happening as far as is possible. Parents are strongly encouraged to be open with them and explain to them truthfully and fully, consistent with the child's ability to understand, the nature of the problem. Children are very sensitive to their parents' behaviour and will know without being told that something is very seriously wrong. Their own imaginations will create, in the absence of explanation, a more frightening reality. Conversation they overhear both in the home and outside may merely feed their imagination, sometimes to intolerable levels. The same arguments apply to being open and truthful with the patient but with even more force. Honesty with the sick child is accepted practice now, but siblings still tend to be forgotten at times.

Brothers and sisters can frequently have their own, unrecognized and barely self-understood, feelings of jealousy and guilt. These often result in behavioural changes which are sometimes for good, but more often for bad. And to make it more complicated they are often reserved for specific people or situations. Being forewarned can make these changes less worrying (at a time when parents have enough to worry about) and easier to deal with. Parents should be advised to let their other children's schools know what is happening in case behaviour problems are manifested there. Extended family members and friends need to be warned that flooding the sick child with gifts while ignoring brothers and sisters can seriously exacerbate problems.

PRACTICALITIES

Practical problems must be tackled now. In the first few days after diagnosis normal family life is disrupted. The social worker will help parents think through arrangements for the care of siblings; organ-ization of home; how family—especially grandparents—and friends are going to be told; whether parents will share the task of staying with their sick child in hospital and, if so, how it will be organized. Parents are thrown into such turmoil by the diagnosis that they often need the calm, objective, third party presence of the social worker to help them consider the problems and then make their own decisions.

Finance can become a problem. Most families operate on a fairly tight budget and many need financial help with the strain imposed by this crisis. Bodkin, Pigott and Mann[5] discovered that for nearly half of a representative group of families who had children with cancer, the cost in lost income plus additional expenses during the first in-patient week of treatment exceeded 50 per cent of their total income. During a later week of outpatient treatment the loss of income plus additional expenditure amounted to more than 20 per cent of total income for more than half the sample families. In another study, Pentol[6] calculated that the total cost to individual families of having a child with leukaemia was over £1000 and that was after allowing for statutory and voluntary grants.

The areas of greatest financial expense during the early stages of the child's illness tend to be travel and subsistence. Most paediatric oncology centres are regionally organized so many families have a lot of travelling to do between home and hospital. Even those living relatively close find that the cost of travelling, often several times a day during inpatient treatment, between home and hospital can quickly add up. Similarly, the extra cost for parents staying in hospital with their child—for meals for parents and for the numerous odds and ends, edible and otherwise, needed to keep the child from boredom—quickly mount up while their normal household expenses continue. Parents, or at least one parent at a time, do not have to pay for the actual accommodation if they are staying with their child in hospital.[7] Families receiving statutory benefit can receive help from the Department of Health and Social Security (DHSS) (see Appendix 2). Application can be rather complicated for parents at a time when they are least able to sort it out—and when money is often the last thing on their minds anyway. The social worker often has a lot of liaison work to do with the appropriate DHSS office to ensure that the family are receiving their entitlement. Most offices are as helpful as the benefit rules allow them to be. Many will go to great lengths to ensure that a family knows about all they are entitled to and will take pains to sort matters out. However, there are exceptions and very occasionally, after all other avenues have been exhausted, a claim may have to go to an appeals tribunal. The social worker who is satisfied about the validity of the claim can act as advocate for parents at a tribunal, if the parents wish it.

VOLUNTARY HELP

Most parents will not be receiving statutory benefit and so will have no recourse to the DHSS for financial help. Thankfully, there are some voluntary organizations providing financial help for such parents (see Appendix 2). The social worker will either make direct application or will refer the family, having discussed it with them, to a particular organization's local representative.

EMPLOYMENT

Many parents take time off work to be with their child in hospital, or to care for siblings at home while the other parent remains in the hospital. Most employers are sympathetic and helpful, especially when kept informed. The social worker can contact employers, with the parent's permission, and seek their support.

Most of what has been described so far is covered both in interview with parents and during the first few days and weeks when the child is an inpatient. Parents' defences tend to be low during this time, and the coping mechanisms are not quite yet in place. It is an ideal time, not only for the social worker but for all members of the unit team, to establish and develop the close relationship with patient, parents and family which will form the basis for all the help the families will need. It is also a time for assessing future possible problem areas. The stress of having a child with cancer is long-term. Husbands and wives often respond differently and can gradually grow apart as a result. If they are unable to communicate or to understand what is happening to each other, or if their relationship is weak to start with, their marriage may be irrevocably damaged. Similarly, the dynamics within the family as a whole, extending to grandparents and aunts and uncles, come under great strain. The management, by parents, of patient and siblings will affect their future behaviour. Over-protectiveness and spoiling can damage personality and hinder return to normality. The social worker—indeed the whole team—can advise parents about all of these things, but they cannot force the parents to accept advice. They cannot, of themselves, change people. They cannot prevent all the problems. There are times when the most they can hope to do is to be around to pick up the pieces.

MAINTENANCE

This phase does not present a crisis for most families. The social work task, however, continues. The social worker maintains contact largely through seeing children and parents when they come to the outpatient clinic. Home visits maintain the relationship but they also help the continuing assessment of how families are coping. Preventive work continues and, of course, where problems persist closer contact is maintained.

SCHOOL

As soon as possible after completing induction, patients of school age are encouraged to resume normal education. Return to school is vital, both as a confirmation to the child that things are returning to normal, and because of the part that school itself plays in enabling a child to grow into a mature, well-adjusted adult. Obstacles to return come from the child, the parents and from the school itself.[8] All need reassurance[9] and it is often the social worker's job to provide this. Younger children need less encouragement and are usually anxious to get back to school. Older children worry more about their appearance, particularly loss of hair. With encouragement and co-operation of parents and school, most problems can be solved. Parents' main worry tends to be that of infection, allied with a natural desire to protect their child. Again, with patient reassurance and the co-operation of the school, the problems can be overcome. Schools themselves are often worried because of their lack of knowledge and understanding of the disease. The social worker will contact the school and reassure them, and will visit if necessary. Written material for schools containing basic information about childhood cancer and advice on handling the children is available and assists the liaison. The fundamental message is that the children should be treated as normally as possible and be expected to play a full part in the life of the school. A protective attitude is firmly discouraged! Seminars for teachers on children with cancer and their problems have proved successful. Local education authorities are able to provide home tutors for children with cancer. However, a home tutor, when provided, often for the best of motives, can cause delay to the child's ultimate return to normal school. For this reason the use of home tutors should be the exception rather than the rule.

GROUPS

Groups, mainly for parents, are being used increasingly in paediatric oncology social work.[10] Some groups are self-help, self-run by their members (see Appendix 3).

Other groups are run by individual units, usually by the social worker, and are more narrowly structured. There may be groups for the parents of newly-diagnosed children—they tend to meet for a set number of sessions only. Other groups may be open to all parents, who join and leave as they wish. Parents normally tend to talk to one another and share their feelings and problems. However, a group offers a more focused environment for doing this, and it offers the presence of some staff to respond to comments the parents make. There are groups for bereaved parents, some running for a specific number of meetings whilst others are open-ended with a changing membership. Most major paediatric oncology centres now organize one or more of these groups.

RELAPSE

When a child relapses, parents face conflicting emotions. Many have been living on edge since their child's illness was first diagnosed, just waiting for the worst. When it comes, they often feel a sense of relief that it has finally happened. At the same time, the hopes they have been building up despite themselves are brought crashing down. The fears and worries of initial diagnosis return with a new intensity. This time around, parents know what to expect from treatment and if their child had a rough time during first induction, they will fear and expect a repeat.

The social worker's involvement will intensify and much of the initial pattern will be repeated. Work will once again be largely on a one-to-one, personal counselling basis. The same communication checks are important now. An advantage, however, is that the relationship between unit and parents and patient is better. People should know each other better and with greater knowledge can come better understanding and deeper trust. One particular assumption that must be guarded against now, however, comes from that closer relationship. It is an assumption that since this is the second time around for parents, and since they know and trust the team so well, there is less need to explain things or to give them information. In fact, the parents are just as confused this time and need just as much, if not more, careful explanation and discussion of what is happening.

Even though there is some limited hope for most patients when they relapse, many parents will soon start thinking seriously about the probability of their child's death. They may feel guilty for having such thoughts and will need reassurance that they are normal.

CESSATION OF ACTIVE THERAPY

Eventually some children reach a stage when, because of progression of their disease, active therapy is no longer serving any useful purpose. A decision must be made to cease such therapy and concentrate on ensuring that whatever time is left to a child is as active, as comfortable and as 'normal' as possible. The decision cannot be made by doctors alone, parents must be included. However, they can and should be counselled, advised and supported during this agonizing process. This is when the quality of the relationship between unit team and parents really begins to bear fruit, for if the relationship is good then unit and parents will work together to make the best decision for the child. Very occasionally, conflict may occur. In seeking to resolve it, the social worker, and all the team, should remember that the parents are the ones who have to live with the decision after their child has died. It is essential for the bereavement process that they can feel they have done their best for their child.

TERMINAL PHASE

It has been said that terminal care begins when a child first comes to the oncology unit and insofar as the work of developing relationships of trust and anticipating problems is concerned, this is true. The possibility that a child might die is there right from the start and how parents may respond to that situation forms part of the continuing assessment. However, when the terminal phase eventually comes, the social work involvement, along with that of most of the team, again intensifies.

Having made the painful decision to cease active treatment, parents have more painful decisions to make. Do they care for their child at home or not? What do they say to their child about what is happening—children will spot any changes in treatment and will want to know why? No-one can make these decisions for them, but they must have help, advice and support in making them. Offering that support and advice calls for great sensitivity to parental feelings. Caring for their dying child is the one last thing that parents can do in the face of a disease that has taken control from them and against which they feel powerless. Most children who die do so at home nowadays and this is as it should be. Sometimes, however, it is not possible for the child to be at home. Parents are not always able to cope at home. Sometimes they feel more secure within the unit, among medical and nursing staff they have come to know and trust. There is an expectation that parents should be able to care for their dying child at home and not living up to that can result in a strong feeling of failure for parents. It needs to be explained to those who do choose hospital that they have done the best for their child. Occasionally, parents may say one thing but reveal through their actions something else. They speak of their desire to nurse their child at home but express through frequent returns to the unit an inability to cope. Very sensitive probing is needed and, if necessary, a willingness by the unit to take responsibility from them by having a 'medical' reason for the child's staying in hospital.

For the majority who die at home, contact with the unit should not, if at all possible, cease. Distance permitting, there can be frequent home visits, usually by the social worker but also by other team members. Liaison with community resources, ideally already well established, is essential now. A good family doctor and district nurse or Macmillan nurse are particularly important at this stage. Material resources are important too.

What to say to their child is a frightening problem for parents. Many fear the question: 'Am I going to die?' and do not know how to handle it. They are often reluctant to volunteer these fears and so the social worker often has to take the initiative in raising the subject and then help parents decide upon their approach. In fact, it is very rare that children will ask such a direct question and if they do, the question can have a variety of meanings. It is more likely to be an expression of their feeling ill rather than a desire to discuss fundamental matters of life and death. It is important that parents know this and are aware of how to find out what is really being asked. It is often helpful to rehearse various responses. Young children, of course, have a different concept of death and their needs will be on the level of their understanding. Their greatest fear may be of separation, of being alone or of pain and these can be relatively easily dealt with if and when necessary.

Older children and adolescents may ask direct questions, but they are also likely to be sensitive to their parents' fears and protective towards them. If they want to talk to anyone about what is happening they are more likely to pick someone else, often a member of the oncology team with whom they have a good relationship. However, they will pick the time and place for such a discussion. It certainly should not be forced upon them. Openings and opportunities can be created, but only if they feel the need to talk about dying will they talk about it—and not everyone has that need. Most children, even some of the younger ones, know much more about what is happening to them than is often appreciated.

Parents often worry about the practical aspects of death at this time—How will it actually happen? What will occur? How do they get a death certificate? How do they register the death? How do they go about organizing a funeral? How much will it cost and can they afford it? They are frequently reluctant to ask these questions—they seem disloyal to the child who has not yet died, as if they could not wait for the death. By gentle probing, the social worker can discover if these things are on their minds and, if so, can deal with them. The cost of funerals is a major burden. The 'death grant' is insufficient, while only parents receiving supplementary benefit will receive more substantial help from the DHSS. That help can be quite substantial, however, but parents will need guidance before the event on how to claim (*see* Appendix 2).

DEATH AND BEREAVEMENT

When a child dies, members of the unit team are affected. Usually there is a close relationship with at least a few of the staff and they grieve too. When families have had a long, close involvement with an oncology unit they suffer a double bereavement when their child dies. They lose their child and they lose the support and involvement with the unit team and with most of the other parents they have come to know. It is important that they can maintain contact with the unit if they want to. They should be encouraged to return, when they feel ready, to talk to doctors, ask questions or just simply visit. The social worker maintains contact by 'phone and letter as well as home visits. He/she provides bereavement support and counselling, as far as possible, and maintains contact as long as is necessary. It is important to remember significant times like birthday and anniversary, particularly the first following the child's death.

Some parents will need further support and counselling and a group for bereaved parents may be appropriate, whether hospital-based or run by a local voluntary organization. More specialized help may be called for—grief counselling or psychiatric help. However, many parents will just want to keep contact, for a while at least, with those who shared with them their child's final illness and death.

CONCLUSION

This chapter has described some of the work of the paediatric oncology social worker. Following the course of a child's illness and concentrating on the key times during that illness, it has demonstrated some of the psychosocial support available to families of children with cancer. Any way of describing such support involves making artificial distinctions between various elements of that support, just as concentrating on the work of the paediatric oncology social worker creates an artificial distinction between the contribution of the various disciplines represented in the oncology team. At its best, of course, the psychosocial support is a seamless part of the total care given to patient and family, and is the responsibility of the whole team.

Appendix 1
Some Useful Publications

Guidance for Parents
Yorkshire Regional Cancer
  Organization,
Secretariat,
Cookridge Hospital,
Leeds 16,
UK
(50p per copy)

Many units now produce their own written material for parents. This short booklet is a good example of something that parents can find very useful during the first few days. It should not replace personal counselling but can supplement it.

Jenny Has Leukaemia
Anne Nicholson and
  Janice Thompson
Paediatric Oncology Unit,
Royal Victoria Infirmary,
Queen Victoria Road,
Newcastle-upon-Tyne,
UK
(Sponsored by the Malcolm
  Sargent Cancer Fund for
  Children. A donation of £1.00
  per copy to the Fund is
  appreciated.)

This well produced and colour-fully illustrated book is aimed at primary school children. However, older children and even parents have found it useful in gaining an initial and basic understanding of leukaemia.

Leukaemia
Allyson Hague
Lederle Laboratories Ltd,
Gosport Road,
Fareham,
Hants,
UK

Similarly aimed at young children, this book uses the 'Mister Men' characters to explain leukaemia and some of the things that happen to children while they are in hospital. The excellent illustrations deliberately lend themselves to being coloured in by children.

When Your Sister or Brother
  Has Leukaemia
John Silkstone and
  Allyson Hague
Lederle Laboratories Ltd,
Gosport Road,
Fareham,
Hants,
UK

This book is similar in style to
the previous one but is for the
young sisters and brothers of the
leukaemia patient. It also has
a very brief but effective
introduction for parents.

Leukaemia in Children
Guide to Treatment and Care
Coping with Childhood
  Leukaemia in the Family
Hodgkin's Disease
Non-Hodgkin's Lymphomas
Multiple Myeloma
Aplastic Anaemia
Chronic Granulocytic Leukaemia
Bone Marrow Transplantation
Leukaemia Research Fund,
43 Great Ormond Street,
London WC1N 3JJ,
UK

These booklets, part of the
range produced by the
Leukaemia Research Fund, are
written for adult readers.
Some parents find them useful.

Neuroblastoma—A Booklet for
  Parents
Jean Simons
The Neuroblastoma Society,
Woodlands,
Ordsall Park Road,
Retford,
Nottinghamshire,
UK

This comprehensive booklet
covers medical details,
psychosocial aspects, practical
problems and sources of help.

In addition, the United Kingdom Children's Cancer Study Group have
produced a booklet for parents.

The Leukaemia Care Society (*see* Appendix 2) publishes a substantial
newsletter (more of a magazine, really) for members three times a
year.
    There are also a number of American booklets of various styles
used by individual units, as follows:

*You and Leukaemia—A Day
   at a Time*
Lynn Baker
W. B. Saunders Co.,
Philadelphia/London, 1978.

This is an excellent, well illustrated (with drawings) and detailed book. It was written for older children but has proved most valuable for parents.

*Children with Cancer—
   a Handbook for Families and
   Helpers*
Merren Parker and David
   Mauger
Cassell Ltd,
London, 1979.

This book is addressed mainly to parents and families of patients. It is well written, easy to read, and sensitive in approach. It is particularly good on the emotional responses of parents.

Living with Childhood Cancer
John Spinetta and Patricia
   Deasy-Spinetta (eds.)
C. V. Mosby Co.,
New York, 1981.

Probably of more help to professionals, this comprehensive book covers all aspects of childhood cancer.

*Coping with Childhood Cancer:
   Where Do We Go From Here?*
David Adams and
   Eleanor Deveau
Reston Publishing Co. Inc.
(Prentice-Hall of Canada),
Toronto, 1984.

Similar to, but more recent than, the Spinetta book, this is also a very comprehensive volume. Both books will be of interest to people concerned with the psychosocial side of childhood cancer.

*The Private Worlds of Dying
   Children*
Myra Bluebond-Langner
Princeton University Press,
Princeton, 1978.

The author, an anthropologist, looks at a paediatric oncology centre and how seriously ill children come to know the implications of their illness when no-one tells them, and how they conceal this knowledge from their parents and the medical staff. Valuable book for anyone working directly with such children.

Appendix 2

Financial Help

TRAVELLING EXPENSES

Families receiving supplementary benefit (SB) or family income supplement (FIS) from the Department of Health and Social Security (DHSS) are eligible for help with travelling expenses to and from hospital. When the patient is admitted or discharged or is attending an outpatient clinic, but is not travelling by ambulance, the full travelling expenses will be paid for the patient and escort usually at actual or equivalent public transport rates.

Those who receive benefit through an order book should be able to claim immediately from the hospital administration by producing the order book and proof of admission, discharge or attendance at clinic. The hospital is subsequently refunded by the DHSS. People paid by giro cheque must claim direct from the DHSS on form H11 'Fares to Hospital'. Copies of the form should be available from the hospital social work department or from administration. Section 2 of the form must be filled in and signed by someone from the hospital. Those attending regular outpatient clinics over a longer period of time (most children with malignant disease fall into this category) can ask their local DHSS to authorize the hospital to make direct payments of expenses rather than submit an H11 for every visit. Parents receiving SB or FIS can also seek help with travel expenses for visiting their child in hospital. However, in this case the DHSS will pay only a proportion of the cost. Application for these expenses must be made separately, preferably by letter (keep a copy), or personal visit to the DHSS office, giving number of visits, travel arrangements and actual cost of travel. It should be accompanied by confirmation from the ward sister that the child is an inpatient.

ATTENDANCE ALLOWANCE

Unfortunately, attendance allowance is a rather fraught area which can cause an amount of bitterness and ill-feeling between sets of parents. The cause of the bitterness seems to be an inconsistency in the awarding of this valuable, non-means-tested allowance. It could well be argued that all parents of children being treated for cancer should receive this allowance, but a reading of the present criteria as set out in DHSS leaflet N1 205 would seem to rule out all but a tiny minority of our patients. Most parents who apply are refused but some, in similar or even identical circumstances, are awarded the allowance. Parents who have been refused feel a deep and understandable sense of injustice, while new parents' expectations are raised, usually to be dashed leaving them, too, with bad feelings. Advice to parents should be, 'You have nothing to lose by applying, but do not build up hopes of succeeding', followed by a full explanation and accompanied by form N1 205 which explains the criteria and includes an application form.

FUNERAL EXPENSES

The death grant is a fixed rate grant available to all on the basis of National Insurance contributions (DHSS leaflet NI 49). The level has not been updated since 1967 and remains at £9.00 for a child under 3 years; £15.00, 3–5 years; £22.50, 6–17 years; £30.00, 18 years and over. Since funerals for even the youngest children can cost an average of £250.00 to £300.00 nowadays, the death grant is not of significant help.

Parents receiving SB can obtain much more substantial help in the form of a single lump sum payment. This will cover such essential funeral expenses as:

1. The cost of any documents needed before a funeral or cremation can take place (e.g. extra death certificate, or additional certificates required for cremation purposes).
2. The cost of a plain coffin.
3. The cost of transport for the coffin and bearers plus one additional car.
4. The reasonable cost of flowers from the person responsible for making the funeral arrangements.
5. Undertaker's fees and gratuities, chaplain's, organist's and cemetery or crematorium fees for a simple funeral or cremation.
6. Expenses, up to a maximum of £75.00, arising from a requirement of the child's religious faith.
7. The cost of transporting the body to the child's home if death occurred elsewhere. If the child died abroad, only the cost of transporting the body within the UK can be met. The child must have normally lived in the UK prior to death and the funeral must take place in the UK if payment for expenses is to be made.

The claim should be made as soon as possible after the child's death, and then followed up with a copy of the undertaker's detailed account as soon as this is available. It is *not* necessary to obtain estimates. The DHSS will not normally contact the undertaker. On the rare occasion when they need to they will obtain the consent of the person making the claim. Families applying to the DHSS for this grant should not make any payment to the undertaker before the claim is made and help received. It is advisable to tell the undertaker on the first meeting that a claim to the DHSS is being made. The DHSS leaflet D49 'What To Do After a Death' is most useful.

Many of the benefit rules which determine what help the DHSS is able to give are being changed and further changes are proposed. Up-to-date advice is available from 'Freefone DHSS', a helpline on 0800 666555. The Child Poverty Action Group publishes annually two guides to benefits; *Rights Guide to Non-Means-Tested Social Security Benefits* and *National Welfare Benefits Handbook*. These are invaluable.

VOLUNTARY HELP

Financial help is available from a number of voluntary sources.

Malcolm Sargent Cancer Fund for Children

14 Abingdon Road,
London W8 6AF,
UK
Tel: 01-937 4548

The Malcolm Sargent Fund will give direct financial assistance to the families of children with any form of cancer.

Grants are usually given towards such things as travelling expenses to and from hospital; fuel bills; winter clothing and bedding for the child; convalescent holidays; telephone installation costs (though the fund will *not normally* help with subsequent regular telephone bills). However, the Trustees will also consider requests for a wide variety of 'one-off' items, so there is never anything to be lost by asking! For children in the final stage of their disease and who are being nursed by their parents at home, the Fund will provide a home nursing grant. This is *not* to provide a home nurse, but is rather to help meet those extra expenses parents have in this situation.

The Fund normally likes parents to make some contribution to the costs, but they accept that this is not always possible. Where large amounts are involved the Fund is very happy to make a partial grant when other organizations, like the Leukaemia Society or Cancer Relief, are also helping. Sometimes the full amount can be met by several organizations working together. Where families are eligible for statutory help, the Malcolm Sargent Fund, like other voluntary funds, will not give aid until all statutory sources have been exhausted.

Any doctor, medical social worker, district nurse or health visitor can make an application to the Fund. An application form is completed with the family, and if the child is accepted he is given a referral number. Thereafter a simple letter quoting the reference number and explaining the situation is sufficient for further requests for help. An accompanying letter with the application form is appreciated. It should make the patients' needs known in simple statements without ambiguity! A breakdown of costs involved helps and a grand total at the end of the letter avoids misunderstanding. When requests for grants are being repeated, the Fund likes to be kept up-to-date, in general terms, on the patient's medical situation. The upper age limit for patients' eligibility for help is 21 years.

The Malcolm Sargent Fund responds very quickly with the minimum of administrative fuss. In cases of very urgent need, they may even respond to a simple telephone call, with the paperwork to be completed afterwards.

Leukaemia Care Society
P.O. Box 82,
Exeter,
Devon EX2 5DP,
UK
Tel: 0392 218514

The Society provides direct financial help (but on a much smaller scale than the Malcolm Sargent Fund), holidays and support for leukaemia sufferers (adults and children) and their families. It also covers allied disorders including lymphomas (Hodgkin's and Non-Hodgkin's), aplastic anaemia, etc. It operates through a network of area secretaries but if you do not know the local one contact the Administrator at the above address.

National Society for Cancer Relief
Benefits Administrator,
Michael Sobell House,
30 Dorset Square,
London NW1 6QL,
UK
Tel: 01-402 8125

The Society will consider giving help to anyone currently suffering from cancer. However, it tends to refer children to the Malcolm Sargent Fund. It has occasionally shared costs with the Malcolm Sargent Fund when the grant sought has been particularly large, but necessary.

The Family Fund—Joseph Rowntree Memorial Trust
P.O. Box 50,
York YO1 1UY,
UK

The Fund will help families with severely handicapped or ill children. They consider each request on its own merits. Notes of guidance are available from the above address.

In addition, many treatment centres have access to local funds which may help families attending their particular centre. The Unit Social Worker will know of these and will be able to advise accordingly.

Appendix 3

Parents' and Voluntary Groups

It might be useful to look at one regional paediatric oncology unit's experience in developing parents' groups.

The groups started, about 10 years ago, as one-off meetings for parents of leukaemic children or parents of children with tumours. Typically, the groups included a talk on some relevant topic followed by a question and answer session. They were held about once every 3–4 months and were attended by some 40–50 parents. It quickly became obvious that they were too large to be anything more than information-imparting meetings. They had a useful social function in enabling parents and unit team to get together over coffee, but there was little or no discussion among parents of shared problems and feelings.

Smaller groups were then started, initially comprising about four meetings, combining parents of newly-diagnosed leukaemics and tumour sufferers and limiting membership to about 10–12 parents. They were overtly therapeutic and encouraged discussion of some of the deepest held fears and worries of parents under the guidance of the social workers. The meetings themselves were successful and those who attended felt they got a lot from them. However, the take-up rate of invitations to the groups was only about 30 per cent and it became clear that some people found the overtly therapeutic nature of the groups quite threatening.

The nature of the groups was again changed to present them as more educative. The take-up rate of invitations rose to more than 60 per cent and the pattern has remained constant, developing only in the detail, for the last number of years. The groups now comprise parents whose children were diagnosed in the preceding 6–9 months and meet for 8 or 9 fortnightly evening sessions. Most sessions are topic-related and are introduced by an appropriate member of the unit or hospital staff who talks informally for about 20 minutes. The rest of the time is devoted to discussion which, initially, is related to the topic, but which usually broadens to include the deeper fears and worries of parents. Discussion is led and, where necessary, guided by the social workers. Topics include the nature of childhood cancer, treatments, drugs, methods of coping, behaviour problems of patients and siblings, and school. This format seems to have worked well. Parents find the idea of the group, with its presented educative function, less than threatening, while the therapeutic part emerges naturally, sometimes with a little guidance, during the course of the meeting. Many members of the unit team are involved in specific meetings of the group, while the social workers provide consistency by organizing and attending every meeting.

Some parents' groups have developed further into independent self-help groups. Many such local groups exist and social workers on individual units work with them, and can put new parents in touch.

Some national groups also exist and can provide information, advice and support. These include:

Leukaemia Care Society
P.O. Box 82,
Exeter,
Devon EX2 5DP,
UK
Tel: 0392 218514

Catering for both adult and child sufferers and their families, the society operates through a network of area secretaries. The paed-iatric oncology social worker will be able to refer parents or they can contact the administrator at the above address. (*See also* Appendix 2.)

The Neuroblastoma Society
Woodlands,
Ordsall Park Road,
Retford,
Nottinghamshire DN22 7PJ,
UK
Tel: 0799 709238

The society raises funds to support British medical research into improving the treatment of neuroblastoma. It also supports parents and seeks to help them understand their child's treatment.

Hodgkin's Disease Association

P.O. Box 275,
Haddenham,
Aylesbury,
Bucks HP17 8JJ
UK
Tel: 0844 291500 (7 p.m.–10 p.m.)

The Association seeks to provide support and information for both adult and child patients and their families.

BACUP

121/123 Charterhouse Street,
London EC1M 6AA,
UK
Tel: 01-608 1661

Cancer Link

46a Pentonville Road,
London N1 9HF,
UK
Tel: 01-833 2451

Both organizations provide information on the telephone and through published material. They are mainly for adult patients. In addition, Cancer Link works with self-help and support groups throughout the country.

Compassionate Friends

National Secretary,
6 Denmark Street,
Bristol BS1 5DR,
UK
Tel: 0272 292778

This is a nationwide organization of bereaved parents offering friendship and understanding to other bereaved parents. It operates through a network of local groups. It runs a central library of books on child bereavement, and publishes a regular newsletter as well as booklets on many different aspects of child bereavement.

THE SUPPORTIVE CARE OF THE CHILD WITH CANCER

Appendix 4

Development of Paediatric Oncology Social Work

It was the growth of the concept of teamwork that led to the development of paediatric oncology as a specialization in social work. Prior to 1976, and with only a few exceptions, social work support to the families of children with cancer was provided on a limited crisis intervention basis from the hospital's social work department. It was not generally seen as having the highest priority. In 1976, the Regional Paediatric Oncology Unit at Alder Hey Children's Hospital in Liverpool got together with the Malcolm Sargent Cancer Fund for Children, Liverpool Social Services Department, and the idea of the 'Malcolm Sargent' Social Worker was born.

A post was created for a full-time, specialist social worker, located in the regional paediatric oncology unit and working as a member of the team, administered and supervised through the local social services department and wholly paid for by the Malcolm Sargent Fund. A need was obviously being met and within a year, a second post was established in Liverpool while other posts were being created, under broadly similar arrangements, in other centres. There are now well over 20 Malcolm Sargent Social Workers throughout the country and the number continues to grow. In other centres local social service departments have established similar specialist posts themselves while the funding of some of the earlier Malcolm Sargent posts has been taken over by the appropriate local authority. Given the growing awareness of, and desire to do something about, the psychosocial problems associated with childhood cancer, it is probable that such posts would eventually have been established anyway—but more slowly and with much more difficulty. The Malcolm Sargent Fund must, therefore, share much credit for the growth, spread and achievements of this new social work specialization in the UK.

1. Adams M. A. (1978) Helping the parents of children with malignancy. *J. Pediatr.* **93**(5), 734.
2. Peck B. (1979) Effects of childhood cancer on long-term survivors and their families. *Br. Med. J.* **1**, 1327–9.
3. Maguire G. P. (1983) *The psychological sequelae of childhood leukaemia.* In: Duncan (ed.) *Recent Results in Cancer Research 88.* Berlin, Springer-Verlag.
4. Ross J. W. and Klar H. (1982) Mental health practice in a physical health setting: social casework. *J. Contemp. Soc. Work.* Family Service Association of America.

5. Bodkin C. M., Pigott T. J. and Mann J. R. (1982) Financial burden of childhood cancer. *Br. Med. J.* **284**, 1542.
6. Pentol A. (1982) *The Costs of Childhood Leukaemia and its Treatment.* Working Paper No. 67; Health Services Management Unit, Dept. of Social Administration, University of Manchester.
7. *See* Department of Health Circular, DS 281/72 *Meals and Accommodation for the Parents of Children in Hospital.* Though dating from September 1972, this circular has not been superceded.
8. Ross J. W. and Scarvalone S. A. (1982) Facilitating the paediatric cancer patient's return to school. *Social Work* **27**, 256–62.
9. Charlton A., Pearson D. and Morris Jones P. J. (1986) Children's return to school after treatment for solid tumours. *Soc. Sci. Med.* **22**(12), 1337–46.
10. Ross J. W. (1979) Coping with childhood cancer: group intervention as an aid to parents in crisis. *Soc. Work Health Care* **4**(4), 381–91.

13. The Psychological Problems of Families of Children with Cancer

J. Culling

Medical advances during the last decade have led to greatly increased survival time and increased cure rate for children diagnosed with a variety of cancers. Along with this go longer periods of treatment, often painful procedures, frequent visits to hospital, disfiguring operations, unpleasant side-effects of irradiation and chemotherapy. The child survivor of cancer can face considerable disruption of social and family life, of education and normal physical and emotional development.

Ahead lies an uncertain future, living with the risk of recurrence and possible consequences of long-standing effects of chemotherapy and irradiation. Medical advances have thus opened doors in the psychological management of children and their families who have to go on living with the consequences of cancer, in spite of cure. The management of the emotional well-being of the child and family and the facilitation of as normal as possible an emotional and social development of the child are important aspects of supportive care.

CHILDHOOD CANCER AS A CHRONIC DISEASE

The literature of 2 decades ago focussed largely on the terminal illness of childhood cancer sufferers and their families. Much was written concerning the psychological adjustment of the dying child and the effects on the family of the loss of a child. During the last decade, some researchers have turned more towards examining the psychological sequelae of being cancer survivors, while others have attempted to understand the child's concepts of illness and death. The challenge for the clinician is, through understanding the emotional and intellectual experience of the child with cancer, to be able to communicate with the child at an appropriate level and thus facilitate the child's acceptance and coping with treatment and its outcome.

The experience of the majority of child cancer sufferers is similar to that of children suffering from other chronic illnesses such as cystic fibrosis, diabetes mellitus and chronic renal failure.

Epidemiological studies, such as the Isle of Wight Survey,[1] indicate that, within a total population of 9–11-year-olds living on the Isle of Wight, the rate of maladjustment as judged by questionnaires based on parental estimates, was higher in the chronically sick group of children. It was also apparent that maladjustment rates varied with the type of disorder and tended to be higher for children with permanent rather than temporary disabilities. Children with chronic illness may suffer long-term psychological problems in a number of areas: in their social adjustment, intellectual functioning and in personal development. Koocher and O'Malley,[2] in their study of cancer survivors, found that 47 per cent of survivors had symptoms indicative of impairment of mental health. While a substantial proportion of these 26 per cent had only mild symptoms, 10 per cent had moderate symptoms and 11 per cent had severe psychological symptoms which impaired their functioning.

Although early studies have tended to point out the negative consequences of chronic illness, where problems in intellectual and social functioning were noted, along with problems in potential marital and occupational status, it is important to recognize that more recent studies concluded that, in some instances, greater achievements and potential have occurred than would have been expected. Maguire[3] gives a more optimistic view of families indicating that sometimes they can become closer emotionally and earlier indications of increased divorce rates in marriage may be misleading.

UNDERSTANDING THE CHILD'S CONCEPT OF ILLNESS

There are practical considerations for having an understanding of children's concepts of their bodies, illness and treatment procedures. Research studies indicate that adults, as well as children, often have a very confused picture of the inside of their bodies and the functions of various organs. The knowledge about their bodies is also frequently erroneous.[4] Without an awareness of these likely misconceptions, there may be a barrier to communication with the child. There is a generally held belief that children of all ages should be informed of their illness, its treatment and consequences, the theory behind this being that even young children will work out for themselves the nature of their illness; but because of their inherent misconceptions about illness, their own theories may leave them feeling confused and frightened. If children can be involved in their illness and treatment, at a level which fits in with their stage of cognitive and emotional development, then the child should experience less anxiety and feel more in control of the situation, as well as being more compliant in following prescribed treatment.

A variety of approaches has been used in an attempt to understand how children acquire their understanding of illness. Explanations of how children view the causality of illness indicate a tendency for children to blame themselves for their illness, or to see it as a punishment for bad behaviour.[5,6] Younger children also frequently hold the view that illness is caused by germs. In their review of the literature, Bibace and Walsh[7] concluded that younger children, not surprisingly, hold a simplistic view of illness relating to external events and changes rather than internal bodily symptoms. Older children, on the other hand, are more able to differentiate between health and illness and are able to provide more realistic explanations based on cause and effect.

Eiser,[8] in her review of the literature, identified two distinct approaches to studying children's ideas about causation of illness. The first approach focuses on sociological influences on acquisition of illness concepts.

Campbell[9] in a study of children aged 6–12 years, compared their definitions of illness with those of their mothers. Campbell identified two processes in the acquisition of adult concepts: (1) patterned similarity, which is defined as an emerging consensus of illness definitions with the child's definitions becoming more like an adult's with age, and (2) developmental changes in illness concepts. Campbell also identified a definitional sophistication, where younger children defined illness in terms of feeling states. Older children became more precise in their definitions of illness using more diagnostically correct information.

Campbell's study was extended to adolescents by Millstein, Adler and Irwin.[10] Although in some ways disappointing and confusing, this study has some important implications for the clinical management of adolescents. It stresses the importance placed by adolescents on the effects of illness on their day-to-day activities and social functioning and less with the actual disease process itself.

COGNITIVE-DEVELOPMENTAL APPROACH

The second approach identified by Eiser[8] is the cognitive-developmental approach, described in the work of Bibace and Walsh.[7] They attempted to draw parallels between children's concepts of illness and the stages of cognitive development—prelogical, concrete logical and formal logical—as described by Piaget.

Prelogical explanations

Children aged 2–6 years of age characteristically view the cause of illness as an external concrete phenomenon that may occur with the illness but is spatially and temporally remote. The child is unable to explain how the external event causes illness. Bibace and Walsh[7] quote the following examples:
'How do people get colds?' "From trees."
'How do people get measles?' "From God."
'How does God give people measles?' "God does it in the sky."
The commonest explanation of illness offered by the child in the prelogical stage of thought is contagion. For example:
'How do people get colds?' "From outside."
'How do they get them from outside?' "They just do, that's all. They come when someone else gets near you." 'How?' "I don't know—by magic I think."[7]

Concrete logical explanations

Between the ages of 7 and 10, the child's ability to differentiate between self and other increases. The child is able to distinguish between what is internal and external to the self. The commonest explanation of illness offered by the younger child at this stage is contamination. The child recognizes that an object, person or action outside himself can cause illness through the child's body becoming physically in contact with the object or person. For example:
'What is a cold?' "It's like in the winter-time."
'How do people get them?' "You're outside without a hat and you start sneezing. Your head would get cold—the cold would touch it—and then it would go all over your body."[7]
The older child, at this stage, may offer a more mature explanation, described as internalization. The child recognizes that the internal effect of illness is linked to the causative agent external to the body. The external agent is internalized, for example, through inhalation or swallowing. However, the child at this stage continues to show confusion about specific functioning of internal organs.

Formal–logical explanations

From early adolescence, the formal–logical stage of cognitive development is reached. The child can clearly differentiate between self and not-self. The child can perceive that the source of illness is within the body while recognizing that the causative agent may lie outside the body. Bibace and Walsh[7] described two sub-stages of formal logical thought in relation to the causes of illness, physiological and psychophysiological. Younger children at the formal logical stage will offer a physiological explanation of illness; the illness will be described as the non-functioning or malfunctioning of a specific internal organ or process. Older children are able to give a psycho-physiological explanation of illness. The illness is still understood as the failure of a specific internal organ or system but, in addition, the child is able to make the association between psychological influences and illness. That is, the child develops an awareness of how thoughts and feeling states can influence bodily functioning.

DEVELOPMENT OF ILLNESS CONCEPTS IN THE CHILD WITH CANCER

We have so far considered how children develop their understanding of disease processes and illness concepts. This raises the question: 'Do children who experience a chronic illness have the same understanding, or does their experience of illness influence their acquisition of illness concepts in any way?' An appreciation of the sick child's understanding of his illness and of treatment procedures, in relation to his experience has important implications for the clinical management of the child and family. It could be speculated that, if the child's understanding of his illness could be enhanced, then the child should suffer less distress at the need for treatment and be more compliant in adhering to and accepting treatment regimes.

Most recent research has tended to indicate that sick children have the same system of beliefs about illness and its causation as that held by well children. A notable study is that of Beales et al.[11] who interviewed 75 patients with juvenile chronic arthritis about the understanding of their illness and its treatment. The patients were divided into 2 age groups, those aged 7–11 years, and those aged 12–17 years. They found that the younger children tended to see their illness in terms of the concrete, outward manifestations of the illness such as swollen joints, pain, restriction of movement. The older group of children was able to make the connection that the external signs were the result of an underlying disease process. The knowledge of the older group was nevertheless restricted to a relatively simplistic description of the disease process. In some cases, children gave an exaggerated account of their pathology which was worse than their actual clinical state. In terms of the implications these findings have for clinical management, Beales et al. concluded that children of different ages require qualitatively different kinds of explanations of their illness. In particular, younger children are more able to make use of explanations or descriptions which draw on specific analogies relative to their everyday experiences; for example, nerves being likened to electrical wiring, or the role of white blood cells in relation to an army seeing off invaders. Younger children also may benefit more through the visual representation of information rather than a verbal description.

Kendrick et al.[12] studied a group of 25 children aged 2–11 years, hospitalized for the treatment of a variety of childhood cancers. Two techniques were used to obtain information about the children's understanding of their illness and treatment. A life-space technique was used for observing the children over a period of time in different situations; in addition, informal interviews with the children were carried out where the children were encouraged to talk about their illness and its treatment. The patients in the study had been given explanations of their illness and its treatment by the clinician in charge, shortly after diagnosis. Kendrick et al.[12] noted that, following this initial explanation, the children without fail entered a phase of increased receptivity to information about their illness. During this 'extra-receptive period' the children were alert to cues from a wide variety of sources, some of them unexpected, for example, domestic staff and other children, as well as parents, teachers, physiotherapists and nurses. Kendrick gives an example of an 8-year-old girl who, when told she had leukaemia, professed to have no knowledge about the functions of the blood in her body. Within a matter of days, she had assimilated a great deal of relevant information about her own illness and her treatment regime. Within a week, she appeared to have grasped the basic concepts of different 'bits' of blood having different functions, and the fact that her own blood was not currently able to perform these functions adequately. These observations highlight the importance of a consensus of information being shared by all personnel caring for the child, and the importance of communication between staff.

Kendrick noted, with interest, that some of the children in the study were showing an understanding of their illness which greatly exceeded their cognitive capacities in other respects. There is a suggestion that these 'cognitive leaps' may occur as a result of experience and the extra-receptive period already referred to. Alongside these 'cognitive leaps', it was also noted that a number of children showed evidence of regression in other areas of their behaviour. For example, reverting to a bottle or dummy, wanting to be dressed and fed, and nocturnal wetting.

Lastly, Kendrick looked at the role of experience in the development of the child's understanding and coming to terms with treatment. In cases where a particular hospital procedure had not yet been experienced but was being anticipated, a considerable level of anxiety was visible. Other, more experienced children sometimes came to the aid of the inexperienced child, giving reassuring explanations and accounts of what a procedure entailed.

In contrast to some earlier studies, the children in this study did not appear to regard their illness as a punishment for some misdemeanour or badness, or to seek to place blame with another person. In general, these children appeared to accept, without question, the fact of their illness and the need for treatment while, at the same time, protesting their distress at the discomfort and pain imposed.

THE PARENTS' UNDERSTANDING OF THE CHILD'S ILLNESS

The clinical management of childhood cancers does not rest solely with the treatment of the child's medical condition. The child is part of a family and, in particular, is the responsibility of parents or a parent. It is therefore important to explore and understand the experience of the parents or parent when their child is diagnosed as having cancer. Without the co-operation and understanding of the parents, the child cannot be properly cared for and supported. The stage of cognitive development, role and position of siblings in the family also need to be given attention.

When a child develops a serious medical condition such as a malignancy, the parents are likely to find themselves suddenly and urgently rushed to a specialist treatment centre, often at some distance from their home and support networks. Family life is suddenly thrown into turmoil, dramatic changes in lifestyle may have to be made at short notice. The parents and child find themselves in an alien environment, amongst strangers and in a situation over which they have little control. The child is torn away from familiar and reassuring surroundings into an environment which is foreign and incomprehensible, and discovers that his parents, to whom in the past he has turned for support and reassurance, are in themselves anxious and bewildered. The diagnosis may not be immediately apparent and there may be a day or two of examinations and investigations which, if not painful, cause discontent to the child and anxiety to the parents who suddenly have to acquire new skills in caring for their sick child. Most families and children experience considerable anxiety and fear during this pre-diagnosis phase. On receiving the diagnosis, the initial reaction is one of shock and numbness which may last for a period from a day or two to several weeks, in which case, it may seriously hamper the parents' acceptance of the treatment programme. When the numbness of shock gives way, the parents are left with feelings of grief at the potential loss of their child. For the majority of parents, still, the diagnosis of childhood cancer is perceived as a death sentence for the child. The parents may hold very distorted ideas and erroneous information about the cause of childhood cancer and its treatment. The task of the physician at this stage is to re-educate the parents and to strike a balance between giving them a too optimistic view of the prognosis which would distract from the seriousness of the situation, and a too pessimistic view which would be equally erroneous. This information may need to be repeated several times on different occasions, as the parents will vary in their receptivity to information, depending on the level of numbness and shock which they are experiencing.

In this early stage following diagnosis, parents will frequently question why their child has become ill and will seek concrete explanations for the illness. They may express feelings of guilt that they are in some way responsible for the illness or that they should have sought medical advice earlier. Frequently, the early symptoms of a malignant condition are of a trivial or insidious nature and, in the early stages, may not, quite rightly, have been viewed with serious- ness by the parents. The parents may also express open anger and hostility at the family doctor who failed initially to make the diagnosis, and at the paediatrician for delaying the diagnosis. There may also be a free-floating anger, produced by the threat of loss of the child, which may be directed at a spouse, nurse or doctor, regardless of innocence.

During this early phase, symptoms of anxiety and depression occur in up to 50 per cent of parents.[13] The symptoms are usually mild to moderate in severity and, in general, subside over a number of weeks as the child begins to respond to therapy, and the parents come to realize that the child's illness is potentially curable.

When the diagnosis has been confirmed and a treatment protocol decided upon, a question asked by the majority of parents is what to tell the child. Many parents find the prospect of telling their child that he has a potentially fatal malignant condition almost unbearable. There is a natural tendency to want to protect the child by withholding information. However, as previously noted, research points to the view that children who are given honest and straightforward information early on in treatment are more likely to make a successful adaptation than those not told or told later in treatment. Parents may need help and encouragement in finding appropriate words and ways of informing their child. An open communication approach, where the clinician talks with the whole family, serves the purpose of pro- viding the parents with a model of how to communicate and also ensures that both parents and child are receiving the same information and that it is not being distorted in any way. However, there are parents who will prefer to tell their child in their own way, in privacy, and these wishes should be respected. In the days following diagnosis, when the child is in the phase of heightened receptivity, and parents are anxious to learn more about the illness, the initial discussion can be expanded on and backed up by suitable leaflets or a visit to the laboratory to view bone marrow smears or peripheral blood films. As the phase of initial treatment proceeds, it is important to continue to educate the parents and to involve them as much as possible in the treatment of their child. This is particularly important for fathers who may be left at home caring for siblings or trying to maintain their income. Many parents, finding themselves in this alien situation, will feel helpless and out of control. To give the parent a role in caring for the child restores confidence and status to the parent, and a reassuring and supportive relationship to the child. Research has indicated that, in preparing young children for hospital treatment, it is of prime importance to prepare and educate the parents, for unless the parent is able to cope, then the task for the child becomes even greater.

Finally, one should not forget the siblings of the sick child who may be left at home, in the care of relatives or friends, feeling bewildered by the sudden changes in family life. The siblings may experience guilt that, in some way, they might be responsible for their brother's or sister's illness, or might feel openly hostile that they have been deprived of parental attention and time. It is important, as much as possible, to involve the siblings during the early stages of diagnosis and treatment in order to relieve their feelings of responsibility and guilt and to prevent the build-up of resentment towards the sick child. Siblings who are kept honestly informed and involved are more likely to remain supportive and understanding during the time of increased family stress ahead.

A situation is described in this chapter where, hopefully and ideally, clinician, parents and child work together as a team sharing a common understanding of the child's disease process, its treatment and prognosis. Inevitably, situations arise where communications become blurred and misconceptions and misunderstandings develop. Mulhern[14] studied communication patterns within families and with paediatricians. Parents, paediatricians and children were asked to rate probable survival times of the child. No significant disagreement was obtained between the prognostic views of mothers and fathers. However, significant misunderstanding between mothers and fathers was found. Mothers generally underestimated fathers' views of the child's prognosis, whereas fathers accurately predicted the prognostic views of mothers.

Paediatricians gave significantly less optimistic estimates of the children's prognosis than did mothers or fathers. Furthermore, paediatricians, as well as parents, appeared to misunderstand each other's views. Paediatricians significantly underestimated the prognostic views of mothers, as well as those of fathers. Mothers and fathers significantly overestimated the paediatrician's view of their child's prognosis. The children's views of their own chances for long-term survival were significantly higher than those given by mothers and paediatricians, but not significantly greater than those given by fathers. Both mothers and fathers accurately estimated the self-reports of their children, whereas paediatricians underestimated the children's prognostic views.

Mulhern[14] went on to make a more in-depth analysis of the independent variables utilized by mothers, fathers and paediatricians to formulate their estimate of prognosis. For paediatricians, age at diagnosis, white blood cell count at diagnosis, acute lymphocytic leukaemia sub-type and duration of remission accounted for $50 \cdot 4$ per cent of the variance. The child's sex contributed no further significance to prediction of paediatrician prognostic views. Mothers' prognostic views were best predicted by the child's sex and duration of remission. Generally, mothers were most optimistic about male children who had longer remissions; age at diagnosis, WBC and ALL sub-type were non-contributory. In contrast, fathers' prognostic views were best predicted by a combination of 4 variables, duration of remission, child's sex, age at diagnosis and ALL sub-type. Fathers were most pessimistic about male children who were diagnosed at an early age and who had common ALL with relatively long remissions.

This study is important as it illustrates the complex nature of patterns of communication between paediatricians and parents. The results suggest that, despite repeated explanations of the disease and its implications, parents consistently differ from paediatricians in their interpretation of information. In the light of other research which points to failure of communication as being the prediction of emotional maladaption in the families of children with cancer, it is of concern to the paediatrician to find ways of assessing interfamilial and paediatrician/parent communication.

LONG-TERM PSYCHOLOGICAL AND SOCIAL SEQUELAE

The increased life expectancy and survival time for sufferers of childhood malignancy has turned attention to the quality of life experienced by child survivors and the long-term effects of psychological and social stress on the whole family. In spite of the improved survival rates, many children still die as a result of their malignancy, even following a period of remission lasting several years. For the parents, this means living with the uncertainty of wondering whether their child will die or survive, for many years. Koocher and O'Malley[2] have described the Damocles syndrome, where the family and child live with the threat of relapse or death constantly hanging over them. Koocher and O'Malley, in their book entitled *The Damocles Syndrome*, describe how, following the diagnosis of childhood cancer, the family experiences many years of continuing stress which waxes and wanes in accordance with the stage of treatment, relapse or remission.

The treatment programme, often of several years' duration, involves the parents and child in frequent visits to clinics or admission to hospital, often at a treatment centre some distance from home. Such visits may cause considerable disruption to home and family life as well as imposing an added financial burden on the family. Removal of the family members from their home base and its social network may leave them feeling isolated and alone without the usual support network of friends and relatives. Isolation may also occur as a result of the stigma attached to having a child with a potentially fatal illness. Friends and neighbours might feel embarrassed or unable to find words of comfort and support and therefore turn away from the family. Primitive and erroneous beliefs that childhood cancer is contagious may cause parents to forbid their children to play with the sick child or siblings, leading to disruption in the social development of the children.

Not infrequently at the time of diagnosis, the child is not feeling particularly unwell nor has any outward sign of underlying disease, beyond a localized lump or bruising. As treatment progresses, the side-effects of chemotherapy, irradiation and surgery may prove more distressing than the illness itself. Given the uncertain prognosis even with treatment, the parents may question the wisdom of allowing their child to suffer when the treatment may be to no avail. This situation may become more acute when the child begins to question the value of treatment and expresses anxiety about the response of school friends to hair loss, or begins to develop anticipatory vomiting prior to chemotherapy.

A major task for parents throughout treatment is in balancing the needs of the sick child against those of the rest of the family. Many parents feel that, when their child is in hospital, they should be there continually to provide support and reassurance. Some parents feel afraid to leave the bedside in case something should happen to the child during their absence. At the same time, parents experience guilt that they are not meeting the needs of their spouse or other children. When the child enters remission or a more stable period in treatment, the task of re-integrating the child back into family life is not always easy. In spite of advice to treat their child normally, parents often find it extremely difficult to impose normal standards of discipline and behaviour on a child who they know might die and who has, at the least, to suffer the stress of unpleasant treatment. The effects of some drugs, such as prednisolone, on the emotional lability of the child make it more difficult for the parents to judge what warrants firm handling or tolerance. Parents also worry about the effects of a double standard of discipline or attention on the other children in the family. However hard parents try not to indulge or spoil the sick child, it is inevitable that the child will receive more attention and be showered with treats and gifts from anxious and well-meaning friends and relations.

PSYCHOLOGICAL PROBLEMS FOR THE CHILD

Intrapersonal problems

With an open approach to communication between paediatrician, child and parents, the sick child will have at least some understanding of the illness, although the extent of this understanding and its implications may be quite variable depending on the age of the child. The majority of children, even those not openly informed, will realize the serious nature of their illness, from the sudden change in their life situations, attitudes and emotional tone of their parents.[15] The majority of children will express some anxiety about their health or their body integrity particularly in the face of hair loss through chemotherapy, weight gain, acne or disfiguring operations. For the younger child, it is the threat to body integrity that is of paramount importance, rather than the long-term issues of survival. For the adolescent patient, it is the change in body image, making the adolescent potentially unattractive to his or her peer group, which gives rise to most anxiety. The adolescent is also more sensitive to the disruption of day-to-day living and social relationships and to the threat of being unable to fulfil expected goals such as career, marriage and having a family.

Intellectual development

Eiser[8] extensively reviews the literature on the intellectual development and academic achievements of children treated for malignant conditions, particularly where prophylactic irradiation of the central nervous system has been a part of treatment. Varying and opposing views on the vulnerability of the brain to irradiation have been put forward. One view holds that, since only developing and dividing cells are vulnerable, and since permanent cells are formed in the brain relatively early, little damage is likely to result from irradiation.[18] Another view is that such brain development continues until at least 5 years of age.[17] Yet another view is that irradiation affects development indirectly through damage to the cerebrovascular system, which results in interference with the blood supply to the brain.[18,19] Research into this area has been, to some degree, hampered by ethical problems in design of research protocols, making the selection of comparison groups and controls difficult. Nevertheless, the findings of a number of retrospective studies have been generally consistent. Investigations carried out prior to the mid-1970s concluded that CNS irradiation did not affect the child's intellectual development. These early studies can, however, be criticized in terms of sample size and poorly matched controls. In addition, more recent work has failed to produce similar findings. Eiser has conducted a number of studies[20,21] comparing the intellectual development of children with ALL, healthy children and children with solid tumours receiving body irradiation but not CNS irradiation. Her initial study indicated that the treatment used to control leukaemia might be too aggressive for the under 5-year-olds. A subsequent study [21] assessed the 3 groups of children. On the measures of assessment used, the children with solid tumours had scores comparable to the healthy controls, suggesting that, despite the aggressive medical treatment and life-threatening nature of their conditions, there were no measurable effects on intellect following recovery. In contrast, the children with leukaemia scored consistently and significantly below their controls. Further correlations were made between the sick child's scores on the different tests with age of diagnosis. Again the correlations were significant for the leukaemic group of children and indicated that scores on the IQ test decreased the younger the age of the child on diagnosis. The results of this study suggest that some aspect of the treatment appears to be implicated in the poorer performance of children with leukaemia compared with those with other life-threatening cancers.

The most recent and extensive investigation is that of Jannoun.[22] Jannoun investigated 129 ALL patients and compared their performance with 67 healthy siblings by means of the British Ability Scales (BAS) and Wechsler Intelligence Scale for Children—Revised (WISC—R). The patients were divided into 3 groups, according to age at diagnosis: those diagnosed aged less than 3 years, those diagnosed aged 3–6 years, and those diagnosed over the age of 7 years. On the WISC—R, the IQ scores for the children in the 2 older age groups were significantly higher than for the youngest age group. On the BAS, the difference approached, but did not reach, significance. Patients' scores were also compared with healthy siblings where possible. The mean scores for patients were significantly lower than those of siblings and in particular on analysis of each separate age group, the difference remained significant for the 2 younger age groups, although not for the older group.

In spite of methodological problems in a number of the papers reviewed by Eiser, the consistency of results is impressive. The literature to date points conclusively to the fact that children treated between the ages of 2 and 3 years of age by CNS irradiation for leukaemia subsequently have lower IQ scores than would be expected.

As a separate issue, apart from the effects of treatment on intellectual development, it is important to consider the influence of having a malignant condition on more general aspects of school life and academic attainment. School attendance is an important part of every child's life, not only in terms of an academic learning experience, but also as a social milieu where the child begins to learn about relationships beyond the family. For the child with cancer, there may be considerable disruption of this aspect of life. To feel an accepted member of a peer group is very important to the majority of children. Repeated absences from school and changes in physical appearance may seriously handicap the sick child's ability to remain a competing member of the peer group. Parents may feel reluctant to encourage their children to attend school regularly because of anxiety that they may be bullied or teased, or through fear that they might be vulnerable to physical injury or exposed to infection. The school teacher also may feel anxious about the responsibility of having a physically ill child in the school and may need guidelines and reassurance about symptoms and side-effects. The school teacher, like the parent, may also be inclined to treat the child as a special child, having different expectations in terms of behaviour or application to work. It is important, however, to recognize that where genuine learning difficulties exist, or where the child is genuinely having difficulty adapting, special support may need to be given in order to help the child maintain a sense of achievement and self-esteem.

Behavioural problems

Behavioural problems develop in a significant proportion of children being treated for malignant conditions. Maguire et al.[13] studied 60 children suffering from leukaemia and discovered that 38 per cent developed behavioural problems compared with only 8 per cent of the control group. The most common problems found included clinging, dependent behaviour, temper tantrums and reluctance to sleep alone. Maguire et al. noted a strong correlation between these behaviour problems and changes in the parents' behaviour towards the child. The changes in parental behaviour in relation to the child included a lessening of discipline, over-indulgence and over-protectiveness. Howarth[23] discovered a similar incidence of behavioural disorders in children with leukaemia. He also studied children with cystic fibrosis and found that a similar proportion (40 per cent) exhibited behaviour problems, suggesting that the problems are related to suffering from a chronic life-threatening disease rather than being disease specific.

Behavioural problems are not only manifest in the family environment but are also reflected in the child's school performance, and in the teacher's appraisal of the child. Eiser[21] found that 2 per cent of the children in her study achieved scores on Rutter Behaviour Questionnaires, completed by teachers, which suggested that they were suffering from behaviour problems. The teachers in the study also reported difficulty in teaching the child who falls behind the peer group through repeated absence from school. A proportion of teachers who felt ill-informed about the illness and its treatment reported a change in attitude towards the child, in terms of becoming more protective and lenient.

Few studies have attempted to answer the question: 'Do behavioural problems and adjustment problems persist over time?' One study, (Slavin et al.[24]) suggests that 1 in 5 of those who survive childhood cancer have difficulties over the longer term. In general, it would seem that the younger the child at diagnosis, and the shorter the length of treatment programme, the less likely are difficulties in emotional adjustment of the child likely to occur.

PSYCHOLOGICAL AND SOCIAL PROBLEMS OF THE PARENTS

Earlier studies investigating the impact of chronic life-threatening illness on the parents of the sick child presented a rather pessimistic picture of how parents coped. The results of these earlier studies have to be reviewed in the light of changes in recent years in the quality of psychosocial support given to families and in changes in treatment protocols which have led to less disruption in family life. More recent studies have been inclined to look more at family resilience and coping mechanisms and have, in general, produced a more encouraging picture of the adaptive skills of families.

Returning to earlier studies, Binger et al.[25] studied 20 families of children with leukaemia and reported a high incidence of problems including family disturbance, difficulties with siblings, depression and divorce. Kaplan[26,27] found profound communication problems in famlies and an increased rate of marital breakdown. A number of studies have investigated the incidence of mental health symptoms in parents. Notably, Maguire[13] conducted a prospective study of the parents of 60 children treated for leukaemia and followed them for the first 12–18 months after diagnosis. Parents were assessed using the Present State examination (Wing, Cooper and Sartorius)[28] and the standardized social interview (Clare and Cairns)[29] and were then compared with a control group of parents where children had been treated for benign disease. Maguire et al. found that, in the period following diagnosis of leukaemia, 30 per cent of the mothers were found to be suffering from an anxiety state. This compared with an incidence of 5 per cent among mothers of children with benign disease. Symptoms of depression were evident in over 30 per cent of mothers of children with leukaemia compared with 9 per cent of mothers of children with benign disease. At follow-up, 12–18 months after diagnosis, 25 per cent of the mothers were suffering from symptoms of anxiety or depression, compared with 8 per cent of the mothers in the control group. Maguire stated the severity of symptoms to be mild to moderate but with a tendency to persist for up to 18 months post diagnosis.

Several investigators have pointed to an increase in marital break-down in families where a child has a chronic life-threatening illness. More recent studies have tended to contradict these earlier findings. Lansky[30] followed up parents of children who were treated in a cancer centre to determine whether they had a greater divorce rate or whether their marriages were under particular strain. Their results indicated that 68 per cent of couples were experiencing marital difficulties. Couples complained about having their own needs unmet, of feelings of helplessness and loss of confidence. Conflicts between parents arose out of differing attitudes to the child in terms of discipline and protectiveness. In spite of these complaints, there was no evidence of an increase in the divorce rate. Kaplan[26] noticed an increase in marital problems following the death of a child. They report that 70 per cent of couples develop problems which lead to divorce or separation in 23 per cent.

This reported divorce rate is, however, lower than in the general population.

PSYCHOLOGICAL PROBLEMS OF THE SIBLINGS

In families where the siblings have been kept openly informed, and have been involved from the time of diagnosis, there is less likelihood that resentment and jealousy towards the sick child will develop. Children are, in general, very sensitive to changes in their parents' behaviour and attitudes. They will soon detect that the parent has become more lenient, over-indulgent or over-protective towards the sick child, and that the child is receiving a considerable amount of attention. Siblings may become angry and bitter towards the sick child as they perceive that they themselves are becoming left out and neglected. Even when the siblings are informed of the diagnosis, their level of understanding may leave them feeling anxious and confused. The children may fear that the disease is contagious and that they, in fact, will develop the symptoms. The sibling may feel guilty or responsible for the illness, particularly if there have been relationship difficulties between the siblings before the onset of the illness, or if the well sibling has secretly harboured a grudge against the sick child. Frequently, the children will not feel able to share their anxieties with their parents because they are sensitive to not wanting to impose more stress or worry on their parents.

The lifestyle for the siblings may be seriously disrupted during the early days of treatment. They may suddenly be left in the charge of friends or relations or, if they are younger, taken away from familiar surroundings to join the rest of the family at a treatment centre away from home.

Binger[25] claimed that 50 per cent of siblings of children with leukaemia developed behavioural problems including abdominal pains, enuresis, school phobias, depression and clinging behaviour. More recent studies indicate that, even siblings of children with a good prognosis can experience difficulties. There is some evidence that siblings' difficulties are related to changes in parents' behaviour. Cairns[31] gave psychological tests to both children with cancer and their siblings. Siblings who perceived parents as more protective and over-indulgent towards the sick child, and who felt the parents had less good feeling towards them, experienced greater anxiety, were worried about their physical health and felt socially isolated. They commonly complained of physical symptoms, including abdominal pain and headache, and felt that their own needs were being neglected. Changes in siblings' behaviour as reflected by their school performance have been investigated in a number of studies. In spite of a high incidence of reported problems in siblings (80 per cent), only in 25 per cent is there reported to be a deterioration in school performance.[32] Eiser[21] records similar findings, her group of teachers assessing that 20 per cent of siblings manifested behavioural disorders at school as judged by ratings on the Rutter Behaviour Scale.

COPING STRATEGIES AND RESILIENCE

In contrast to early literature, increasing interest has been turned towards investigating how many families and children cope surprisingly well with the stress of malignant disease. There is now a wealth of evidence accumulating that would suggest that the reports of high levels of emotional disturbance found in the earlier literature may not be comparable to more recent findings. The reason for this may be two-fold; firstly, the prognosis for many malignant conditions in childhood has improved considerably in recent years and, along with this, treatment protocols, although sometimes more intense, have tended to become of shorter duration. Secondly, treatment centres have become more aware and sensitive to psychosocial issues, thus providing a higher degree of psychosocial support. Recent studies have also perhaps been designed to look for positive functioning in families as well as for signs of maladaptive functioning.

Any threat to an individual's body integrity or psychological functioning will be met by an alteration in behaviour designed to protect the integrity of the individual. Mattson[33] describes coping strategies as 'adaptational techniques used by an individual to master a major psychological threat and its attendant negative feelings, in order to allow him to achieve personal and social goals'. The recognition of the individual's or family's coping strategies has important clinical implications for the management of families of children with a malignant condition. Recent research has investigated ways of detecting maladaptive functioning in families in the early weeks following diagnosis. The expectation is that, by offering early intervention to non-coping families, it should be possible to prevent maladaptive behaviour becoming too rigidly set.

The child has a number of coping techniques which enable him to come to terms with the illness and its effects, while continuing to lead a rewarding life and maintain social and emotional growth. The first task for the child is to accept the limitations imposed by the illness. The child must accept that the illness is a part of him and he has to learn to take some responsibility for the management of the illness, and to comply with the medical treatment. Secondly, the child must learn how to manage the anger and frustrations produced by the illness in a socially acceptable manner. Some children may develop compensatory physical or intellectual skills to balance the loss imposed by the illness. Finally, the child may utilize the common defence mechanisms of denial and suppression in order to keep anxiety manageable, so that other tasks may be achieved.

The child's coping strategies cannot be considered in isolation. The child is part of the family system. The family is a unique system of relationships whereby stress imposed on any member of the system will be transmitted directly or indirectly to other members. It is therefore important to consider the coping strategies used by the parents. Several workers[26] have described a number of coping tasks imposed on the family following the diagnosis of a potentially life-threatening illness in a child. These coping tasks vary with the nature of the illness, for example, if it is a chronic but not life-threatening illness, as opposed to a relatively short-term but fatal illness. Much of the earlier literature has focused on the tasks facing the families of children fatally ill with leukaemia, but are nevertheless applicable to situations where the prognosis is more favourable.

The coping tasks for the parents follow a specific sequence dependent on the stage of illness. These stages are as follows: diagnosis, remission, relapse leading to terminal illness or, in cases where there is a favourable outcome, to termination of treatment. The task at diagnosis is for the parent to accept the reality of the diagnosis, to express feelings of sadness and grief and to communicate these feelings with spouse and family. The task during remission is, to some extent, utilizing adaptive denial to suppress anxiety in order to enable the child to reintegrate into family and social life. Should the child relapse and enter the terminal phase of the illness, the task for the parents is to begin the process of anticipatory mourning and loosening of the relationship bond with the child, in order that following the loss of the child, reorganization of family relationships may proceed. Should there be a more favourable outcome, the family and child must face the crisis of termination of treatment. During the often long period of treatment, the family can become dependent on the treatment, seeing it as security against relapse, in spite of explanations contrary to this. The parents and child may also have become quite dependent on relationships with hospital staff and have grown accustomed to the unique status bestowed upon them as regular visitors to the specialist centre. The task at this stage is to loosen the dependency on the hospital and to reinvest in relationships and social activities in the outside environment. This task is not always made easy by the constant reminder of the threat of relapse or long-term side-effects, brought about by continuing follow-up appointments.

It is believed that successful psychological intervention depends on detecting maladaptive coping strategies soon after diagnosis. Kaplan et al.[26] studied 40 families in which a child had leukaemia and reported on the relation between different family coping reactions and stress outcome. The families' early coping reactions were classified as either adaptive or maladaptive. Coping responses were classified as: (1) the ability of the parents to comprehend the nature of the disease—that leukaemia is a serious, chronic illness with a poor long-term prognosis, (2) the ability of the parents to communicate the seriousness of the illness to all members of the family, including the patient, and (3) the ability of the parents to respond to the diagnosis with appropriate feelings of grief and sadness without inhibiting the expression of these feelings in themselves or in any family member. Families rated as showing adaptive coping had significantly fewer problems and stress factors at follow-up.

Maladaptive coping strategies believed to be good predictors of later family dysfunction are a persistence of denial in acknowledging the diagnosis. Frequently, these families will seek alternative medical opinions or seek out alternative treatments. A suppression, or denial of feelings of sadness and grief at the threatened loss of the child or future goals occurs; sometimes this is accompanied by a 'flight into activity' where ill-judged major decisions on family life may be made, such as a move of house, or a pregnancy. Finally, there may be a failure of open communication in the family where the parents insist on the child not being told the reality of the diagnosis or keeping the diagnosis a secret from friends and family. Particular difficulties may arise where mothers and fathers adopt different coping strategies, thereby blocking open communication between them and denying each other mutual support.

PSYCHOSOCIAL SUPPORT AND METHODS OF INTERVENTION

Two questions need to be addressed in considering the issues of psychosocial support and intervention. The first is, 'Why should we offer psychosocial support; what do we hope to achieve?' It is evident, from the wealth of research material available, that the consequences of surviving and living with childhood cancer produce, in a substantial proportion of patients and their families, significant psychological disturbance or behavioural problems. In offering psychosocial support to families, our aim would be to minimize the development of psychological dysfunction and to maximize the coping abilities of the child and family, so that the child's emotional and social development will continue throughout, and in spite of, treatment.

The second question to be addressed is, 'How should we intervene? How can we effectively help the child and family?' Several researchers have commented on the reluctance of parents to admit to feeling stressed or to discuss openly their emotional reactions in response to their child's illness. Parents faced with a seriously ill child find it hard to admit that they are having difficulty coping, for a number of reasons. Firstly, they often receive non-verbal cues from people around them, medical staff, general practitioner and family that it is their duty to cope. Secondly, the parents may feel that it is inappropriate to raise their own problems with the medical staff caring for their child. They may feel that they will be considered to be difficult and troublesome. The parents then have the difficulty of whom to turn to. Social workers sometimes take on the role of counsellor to the parents, but, not infrequently, parents perceive the social worker as being helpful in sorting out financial problems but not qualified to deal with emotional problems. When parents are asked what kind of help they would like, they tend to ask for someone who has specific knowledge of the child's illness and treatment, an understanding of the stresses and emotional difficulties, plus a knowledge of counselling skills.

Given that parents are unlikely to ask for help themselves, some centres advocate the inclusion of a specially trained counsellor in the treatment team who will routinely approach and assess families. This counsellor may come from a variety of professional backgrounds, for example, child psychiatrist, psychologist, specialist social worker or nurse. It is important that the person is seen to be an accepted member of the team and has the respect of the consultant paediatrician, otherwise the parents are unlikely to respond to the approach. The advantage of making the counsellor available routinely removes the threat of stigma from parents who have difficulty in admitting to their emotional difficulties.

The importance of teamwork

To provide the very best medical and psychosocial care for the child and family, it is very important that the caring professionals work together as a cohesive team. The hospital team provides stability and consistency to the family, helping to develop trust and a feeling of being cared for and supported. It is essential that the team achieves a level of good communication and provides a consensus of information to the child and family. It is also important that there is sufficient trust within the team to discuss openly controversial issues such as the use of experimental treatment protocols, or the decision of termination of therapy following repeated relapses. For nurses in particular, who have more face-to-face contact with patients, it is important that they have an avenue for expressing their opinions and feelings about treatment. It is advantageous to the patient and family if a key medical person can be assigned to a particular patient and a system of multiple carers avoided. The family are able to develop, over a period of time, a trusting relationship with their key doctor and will feel more able to express their concerns openly. Reciprocally, the doctor will develop a unique understanding of how the family functions and will be in a position to anticipate difficulties which may arise.

Other members of the team, such as teachers, occupational therapists and play leaders, have an important role beyond that of their professional training. It is the carers who have most physical or face-to-face contact with the child who are likely to receive their confidences or worries and anxieties. These carers should have an opportunity to share these confidences with the rest of the team. It is important that the child realizes that such information will be shared, otherwise the child may feel that trust has been broken.

When talking about the fears, we are referring largely to the hospital team. However, the primary health care team should not be forgotten as they play an important role in the longer term care of the child, particularly if the child dies at home. The majority of general practitioners and health visitors will have had no experience of caring for a child with a malignant disease. In general, a programme of education for the general practitioner is useful. This could take the form of a leaflet or fact sheet giving information about the disease and its treatment, the drugs used and their side-effects. Failure to educate the primary health team may result in conflicting and potentially harmful information being given to the family. An opportunity for the general practitioner to visit the hospital and discuss the management can also be of value. Many general practitioners will not have cared for a terminally ill child and may need considerable support if they are to be involved in the terminal care of a child dying at home. The support may be in terms of management of pain relief and other symptoms, but also in relation to communicating with the family about the prospective death of their child.

The role of the counsellor

It is useful if the team counsellor can be introduced to the family at an early stage, preferably shortly after the diagnosis has been made. At this stage, the family are unlikely to want or be able to discuss their emotional responses, but will welcome the interest shown by the counsellor and acknowledgment that this is a difficult and painful time. It is not advisable to confront the family with their underlying feelings at this stage as they are likely to back off or become hostile to further approaches. Once treatment is under way, the family will have settled into a routine and will be more receptive to talking about their reactions and feelings. The aims of the counsellor at this stage should be (1) to acknowledge and anticipate on behalf of the family the reactions and feelings they are likely to experience, (2) to facilitate communication between family members and to encourage the expression of their feelings, (3) to educate the parents about the difficulties the child might encounter in coming to terms with the treatment, about how to respond to questions posed by the child and siblings, and (4) to recognize and acknowledge the family's positive qualities and strengths and their ability to cope with the situation.

The family may find it helpful to meet with the counsellor at regular intervals or sometimes only at particularly critical times. Many families, once the child is established in remission, will want to return to as near normal life as possible and will use adaptive denial as a means of coping with the uncertainty ahead. If this is the case, it would perhaps be prudent for the counsellor to withdraw somewhat, as it would not be helpful to the family at this stage to confront them with their underlying anxieties. The critical times at which the counsellor might again become more actively involved are, in the case of a relapse, when the initial feelings of shock and grief may return. In this situation, the counsellor, whilst acknowledging the seriousness of the problem, can enable the family to retain hope. Other critical times are in the event of the child becoming terminally ill or, more hopefully, at the end of the treatment period when the child is well. The counsellor can play a vital role in enabling the family to detach themselves from their dependency on the hospital and staff and begin to re-integrate their lives outside the hospital setting. It is helpful to hold a systems view of family functioning and, from time to time, the counsellor may have to switch attention from working with the whole family, to working with the parents, siblings, sick child or even members of the extended family.

An additional role for the counsellor may be in liaising between the hospital and other agencies. For example, it is very important that the school is kept informed of the child's illness and progress. The teacher will often welcome advice on how to manage the child on return to school, and what expectations to have in terms of behaviour and learning.

The role of play

Much has been written on the role of play in relation to children in hospital. Play is an important aspect of every child's life. It is a preparation for life, giving the child an opportunity to practise and acquire both practical and social skills. Play is also a good indicator of the child's response to life. It is a vehicle through which the child can express his reactions and emotional responses to events. This is particularly important for the child who is undergoing stressful treatment in hospital. Play can be used as a useful tool in preparing the child for treatment, by showing how something will be done, and how bravely the doll can cope. Play can bring more normality into the child's life in hospital, and the playroom can provide a sanctuary away from the ward and clinical procedures.

The play teacher can become friend and counsellor to the child, and will often be the person in whom the child confides. The role of the play leader may extend from providing constructive diversionary activity to facilitating the expression of feelings through use of play A wide variety of play materials, including projective materials, is useful, but the sick child should not be allowed to feel overwhelmed by too much choice or activity.

The adolescent patient has special needs which challenge the play leader. Adolescents often resent the intrusion into their privacy which comes through being in hospital. A separate day room or area for adolescent patients can be very valuable. Access to appropriate music, a computer, cooking facilities or games like snooker are usually appreciated.

PREPARATION FOR TREATMENT

It has long been recognized that admission to hospital and the subjection to hospital treatment procedures and investigations causes considerable distress to young children. Much has been done to alleviate the stress of separation from home and family by admitting children for as short a period of time as possible and by involving parents in their care. In recent years, attention has turned towards examining the stress induced by medical procedures, and how this stress might be ameliorated. Katz and Kellerman[34] found that anxiety in relation to procedures was commonplace amongst hospitalized children and was particularly so in younger children. Younger children also tended to be less inhibited in their reactions to stress and would protest both physically and vocally. Katz et al.[34] also noted a variation in response in girls and boys; girls being more likely to show distress, cry and seek support, while boys would use stalling or delaying tactics. Children who were inquisitive and sought explanations for their treatment had reduced levels of anxiety.

Katz[34] reviews the psychological effects of treatment and a variety of approaches to preparation. She concludes that there is insufficient evidence to suggest the best single method for preparing children for medical treatment. She suggests instead a model which can be adapted to meet any medical event experienced by paediatric cancer patients. The model proposed describes 4 stages: *Stage 1—Introduction and Assessment,* where the child is given information about the medical event and an opportunity to express feelings about it; *Stage 2— Education Session,* where the procedure is explained in detail and is demonstrated to the child using real equipment or play material; again, time is given for the child to express feelings; *Stage 3—Medical Event,* where the preparer continues to explain the procedure, and attempts to include the child in it; *Stage 4—Post Procedure,* where the procedure is discussed and expression of the child's feelings is facilitated with an emphasis on coping and mastering.

Other methods of preparation generally used are information leaflets about procedures, supported by drawings or photographs of equipment. Video recordings of child models undergoing treatment are useful to provide a model for responses, reducing fear and anxiety and increasing co-operation.

The use of relaxation techniques in combination with hypnosis have been generally found to be helpful in the control of pain and management of anticipatory vomiting. Children make very good hypnotic subjects due to their level of trust, vivid imagination and ability to move readily between fantasy and reality. The teaching of auto-hypnotic techniques to children gives them a sense of mastery and control over their bodies, particularly useful to adolescents who strongly resent the loss of control over their lives and bodies as a result of their illness.

THE ROLE OF GROUPS

A number of workers have described the value of group meetings as a means of providing peer group support and education to parents and siblings of child cancer patients. Kellerman[35] described in detail a group for the siblings of children being actively treated for leukaemia and solid tumours. Siblings were selected on the grounds that they were presenting regressive or angry interpersonal behaviour at home, or problems in school. In this way, 10 siblings aged 9–12 years were selected and met together, with two counsellors, for 1½ hours over a period of 5 consecutive weeks. The time was structured into a discussion period, a tour of a hospital area related to treatment of the patient and a light refreshment break. Over the 5-week period, discussion centred on 3 main areas: (1) resentment at the special attention given to the sick child by the parents, and feelings of being neglected or left out by the siblings; (2) embarrassment in discussing the patient's illness and in using taboo words like cancer; (3) variation in levels of learning and knowledge or information about the illness. Kellerman concluded that the sibling group was successful in helping the members define and discuss common problems; in minimizing anxiety and in mobilizing positive coping strategies. Follow-up at one year, in the form of interviews with the parents, confirmed the ongoing positive effects of the group. Attention-seeking behaviour was essentially non-existent either at home or at school and, of major importance, the siblings were able to verbalize their attitudes about the illness and hospital-related matters.

Groups for parents can serve a similar function, giving the parents a forum where they can share their experiences and reactions, along with discussing coping strategies and ways of managing siblings. Parent groups can also be an effective means of educating parents about the illness and its treatment and providing parents with a forum for asking questions without the anxiety that they are encroaching on the clinician's time. It is important to consider the possible negative consequences of groups for parents. There is a danger that the group could be taken over by particularly vocal parents with strong views which are contrary to the majority's beliefs. Also, parents who have had particularly bad or atypical experiences may cause unnecessary anxiety to other parents. In view of these possibilities, it is important that the group is run by workers skilled in group processes as well as being knowledgeable in the field of paediatric oncology. Groups in general should aim to be time-limited and held for a fixed number of sessions. This avoids the danger of parents being too dependent on each other for support and not maintaining normal social supports and relationships in their lives.

In considering psychosocial support and intervention, it is important to acknowledge the needs of the staff who are providing the support to child, patient and family. It can be enormously stressful to work in close contact with the families of seriously ill children. Often, the child and family attend the hospital for treatment over a period of several years and very close relationships with staff can develop. When a child dies, the sense of grief of the staff can be very great. Particularly for the nurses working in the inpatient setting, it is important that they have opportunities to see the children who are progressing well in the outpatient department, as this balances the stress of constantly caring for seriously ill children in the early stages of treatment or relapse.

A staff group can be an effective way of providing a forum for sharing the stress of the work. A group also provides an opportunity to share attitudes and feelings about clinical decisions, and facilitates good communication and understanding within the treatment team. A group which meets regularly and has a stable membership is the most effective, as trust is more readily developed. An outside facilitator to the group is helpful in allowing senior members of the staff to become equal members of the group and not take the role of leader. The facilitator can also bring an independent and objective viewpoint to the discussion.

Although there is much in the literature on methods of psychosocial intervention, there is a relative sparseness of information on the evaluation and effectiveness of intervention. More work needs to be directed into these areas before we can fully justify the setting up of costly intervention programmes, although an intuitive response is that, generally, child and family find such interventions useful and helpful.

TERMINAL CARE

In spite of improvements in survival rates for children suffering from malignant conditions, childhood cancer remains one of the commonest causes of death in childhood. No account of the supportive care of the child with cancer would be complete without consideration of the management of the dying child and his family. Professionals involved in the care of dying children have long debated how much young children are aware of the seriousness of their illness, or how aware they are of the approach of death. Others have debated what the dying child should be told as he approaches death. Should he be protected by a veil of secrecy and silence? In more recent years, attention has turned towards where the child should die, and more children have been allowed to die at home or in the community as opposed to in hospital.

The child's concept of death

Before considering the management of the dying child, it is necessary to understand how children of different ages develop concepts of death. In the healthy child, the concept of death is age-related and depends also on the child's intellectual ability and stage of emotional development. For children in our own western culture, and it is important to recognize that there are cultural differences, the following broad scheme generally applies. The child aged 0–3 years has no understanding of death as conceptualized in adult terms. For the child of this age, it is the threat of separation from the mother or mother figure, and threat of isolation which gives rise to profound anxiety. From the age of 3 years, the majority of children have the word 'dead' as part of their vocabulary and are beginning to develop a curiosity about the concept of death. Very young children will develop an awareness of death through their everyday experiences of living things—plants and animals. Nevertheless, at this age, death remains a very vague concept associated with sleep, loss of movement, darkness; it is not conceptualized as a permanent state or a universal inevitability. The young child's love of cartoon characters who endlessly bounce back to life is perhaps a good illustration of the level of understanding. From the age of 6 years, there is a gradual development of understanding death as a final, irreversible, universal and permanent event. Children from the age of 6 years to adolescence vary widely in their understanding of death. This is based on their everyday experiences, whether they have been involved in a death, and on family attitudes to death. Until the age of about 10 years, there will continue to be uncertainties about death as a process but the child becomes increasingly sophisticated in understanding death as a biological process. From the age of 10 years upwards, the child's cognitive development reaches the stage of adult reasoning and capability of abstract thought. This stage varies considerably with intellectual ability. In general, the young adolescent will have an adult understanding of death as a universal and permanent end to life. An awareness of one's own mortality develops, although the majority of adolescents will defer exploring this issue through the use of denial.

The dying child's awareness of death

In the management of the seriously ill child, the question arises: 'Do seriously or terminally ill children have an awareness of the situation in relation to their level of cognitive development, or do seriously ill children somehow develop an increased awareness of their approaching death?' For many years, it was felt that dying children below the age of 10 years were not aware of their approaching death and, therefore, there was no need to inform them of the reality of their situation. Recent studies have questioned this position and have thrown new light on our understanding. Waechter[36] used projection techniques and a general anxiety scale for children to measure anxiety levels and awareness of death or threat to body integrity in 4 groups of children; those with a fatal illness, those with a chronic but not fatal illness, those with a brief illness and healthy, non-hospitalized children. Waechter concluded that children under the age of 10 years with a potential fatal illness showed higher general levels of anxiety and an increased sense of isolation than children in any of the other groups. She also observed that, where parents had sought to protect their child by avoidance of discussing the diagnosis and its prognosis, the child nevertheless, in some way, perhaps from alteration of parents' behaviour or emotional tone, developed an awareness of the seriousness of the illness, and his imminent death, although this might not have been at a level which could be verbalized.

Spinetta[37] supported these findings in a study of the dying child's sense of isolation using interpersonal distance measured as an indication of sense of isolation. In this study, an experimental group of 25 children with leukaemia, aged 6–10, was compared with a matched group of chronically ill, hospitalized children. The children were asked to place each of 4 significant figures (nurse, mother, father, doctor) at their usual place in a three-dimensional hospital room replica. The leukaemic children consistently placed figures at a greater distance than the control group, giving some indication that the fatally ill child develops a sense of isolation and psychological distance as death approaches. Spinetta suggests a number of possible reasons why the fatally ill child might perceive an increased physical distance between himself and key figures. An awareness of impending death at a preverbal level might lead a child to distance himself. The child might be picking up non-verbal cues from adults around who, aware of the child's approaching death, reduce the frequency and intensity of their physical and verbal contact with the child. Is separation a normal part of preparation for death by the child, as has been observed in adults?

These studies and others give increasing support to the impression that even very young children can have some sense of their impending death, even if they are not able to verbalize it. For the child at this stage, it is perhaps not necessary to confront him with the fact that he is dying, but it is more important to respond to his underlying anxieties, feelings of isolation and threat to body integrity.

Communicating with dying children

A wealth of evidence now exists supporting the belief that children from as young an age as 5–6 years old should be honestly and openly informed of the seriousness of their illness and, when the time comes, the fact that they are dying. We know now that even children who are not informed, in the belief that they are being protected from unnecessary emotional pain or anxiety, in some way work it out for themselves but, because of the conspiracy of silence around them, are left feeling isolated and alone. To talk with a child about the fact that he or she is going to die is far from an easy task and many will prefer to avoid it, or feel unskilled in finding an appropriate language with which to communicate with the child. It is impossible to give a correct solution, or formula, to be used when talking with a dying child. Each child is unique in terms of personality, development and coping skills. Some will want to talk openly about their approaching death, while others will wish to remain silent. Individual differences should be respected and understood. Of prime importance is to talk to the child truthfully and honestly at a level appropriate to the child's level of cognitive and emotional development.

There are some fundamental rules which can facilitate talking with the dying child. Firstly, it is essential to obtain the parents' permission before talking to a child about his death. Some parents will prefer initially to deal with the task of informing their child themselves in their own way. Other parents will prefer to delegate this task to the physician or request that their child should not be informed. The parents' wishes should always be respected, although it is often possible, through support and explanation, to enable parents to change their stance. An understanding and acceptance of the parents' philosophy of life and death is important. Even if the clinician strongly disagrees with the parents' views, this is not the time to challenge them, the aim being more to support the parents and increase their coping skills by exploring with them past experiences of death.

In talking to the child, it is important to listen to his cues about underlying anxieties, and to give information as questions arise, or to watch for non-verbal cues indicating an area of concern. For example, a child saying he will not have another birthday may be asking indirectly how long he has left to live. Children can find it helpful to have it explained to them that death is a natural process that comes to us all. That, although it is a separation, the loss is not complete and, for their families, they will live on as memories and will not be forgotten. The majority of children have some fear of being alone at death and welcome reassurance that they will be supported to the end and not left alone even after death. Another fear is the fear of pain and how they will die. It is reassuring to the child to know that the pain of the dying process will be controlled and that, after death, there will be no pain, their suffering will end.

Older children, in particular, may wish to organize their time in the last weeks, to complete unfinished business or say goodbye to friends. Some children will keep a diary of things they wish to do and complete. This may involve visiting school for the last time, attending a football match or making arrangements for the dispersal of valued possessions. Some children will wish to discuss arrangements for their funeral and burial. Having completed these tasks, it is not unusual for the child to enter rapidly into the terminal phase. Other children will prefer to be less open and may continue their lives as normal within the limits of their condition. With effective management of pain and other symptoms, many children continue to lead a satisfying and happy existence to within days of their death.

There should be no expectation that the child will accept the fact that he is dying without initially being distressed and upset. The child should be told that it is acceptable to feel sad and angry and that it is all right to cry and express the angry feelings. The child should not be forced to talk when he does not wish to, but it is helpful to say that, when he does want to talk, someone will be there to listen. Finally, in communicating with a child about death, what is most important is not what is said but how it is said; the sense of feeling understood and supported is much more important to the child than the words used. To sit in silence, communicating an understanding and care, can mean infinitely more than carefully thought out words said without feeling.

The family of the dying child

For the family of the dying child, the grieving process usually commences when the parents are first told of the diagnosis of a malignant condition. The grieving process goes into abeyance when the child enters remission but generally returns when the child relapses or active treatment is withdrawn, and it is acknowledged that the child will die.

To a varying extent, when informed that there is no further effective treatment available to their child, and that their child should be allowed to die, the parents will enter a phase of anticipatory mourning. Futterman[38] has defined anticipatory mourning as 'a set of processes that are directly related to the awareness of the impending loss, to its emotional impact and to the adaptive mechanisms whereby emotional attachment to the dying child is relinquished over time'. The stages of this process begin with the acknowledgement by the parents that the death of the child is inevitable. Acknowledgement is not instantly complete, but involves a struggle between hope and despair, awareness deepening as the time of death approaches. Acknowledgement is followed by grieving over the expected loss of the child and is accompanied by the physical and psychological manifestations of the grieving process. As the parents come to terms with their grief, a stage of reconciliation follows, where they seek to find strength in viewing the child's life positively. As death approaches, a process of emotional detachment occurs in relation to the child, by which the parents begin to withdraw emotional invest-ment in the child, and come to see him as having no future. This process is often intermittent and interspersed with a clinging dependency on the child. The final stage is one of memorialization, whereby parents develop a relatively fixed, idealized mental representation of the dying child which will endure beyond death.

The course of anticipatory mourning is adaptive in allowing the parents to prepare themselves for the tasks of post-bereavement mourning and in beginning the reinvestment in relationships which will endure beyond the death of the child. It also serves to enable the parents to turn their energies towards supporting and caring for the child during the terminal illness. For the parents to feel that they are involved in their child's care at this time increases their feelings of worth and confidence, giving them more strength to cope with the emotional impact of the loss. The majority of parents prefer their child to die at home rather than in hospital. For the child, it is preferable to be in familiar surroundings where family and friends can offer support, and where the child can continue to live as near normal a life as possible. The parents feel they have more control over the environment and do not have the anxiety that the child will be upset by unnecessary medical interventions at the time of death. The parents are able to spend as much time as they want with the child after death and do not need to feel hurried.

Most parents will require medical and nursing support when the child is to die at home. No parent likes to see their child in pain and will require ready access to pain-relieving drugs and reassessment of needs. A fear often unspoken by parents is how the child will die, what they can expect at the moment of death. It is a great relief to the parents if this fear can be anticipated and the parents told simply how their child is likely to die and what are the signs of imminent death. Preparation in this way avoids the panic of rushing a dying child into hospital because the parents are afraid that they will not be able to cope.

Bereavement reactions following the death of the child
Every family grieves the loss of their child in a unique and individual way; there is no correct formula. The family should be supported in

grieving over their loss in whatever way seems right for them. Some parents will wish the child to remain with them at home until the funeral. It is not unusual for a parent to sleep with the dead child for one or two nights after the death. If possible, siblings should be allowed to be present with the child during the terminal phase and to see their dead brother or sister after death. This helps to dispel any anxieties and fantasies about the death event. The majority of parents welcome an opportunity to meet with the consultant paediatrician a few weeks after the death, to ask questions about the illness, the death and postmortem findings. Parents welcome the continued support and interest shown by the hospital staff following the death of the child. The time of the first anniversary of the death is a very poignant time and the majority of parents will welcome contact at that time. Visiting by the social worker or counsellor for a period of time after the death to give the parents an opportunity to ask questions and share their experience is very important. However, there is a time when the family has to let go of the links with the hospital and begin to reorganize their lives into new avenues. This time of saying goodbye can be difficult for both parents and hospital staff, but is necessary if the family are to proceed normally through the grieving process.

Pathological grief reactions

As already stated, the experience of grief is unique in each family. Variations in the grieving process are enormous and no attempt should be made to force a family to behave differently. It is when the grieving process becomes stuck or the parents fail to complete the individual tasks of grieving that we consider that grief has become pathological in the sense that emotional growth of the family comes to a halt. The 4 tasks of mourning are: (1) to accept the reality of the loss, (2) to experience the pain of grief, (3) to adjust to an environment without the dead child, and (4) to withdraw emotional energy and reinvest it in other relationships. Grief cannot proceed satisfactorily unless each task in turn is dealt with; parents can become stuck at any point in this process. Experience and research show us that the death of a child is the most profound of all grief experiences and is more likely to lead to emotional disturbance than any other form of bereavement. The majority of parents will tell us that they never completely recover from the loss of a valued child, only that as time goes on, the pain lessens.

REFERENCES

1. Rutter M., Tizard J. and Whitmore K. (1970) *Education, Health and Behaviour.* London, Longman.
2. Koocher G. P. and O'Malley J. E. (1981) *Damocles Syndrome.* New York, McGraw Hill.
3. Maguire D. P. (1983) Psychological and social aspects of childhood malignancy. *Ann. Nestle* **41**(2), 32–43.
4. Pearson J. and Dudley H. A. F. (1982) Bodily perceptions in surgical patients. *Br. Med. J.* **284**, 1545–6.
5. Langford W. F. (1948) Physical illness and convalescence: their meaning to the child. *Pediatrics* **33**, 242–50.
6. Brodie B. (1974) Views of healthy children toward illness. *Am. J. Pub. Health* **64**, 1156–9.
7. Bibace R. and Walsh M. E. (1981) Children's conceptions of illness. In: Bibace R. and 'Walsh M. E. (eds.) *New Directions for Child Development* Vol. 14, San Francisco, Jossey-Bass, pp. 31–48.
8. Eiser C. (1985) *The Psychology of Childhood Illness.* New York, Springer-Verlag.
9. Campbell J. D. (1975) Illness is a point of view: the development of children's concepts of illness. *Child Dev.* **46**, 92–100.
10. Millstein S. G., Adler N. E. and Irwin C. E. (1981) Conceptions of illness in young adolescents. *Pediatrics* **68**, 834–9.
11. Beale J. G., Holt P. L. J., Keen J. H. et al. (1983) Children with juvenile chronic arthritis: their beliefs about their illness and therapy. *Ann. Rheum. Dis.* **42**, 481–6.
12. Kendrick C., Culling J., Oakhill A. et al. (1986) Children's understanding of their illness: its treatment within a paediatric oncology unit. *Assoc. Child Psychol. Psychiatry Newsletter* **8**, 2.
13. Maguire P. (1983) *The Psychological Sequelae of Childhood Leukaemia: Recent Results in Cancer Research 88.* Berlin, Springer-Verlag.
14. Mulhern R. K., Crisco J. J. and Camitta B. M. (1981) Patterns of communication among paediatric patients with leukaemia. Parents' and physicians' prognostic disagreements and misunderstandings. *J. Pediatr.* **99**, 480–3.
15. Spinetta J. J. and Maloney L. J. (1975) Death anxiety in the outpatient leukaemic child. *Pediatrics* **56**, 1034–7.
16. Furchgott E. (1963) Behavioural effects of iodizing radiations 1955–61. *Psychol. Bull.* **60**, 157–99.
17. Dobbing J. (1968) Vulnerable periods in the developing brain. In: Davidson A. N. and Dobbing J. (eds.) *Applied Neurochemistry,* Oxford, Blackwell, pp. 287–316.
18. Allen J. C. (1978) The effects of cancer on the nervous system. *J. Pediatr.* **93**, 903–9.
19. Price R. A. and Jamieson P. A. (1975) The central nervous system in childhood leukaemia. II: Subacute leukoencephalopathy. *Cancer* **35**, 306–18.
20. Eiser C. and Lansdown R. (1977) Antrospective study of intellectual development in children treated for acute lymphoblastic leukaemia. *Arch. Dis. Child.* **52**, 525–9.
21. Eiser C. (1980b) How leukaemia affects a child's schooling. *Br. J. Soc. Clin. Psychol.* **19**, 365–8.
22. Jannoun L. (1983) Are cognitive and educational development affected by age at which prophylactic therapy is given in acute lymphoblastic leukaemia? *Arch. Dis. Child.* **58**(12), 953–8.
23. Howarth R. V. (1972) The psychiatry of terminal illness in children. *Proc. R. Soc. Med.* **65**, 1039–40.
24. Slavin M. A., O'Malley J. E., Koocher G. et al. (1982) Communication of the cancer diagnosis to pediatric patients: impact on long-term adjustment. *Am. J. Psychiatry* **139**(2), 179–83.

25. Binger C. M., Ablin A. R., Flurestein R. C. et al. (1959) Childhood leukaemia: emotional impact on patient's family. *N. Engl. J. Med.* **280**, 414–8.
26. Kaplan B. M., Smith A., Grobstein R. et al. (1973) Family mediation of stress. *Soc. Work* **18**, 60–9.
27. Kaplan B. M., Grubstein R. and Smith A. (1976) Predicting the impact of severe illness in families. *Health Soc. Work* **1**, 72–82.
28. Wing J. K., Cooper J. E. and Sartorius N. (1974) *Measurement and Classification of Psychiatry Symptoms.* Cambridge, Cambridge University Press.
29. Clare A. W. and Cairns V. E. (1978) Design, development and use of a standardized interview to assess social maladjustment and dysfunction in community studies. *Psychol. Med.* **8**, 589–604.
30. Lansky S. B., Cairns N. U., Hassanein R. et al. (1978) Childhood cancer: parental discord and divorce. *Pediatrics* **62**, 184.
31. Cairns N. U., Clark G. M., Smith S. D. et al. (1980) Adaptation of siblings to childhood malignancy. *J. Pediatrics* **95**, 485.
32. Tiller J. W. G., Ekert H. and Rickards W. S. (1977) Family reactions in childhood acute lymphoblastic leukaemia in remission. *Aust. Paediatr. J.* **13**, 176–81.
33. Mattson A. (1972) Long-term physical illness in childhood: a challenge to psychosocial adaptation. *Pediatrics* **50**, 801–11.
34. Katz E. R., Kellerman J. and Siegel S. (1980) Behavioural distress in children undergoing medical procedures: developmental considerations. *J. Consult. Clin. Psychol.* **49**(3), 470–1.
35. Kellerman J., Zetter L., Ettenberg L. et al. (1980) Psychological effects of illness in adolescence. I. Anxiety, self-esteem and perception of control. *J. Pediatr.* **97**, 126–31.
36. Waechter E. H. (1971) Children's awareness of fatal illness. *Am. J. Nurs.* 1168–72.
37. Spinetta J. J., Rigler D. and Karon M. (1974) Personal space as a measure of a dying child's sense of isolation. *J. Consult. Clin. Psychol.* **42**, 751–7.
38. Futterman E. J. and Hoffman I. (1973) Crisis and adaptation in families of fatally ill children. In: Anthony E. J. and Koupernick C. (eds.) *The Child in His Family. The Impact of Disease and Death.* New York, Wiley.

14. Terminal Care

P. Ward and A. Oakhill

INTRODUCTION

It is an unfortunate fact that approximately one third of all children presenting with malignant disease will die whilst still within the paediatric age range. A few children die suddenly and unexpectedly in hospital as a result of complications of the disease or its treatment. The majority of deaths, however, are due to uncontrollable malignant disease following unsuccessful attempts at curative treatment. In these circumstances, death is usually predictable and can be prepared for. Following the decision to abandon further curative treatment, a period of 'terminal care' usually follows, during which the emphasis of care changes from cure to the relief of physical, emotional, social and spiritual distress. The duration of such terminal care is extremely variable but is usually measured in weeks rather than days or months.

It is never an easy decision to give up the struggle to save a child's life but, if terminal care is to be successful, it is essential that everyone involved—parents, doctors, nurses and the child himself, if old enough to understand—should accept that further 'curative' treatment is inappropriate. Repeated attempts at experimental treatment only serve falsely to raise hopes of success, may cause further distress to the child, and delay the instigation of effective palliative measures. Conversely, it is not acceptable to permit a child to endure unpleasant symptoms because the decision to withdraw curative treatment has not been made. For example, some doctors may be reluctant to prescribe regular opiate analgesia for children who have not been deemed 'terminal' for fear of inducing opiate addiction.

Even when active cancer therapy has been discontinued, it is never true to say that nothing further can be done. Distressing symptoms can usually be relieved and it is frequently possible to allow the child to return home. With appropriate use of resources and proper use of analgesics and other medication, the child can live his remaining life comfortably and free from pain. For the dying patient is not dead.

Death may be the final event, but dying is part of living and terminal care is concerned not with death itself, nor with the quantity of life remaining. The emphasis should be on the quality of life enjoyed by the patient and on the support of the child's parents and family during this distressing period.

A PLACE TO DIE

Where should the child be cared for during his final illness? A century ago people were born and usually died in their own homes with the majority of care being provided by members of their family. More recently, it has become usual both to be born and to die in hospital, surrounded by professional attendants and with only minimal active participation by relatives. The pendulum is now swinging back.

In a recent unpublished review of 100 consecutive deaths of children with malignant disease under the care of the Bristol paediatric oncology service between 1978 and 1983, 53 died in hospital, 45 died at home, 1 died in a hospice for the terminally ill and 1 was taken on a pilgrimage to India where the child died.

The appointment of a nurse experienced in terminal care in 1983 allowed the expansion of domiciliary care. The improvement in communication with the community services has increased considerably the proportion of children dying at home. We discovered difficulties, however, in knowing the appropriate time to introduce this nurse to the families of children in whom we had decided not to continue with attempts at curative treatment. It seemed a logical step, therefore, to appoint a 'community paediatric oncology nurse' who would be introduced at the time of diagnosis. She is involved in liaising with the community services and the patient's school, continuing the education of parents and patient into the nature of the disease and its treatment and counselling. She is also capable of practical help such as taking blood, care of long lines etc. This role allows her to be accepted early in the management and it therefore allows her more easily to take on the role of co-ordinating terminal care if this becomes necessary.

Following the success of this broader role, in one of our joint clinical services in Gloucestershire, which was charitably funded, it has been decided to appoint similar positions throughout the area covered by the Bristol oncology service. Because of the great distances involved for families to travel, we have for several years used a system of shared care with referring paediatricians. Diagnostic investigations, surgery and intensive therapy is instituted at the central unit, whilst maintenance treatment and follow-up is provided at the referring centre. The appointment of community oncology nurses to each of these centres will, we feel, improve our clinical service considerably.

Most doctors and nurses caring for the dying currently believe that children should have the option to die in their own homes, surrounded by family, friends, pets and familiar belongings. Domiciliary terminal care is not easy, however, and demands enormous support from the community and hospital medical and nursing services. It will not be suitable for all families. Practical problems may be insuperable, for example, if the parents are themselves unwell or possibly if one parent must care for the child without the help and support of a spouse. Some parents feel that they would be unable to continue living in their house after their child had died at home. Undoubtedly most children would prefer to be at home and most parents who choose to nurse their child at home do so because they believe that home is where their child would prefer to be. Practical objections to home care can usually be overcome by the intelligent mobilization of resources but the wishes of the parents should be listened to and they should not be put in a position where they feel compelled to take their child home. In some cases, an alternative to home and hospital may be a hospice. Hospices now commonly care for dying adults and the hospice movement has been responsible for many advances in symptom control. At the time of writing there are very few hospices specializing in the care of children. The best known is Helen House, in Oxford, England, which was the first hospice in the world to be established specifically to look after dying children.[1] The role of hospices in the care of dying children is as yet uncertain. The number of children likely to require hospice care is small and for hospices to care for sufficient patients to maintain and develop their skills they are likely to need large catchment areas. Children and families might then be faced with long journeys and be far from home at a time when they are most likely to need the support of their friends and neighbours. Children's hospices will undoubtedly have a role in the care of some dying children but most are likely to be cared for by the hospital or family doctor services working separately or, preferably, in combination. The work of Helen House is being carefully monitored and the efficacy, advantages and possible undesirable side-effects of hospice care for children are under evaluation. For the time being Baum[2] has urged restraint on those considering the establishment of further hospices for children.

THE ORGANIZATION OF DOMICILIARY TERMINAL CARE

Fortunately, malignant disease in children is relatively rare and it is now uncommon for children to die. This means, however, that outside paediatric oncology departments, doctors and nurses may have little experience of children dying with cancer or leukaemia. It has been estimated that family doctors may only see one or two children with malignancies in the course of their career. Many general practitioners feel that they have insufficient training and experience in caring for terminally ill adults;[3] how must they feel when confronted with a dying child? Even general paediatricians may only see a handful of children with cancer each year so that their experience of terminal care may also be limited. For terminal care to be carried out effectively, therefore, there is the greatest need for flexibility in working practices and traditional barriers between hospital and community care need to be overcome.

Once cancer or leukaemia has been diagnosed, it is not uncommon for the child's family to bypass the family doctor and, instead, turn directly to the hospital for medical advice whether or not their child's current problem is related to the malignancy. Commonly, direct access to the hospital is not inappropriate. For example, when a child receiving chemotherapy or radiotherapy develops a febrile illness, it is vital that the neutrophil count be known before a course of action is decided upon. The danger, however, is that the family doctor may lose contact with the child. It is clearly inappropriate, then, to return the child to the general practitioner for terminal care unless he has been kept informed of progress throughout the entire illness. The success of terminal care, therefore, depends upon communication between the hospital and the family doctor at diagnosis, throughout treatment and, in the event of treatment failure, during the period of terminal care.

In the last few years, the Bristol paediatric oncology service has made strenuous efforts to realize these ideals. At diagnosis, family doctors are sent details of the child's illness, the drugs likely to be used during treatment and the side-effects which might be anticipated. This information is posted whilst the child is still in hospital and is separate from the hospital discharge summary. On several occasions, a member of the oncology team has met with family doctors, either at the hospital or in the surgery, to discuss the case and the organization of care. Letters and discharge summaries are sent out as promptly as possible after each hospital attendance but especially after any new developments or change of treatment. In the event of treatment failure, a member of the oncology team, consultant, senior registrar or clinical assistant, is designated to liaise with the family doctor in the organization and delivery of terminal care. The hospital doctor, community oncology nurse, sometimes accompanied by a medical social worker, visit the child at home and maintain regular contact by telephone. Practical advice concerning, for example, analgesia, may be offered to the family doctor and the hospital is able to act as a resource centre for the provision of certain items of equipment. Day-to-day medical care is provided by the family doctor and his colleagues and practical nursing help is provided by regular visits from the district nursing service. In some areas, MacMillan nurses may be able to provide residential nursing cover. The district nursing service may also be able to supply items of equipment including incontinence pads, sheepskins, ripple beds, bedpans and bottles, hoists and even King's Fund beds. Specialist nursing advice is available from the community oncology nurse, based at the hospital but able to move freely within the community. She has special experience of terminal care and bereavement counselling and is able to offer practical advice and undertake training of health visitors and district nurses in the care of dying children. It is hoped that this combined approach will allow the child to be cared for at home, with the majority of care being provided by the family and the primary health care team but with the experience and resources of the oncology department available to encourage a high standard of terminal care.

Clearly, terminal care at home requires some alteration of roles and working practices. The parents become the principal care-givers, assisted and advised by professionals. In practice, the burden of care usually falls on the mother whilst the father frequently remains in whole-time employment, although this pattern is variable. The parents must accept that their child is dying and they need to realize that a sudden change in the child's condition is not a reason to rush back to the hospital. Hospital and family doctors need to accept the need to work together and not become hidebound by traditional 'territorial disputes'. Physicians need to be flexible in the prescription of drugs, allowing the parents or nurses to vary the dose and scheduling as necessary within previously agreed limits. All of the key personnel involved, the child, parents, doctors and nurses, must see home care as being desirable. The commonest causes of failure are the fear of uncontrollable symptoms, especially pain, ambivalence by the parents, lack of co-operation by doctors and lack of flexibility by nurses.[4]

How does home care work in practice? Martinson et al.[4] studied 32 families with a child aged less than 17 years who was dying with cancer. The majority of the nursing care was given by the parents under the guidance of one or two nurses who were available on 24-hour call. The nurses instructed the parents in specific practical procedures and performed any which the parents were unable to manage. Specialized equipment was provided by the nurses who also acted as intermediaries between the family and the physician in obtaining medication. When the child died, the nurses assisted the family with the necessary formalities and maintained contact with the parents afterwards to provide bereavement counselling. The mean age of the children studied was 8.7 years with a range from 1 month to 17 years. Twenty-seven of the 32 children died at home. Five were readmitted and died in hospital. The period of terminal care, defined as the interval between entry into the study and death, was variable with a median of 20 days and a range from 2 to 104 days. Equipment and supply needs included bedpans, basins, ripple beds, wheelchairs and hospital beds. A few children required more specialized equipment including home oxygen, urinary catheters, suction machines and intravenous equipment. The principal needs were for incontinence pads and oral hygiene packs. Analgesics were used by 18 children, 10 needed opiates, either morphine or methadone, and 19 received tranquillizers or sedatives. Of the 5 children who died in hospital, 2 were admitted for pain control, 1 because of bleeding and 1 because of a painful, non-healing wound that distressed her parents. Similar experiences have been reported by Lauer and Camitta.[5]

Kohler and Radford[6] described their experience with 18 children who had died from cancer. The mean age at death was 5 years 11 months. All the families decided to take their child home after curative treatment had been stopped. In most cases the quality of life during terminal care was described as 'good'. Six children experienced pain which was subsequently controlled in 5 with oral medication. Fifteen children received diamorphine elixir. Gastrointestinal problems included mainly anorexia and constipation. A third of patients had respiratory problems and 2 children had bleeding problems, one melaena and the other haematuria. Three children suffered from seizures. Of the 18 children, 13 died at home, 4 eventually died in hospital and 1 died in a hospice. Two children were readmitted at their parents' request and the remainder because of uncontrollable symptoms. Fourteen families needed special equipment, particularly sheepskins and wheelchairs. Seventeen of the 18 children died following a period of progressive deterioration so that death was not unexpected. Half of the families believed that their family doctor was medically in charge whilst the other half maintained contact with the hospital.

THE DESIRABILITY OF DOMICILIARY CARE

Home care for dying children is clearly a feasible option but is it desirable?

It is easy to believe that the dying child may benefit from being nursed at home. Home is the normal place for a child to live and it seems the natural place for him to die. Simply being at home seems to bring some relief from stress and may help to raise the child's tolerance of symptoms. After a prolonged course of anti-cancer treatment, some children may develop a morbid fear of hospitals and they may even minimize their symptoms for fear of being readmitted for further treatment. Most children old enough to express an opinion prefer to be cared for at home if the option is available. Similarly, most parents will select home care because they believe that their child would prefer to be at home. However, the death of the child in the home has implications for other members of the family, especially parents and siblings.

Whilst a child is being nursed in hospital, the role of the parents is traditionally a passive one. Most of the care is provided by the nurses. Parents have little direct control over the immediate environment and feelings of helplessness are common. In Martinson's series,[4] one reason given by parents for choosing home care was that it enabled them to be actively involved in caring for the child and gave them constant and unrestricted access. One tentative finding of this study was that parents who participated in home care returned to 'normal' sooner after the child's death than parents of children who died in hospital. This view is supported by Lauer et al.[7] who found that parental adaptation following home care appeared to be more favourable than following terminal care and death in hospital. Parents who had cared for their dying child at home had more positive views of the ways in which the death had affected their marriage, social reorientation, religious beliefs and views on the meanings of life and death. There was a significant reduction in parental guilt feelings during the home care experience which was maintained 6 and 12 months following the child's death. In contrast, parents whose child was cared for in hospital reported increased feelings of guilt during their child's terminal hospitalization which were unresolved 12 months after the child's death.

Domiciliary terminal care must inevitably result in some disruption of normal family routine and functioning. However, it is unlikely that hospital care would be less disruptive with the attendant demands of frequent hospital visiting or residence. Where hospitals serve a large geographical area, one parent may remain at the hospital whilst the other stays at home, perhaps many miles away, with the rest of the family. At least with home care all the family can be together at the time when they need mutual support and companionship.

Parents' greatest fears about terminal care at home relate to difficulties in controlling symptoms, especially pain, lack of co-operation by medical and nursing staff and anxieties about the events at the time of death and immediately afterwards. If these fears can be anticipated and allayed, most parents will select home care for their child if the option is offered.

Another implication of domiciliary terminal care which must be considered is the effect of the child's death on siblings. It is inevitable that siblings will be distressed by the death of a brother or sister, but there is evidence to suggest that the incidence of abnormal reactions is reduced when the child dies at home. In a moving article written by a paediatrician and the parents of a boy who died with a Wilms' tumour, Cotton et al.,[8] relating their personal experiences, maintained that there were clear benefits for the other children in the family resulting from their inclusion in the preparations for their brother's death and in the process of bereavement which followed. The siblings were involved with the care of the boy throughout his final illness and were frequently able to play with him on his bed. When he died they were able to say goodbye to him and afterwards were able to share in grieving with their parents. They were subsequently able to talk freely with parents, teachers and peers about what had happened. Martinson et al.[4] reported that siblings were not adversely affected by the terminal care and death of a brother or sister at home. Short-term disruption of schooling, conflicts over feelings towards the dead sibling and a need for reassurance that they themselves were not going to die were common but no long-term reactions were observed. This is in contrast to the siblings of children who died from leukaemia in hospital where behavioural problems, including severe enuresis, headaches, poor school performance, school phobia, depression, severe separation anxieties and persistent abdominal pains were present in one or more siblings in half a series of 20 families reported by Binger et al.[9]

Domiciliary terminal care seems, therefore, to be both feasible and desirable. There appear to be advantages for the child, his parents and his siblings. It is also cheaper. Martinson et al.[4] estimated that the mean cost of home care for their 27 children was $827 compared with $13 022 for hospital care (1978 figures).

SYMPTOM CONTROL FOR DYING CHILDREN

The relief of pain

Although not all children with advanced cancer or leukaemia suffer from severe pain, it is the symptom most dreaded by parents. The incidence of pain in children dying with malignant disease is difficult to determine but in one series (Kohler and Radford)[6] 6 of 18 children suffered from pain. This is comparable to the 34 per cent incidence of moderate to severe pain in adults with advanced cancer described by Woodbine.[10]

The principles of pain control include accurate assessment of the cause and severity of symptoms, regular use of an adequate dose of an effective analgesic, and regular review of the efficacy of treatment.

The commonest reasons for failure include inability to recognize that the child is in pain, underestimation of severity, reluctance to use opiate analgesics for fear of causing addiction and failure to review efficacy frequently and alter the dose or treatment if necessary.

The aetiology of cancer pain

The cause of cancer pain may be directly related to the tumour itself, a consequence of previous anti-cancer treatment, or coincidental and unrelated to the malignancy. It has been estimated that 75 per cent of cancer pain in adults is due to the tumour and 20 per cent is due to previous treatment. Cancer may cause pain by compression or invasion of pain-sensitive structures such as bone, nerves and visceral organs. Pain due to treatment may follow surgery, chemotherapy or radiotherapy. Damage to nerves at operation may result in numbness, dysaesthesiae, paraesthesiae or shooting pains. The problem of phantom limb pains in amputees is well known. Vincristine and vinblastine can cause peripheral neuropathy which may present with pain in the hands, feet and jaw. Methotrexate may produce mucous membrane ulceration which may be painful. Radiation necrosis or post-irradiation scarring may produce burning pain resulting from deafferentation. Not all symptoms experienced by the child dying with cancer are attributable to the malignancy or its treatment. Immobility may lead to pressure sores, constipation or urinary retention, all of which may be uncomfortable. Even children with cancer may suffer from tension headaches or otitis media!

Assessment of pain

As in all fields of medicine, careful assessment should precede treatment. This is particularly true of cancer pain since symptoms of different aetiologies may require different approaches to treatment.

It is not always obvious that a child is in pain. Older children are usually able to report their pain but young, prelingual children are dependent on their caregivers, usually the parents, to recognize their distress. Eland[11] has described some of the difficulties and misconceptions surrounding the assessment of children's pain. These include the myth that children's nervous systems are different from adults' such that they do not feel pain with the same intensity and the false belief that an active child cannot be in pain. Certainly, restlessness, apathy, refusal to eat or participate in normal activities may indicate that the child is in pain but some children remain active as a way of escaping from their symptoms or of denying their presence. Children do not always tell the truth about their pain. They may deny its presence for fear of the consequences if the response is a pain-relieving injection. When the onset of pain is gradual, children may sometimes not appreciate how much pain they have until it has been relieved and they realize how much better they feel.

Adults may have difficulty describing the nature and severity of their pain. Children may be unable to describe their pain but may be able to say whether it is a 'big hurt' or a 'little hurt' and point to where it is worst.

To try to overcome these difficulties, a number of techniques of pain assessment has been devised. The Eland Color Tool uses body outlines on which the child indicates where and how much they hurt by drawing with different coloured crayons.[11] The child is asked to imagine the worst pain he has ever experienced and choose a coloured crayon which he feels best represents that feeling. A further 3 colours are chosen to represent pain of decreasing intensity with the 4th crayon representing freedom from pain. The crayons are then used by the child to draw on the body outline indicating areas of severe, moderate, mild and no pain. The language used to present the Color Tool to the child is chosen to be appropriate to his level of understanding. Another approach is the use of visual linear analogue scales. One end of a 10cm line represents freedom from pain whilst the other represents the worst pain imaginable. The patient makes a mark on the line at the position which he feels best represents his current pain. This technique may be usable by older children and provides a semiquantitative measure which may be useful in serial assessments. It does not, of course, give any indication of the site of the pain. Savedra et al.[12] have concentrated on the language children use to describe their pain. They found that children aged 9–12 years were able to describe pain clearly with no appreciable differences by age groups within the limited age range studied. Levine and Gordon[13] have studied pain-induced vocalization in prelingual children and have confirmed what every mother and children's nurse knows, that is that the cries of stress, hunger and pain are distinguishable both aurally and spectrographically. Another approach is to use the patient's spontaneous behaviour as an indicator of his symptoms. Richards et al.,[14] describing the UAB Pain Behaviour Scale, scored such items as vocal complaints, 'down time', facial grimaces, standing posture, mobility, body language, use of visible supportive equipment and medication. Although standardized for adults, this approach could be adapted for children. Finally, a method used in adults, and possibly useful for older children and adolescents, is a pain questionnaire such as the McGill pain questionnaire.[15]

Many of the techniques described above are used informally, consciously or subconsciously, in the clinical assessment of children in pain by doctors, nurses and parents. An experienced children's nurse or the child's mother will usually 'know' when the child is in pain although sometimes the parents may have never seen a child in pain before and will rely on professionals to recognize their child's distress. Formal clinical assessment should follow the traditional approach of history, examination and investigation. The history will include details of site, intensity, radiation and aggravating and relieving factors and will be considered in the knowledge of the underlying malignancy and its distribution. Should investigations be necessary, they should be performed with sedation, local or general anaesthesia, if there is any likelihood of the procedure causing discomfort. If the child is carefully assessed, it should usually be possible to determine the probable cause of pain and decide upon a management strategy likely to succeed in its relief.

Management of pain

Chronic pain in terminally ill children may be persistent, unremitting, and come to dominate the entire attention of the child and those around him. The object of treatment is to relieve pain and then prevent its return so that the fear of pain may be allowed to subside. In some situations, specific measures will be required and these will be considered later. Frequently, treatment will revolve around the use of non-specific analgesics.

General principles

Route of administration

Cancer pain can usually be controlled with oral medication and this should be the route of first choice. Many children cannot or will not swallow tablets but most analgesics are available in liquid formulations. Occasionally, oral drugs cannot be used because of drowsiness, malabsorption, dysphagia or stubbornness! In this situation some analgesics, particularly morphine, may be administered as suppositories. Traditionally, the rectal route has not been popular in Great Britain but it is widely used elsewhere. We have found children to be surprisingly accepting of suppositories provided they are lubricated with water soluble jelly and inserted gently after carefully explaining what is to happen. Parents may initially find the procedure distasteful but they are usually able to insert the suppositories after a few demonstrations by the nurses.

Parenteral analgesics may occasionally be needed but can usually be avoided. Intramuscular injections are painful, may lead to haematoma formation if the child is thrombocytopenic, and should not be used. Subcutaneous injections and infusions are a more suitable alternative. Small, battery driven syringe drivers are available to deliver analgesic solutions through fine gauge 'butterfly' needles into the subcutaneous tissues of, for example, the abdomen. This technique is well established in other areas of medicine and seems to be suitable for the administration of opiate analgesics.[16] There may be problems, however, in children who have anaemia and oedema when there may be poor absorption from the subcutaneous site. Intravenous injections are not usually practicable for home use because of the difficulties of securing and maintaining venous access. However, an increasing number of children with cancer have tunnelled central venous catheters inserted for blood sampling and the administration of chemotherapy. Parents become very adept at caring for central venous catheters and, if they are still in situ when curative treatment is discontinued, they may offer a more practicable route for the administration of intravenous drugs. If venous access can be secured, Miser et al.[17] have demonstrated that continuous morphine infusions are effective and may be preferable to intermittent bolus injections.

Scheduling of analgesics

There is no place for 'as required' or 'PRN' prescriptions in the management of terminal cancer pain. Analgesics must be prescribed and administered regularly. The next dose should be given before the previous one has worn off in order to prevent the pain returning. Only in this way can the child's fear of the pain be abolished. Provided that a sufficient dose of an appropriate drug is used, it should not be necessary to give analgesics more frequently than 4-hourly. Should pain return before the next dose is due, the child should not be kept waiting. An additional, larger dose should be given immediately or a more potent analgesic may be substituted. Initially, a period of 'dose finding' is likely to be necessary but it should be possible rapidly to find a regime which provides freedom from pain for at least 4 hours at a time. Newer, sustained release analgesics are available which may reduce the frequency of drug administration. They will not be suitable for everyone, however, since they offer less flexibility than the shorter acting liquid formulations and may be more difficult to titrate against the child's pain, particularly if it is rapidly evolving. They are useful at night, however, perhaps allowing undisturbed sleep for the child and his parents. If sustained-release formulations are used, then a supply of a rapidly acting analgesic should also be available for the prompt relief of breakthrough pain should it occur.

Regular assessment

It is not sufficient to prescribe an analgesic and assume that the pain will be relieved. It is essential that the efficacy of treatment is repeatedly reviewed. Initially, this will mean reviewing the child after each dose before the next one is given. If pain control is unsatisfactory, it will be necessary to increase the dose, change to a more potent analgesic or consider some alternative measure. Success depends on attention to detail and a flexible approach to management.

Additional measures

Although analgesics are the mainstay of pain relief, additional measures are sometimes required. Palliative oncological treatments may play a role in the relief of symptoms. Radiotherapy is particularly effective for the relief of bone pain due to leukaemic infiltration and neuroblastoma. Intrathecal methotrexate may rapidly relieve headache due to meningeal leukaemia. When palliative radiotherapy or chemotherapy is employed, care should be taken to ensure that the treatment is not more unbearable than the symptoms. Nausea and vomiting in particular should be managed aggressively rather than expectantly.

Many hospitals offer a pain relief service staffed by anaesthetists with a special interest. The services of such a clinic can be invaluable. We have witnessed spectacular results with local anaesthetic or phenol nerve blocks and long-term epidural analgesia. The use of transcutaneous nerve stimulators by children has been reported by Mannheimer and Lampe[18] who found them to be useful and liked by the children. When these physical methods of pain control are successful, it is frequently possible to reduce the dose of analgesics or even discontinue them completely.

Distraction

Play and diversional activity may be useful in diverting the child's attention away from his symptoms and improving morale. In hospital, a play leader, occupational therapist or nursery nurse may be available to organize recreational activities and the hospital teacher may be able to continue some form of schoolwork. If the child is cared for at home, it is not inappropriate for him to go to school so long as he is able. The social contact of school attendance is important in maintaining as normal a life as possible. Once school attendance becomes impracticable, visits from schoolfriends and teachers maintain contact and help to reduce feelings of isolation. Even when the child is confined to bed, he may still be able to play with his siblings and take part in family activities.[8]

Choice of analgesics

Pharmacopoeias list a great variety of different analgesics but not all

Table 14.1. Analgesics for routine use in the management of cancer pain in children

Drug	Presentation	Dosage (4-hourly)		
Paracetamol	tablets 500mg soluble tablets 500mg liquid 120mg/5ml liquid 240mg/5ml	< 1 year 25mg/kg 1–5 years 240mg 6–12 years 250–500mg		
Dihydrocodeine	tablets 30mg liquid 10mg/5ml injection 50mg/ml	1mg/kg		
Diamorphine	tablets 10mg liquid 5mg/5ml injection 5, 10 and 30mg amps	Oral: Parenteral:	1–7 years 7–12 years > 12 years 0·1mg/kg	1–2·5mg 2–5mg 5–10mg

are suitable for terminal care. We believe that it is better to be thoroughly familiar with a small number of drugs and we have therefore deliberately restricted our choice of analgesics for routine use. The initial choice will depend on the clinical situation and the apparent cause and intensity of the pain. If there is any doubt, it is more humane to overestimate the severity of the symptoms and begin with a strong analgesic rather than work through a hierarchy of increasingly potent drugs whilst the child remains in distress. Failure to adopt an aggressive approach to pain control may result in the child and parents losing confidence in their physician and in their own ability to cope.

When pain is considered to be moderate or severe, there is really no alternative to opiate analgesics. Paracetamol and sometimes aspirin are usually sufficiently potent to control mild pain. Although a number of analgesics of intermediate potency are marketed, few are really suitable for the relief of chronic cancer pain. Many doctors feel that there is no need for an intermediate drug and if simple analgesics fail, then opiates should be commenced. Of the various alternatives available, we have selected dihydrocodeine as our intermediate drug of first choice. *Table* 14.1 offers suggested initial doses of the drugs we use routinely. The final doses will be found by titrating the dose against the child's symptoms.

Simple analgesics
Paracetamol is the most widely used simple analgesic in children. the proprietary formulations 'Calpol' and 'Calpol 6 Plus' (Wellcome Foundation Ltd) seem to be more palatable and cause vomiting less frequently than paracetamol elixir BP. Aspirin is useful for the relief

of bone pain, probably because of its anti-inflammatory action. Special care is needed in thrombocytopaenic children as bleeding may occur. Because of an epidemiological association with Reye's syndrome, aspirin is now contraindicated for the relief of pain and fever in children under 12 years of age.

Intermediate analgesics

Dihydrocodeine is available as tablets, elixir and injection. The elixir is rather unpalatable and many children will not take it. Being a weak opiate, dihydrocodeine frequently causes constipation when taken regularly. A laxative should be prescribed routinely. Pethidine and pentazocine have no place in the management of chronic pain because of their short duration of action and, in the usual oral dose, are ineffective.

Buprenorphine initially seems to be an attractive intermediate analgesic because of the ease of administration by the sublingual route. However, this drug binds strongly to opiate receptors rendering them inaccessible to other, more potent opiates. It is only partly reversed by naloxone. The authors experienced great difficulty in relieving the abdominal pain of a boy with a gastric lymphoma in whom sublingual buprenorphine did not provide relief and rendered other opiates ineffective for many days afterwards. Whilst buprenorphine may be effective in some patients, we would counsel special care in its use, particularly if the child's pain is still increasing in intensity.

Opiate analgesics

The most widely used opiate analgesics are morphine and diamorphine; both are suitable for terminal care. Diamorphine is not available in some countries and morphine has become the drug of choice in many centres. However, provided equianalgesic doses are used, they are equally effective in relieving chronic pain. Orally administered, diamorphine is metabolized to morphine and 6-acetyl morphine.[19] The main differences between the two drugs are solubility and potency.

Diamorphine is more soluble than morphine and is consequently more suitable for parenteral use. Oral diamorphine is 1·5 times as potent as oral morphine, therefore 1mg oral diamorphine has the analgesic effect of 1·5mg oral morphine. Parenteral diamorphine is twice as effective as parenteral morphine; 1mg parenteral diamorphine has the analgesic effect of 2mg parenteral morphine. The bioavailability of oral diamorphine is half that of parenteral diamorphine, therefore to obtain the same analgesic effect, the dose should be doubled if changing from parenteral to oral diamorphine.

To avoid confusion and reduce the likelihood of mistakes being made when changing from one drug or route to another, we usually use diamorphine both orally and parenterally.

Oral diamorphine is best administered in simple solution in water or chloroform water which acts as a preservative to prolong the stability of the solution. The traditional 'Brompton's cocktail' of morphine or diamorphine, cocaine, chlorpromazine and alcohol, is no longer considered appropriate. Children frequently dislike the taste of alcohol and cocaine and chlorpromazine may have adverse central side-effects which are inappropriately attributed to the opiate.[20] Diamorphine solution can be made up in an initial concentration of 5mg in 5ml and the concentration may be increased as necessary. The solution may be flavoured with fruit juice or squash according to the child's taste. The potency of the solution may diminish with storage. It may be necessary to reduce the dose slightly when a fresh solution is dispensed, otherwise unexpected drowsiness may occur.

Morphine may also be administered in simple solution and is also available as sustained-release tablets and suppositories. The sustained-release preparation (MST Continus, Napp Laboratories Ltd) is available in 10, 30, 60 and 100mg tablets. When changing from diamorphine or morphine solution to sustained-release tablets the same total dose of morphine should be given, divided between the morning and evening doses. Peak plasma free morphine concentrations are not achieved until 3–4 h after taking sustained-release morphine tablets. It is wise, therefore, to have an opiate solution available for the rapid relief of breakthrough pain should it occur. If morphine or diamorphine cannot be given by mouth, then morphine is commercially available as 15mg and 30mg suppositories. Hospital pharmacies may be able to prepare other strengths. If changing from oral diamorphine to rectal morphine, the dose of morphine should be 1·5 times the previous dose of diamorphine to achieve the same effect.

Both morphine and diamorphine may be given by injection. Miser et al.[16,17] have reported the use of continuous intravenous and subcutaneous infusions of morphine in children with cancer pain and have found both methods to be effective and well tolerated.

Adverse effects of opiate and analgesics

Constipation is an almost inevitable consequence of regular opiate administration. This problem should be anticipated and ameliorated by the routine prescription of a laxative. One approach is to use lactulose and sennakot to soften the stools and stimulate colonic motility respectively. Lactulose may be diluted in unsweetened orange juice or grapefruit juice to reduce the sweetness which some children may find nauseating. Many patients may also need bisacodyl (Dulcolax) suppositories from time to time.

Nausea and vomiting are not a frequent problem in children receiving morphine or diamorphine. If vomiting develops, another cause, for example intestinal obstruction or raised intracranial pressure, should be searched for. If symptomatic relief is necessary, a variety of drugs are available. Chlorpromazine has a small incidence of extrapyramidal reactions but is sedative which may or may not be desirable depending on the clinical situation. Prochlorperazine and metoclopramide are less sedative but have a higher incidence of dystonic reactions. Domperidone rarely causes adverse central effects and can be given orally or rectally.

Drowsiness frequently occurs when morphine or diamorphine are first administered. This effect is usually temporary and declines as tolerance develops. It is wise to warn parents that the child may be sleepy initially, otherwise they may fear that pain relief can only be provided at the cost of impaired consciousness. It is usually possible to find a dose which provides relief from pain without clouding the sensorium excessively. When the dose of opiates is increased, there may be a temporary recurrence of drowsiness until the child becomes accustomed to the new dose.

For whatever reason, physicians seem to be more reluctant to prescribe opiates for children than for adults.[21] One possible reason is the fear of causing opiate addiction.[22] All narcotic analgesics given regularly for a period of time will result in the development of tolerance and physical dependence. Tolerance is the phenomenon whereby an increasing dose is required to obtain the same effect. Tolerance to both the analgesic and respiratory depressant effects of opiates develops with regular usage. However, tolerance to central nervous system excitation does not develop,[23] so that somnolence and respiratory compromise do not present practical problems when narcotic analgesics are administered regularly to control chronic pain. When commencing treatment, it is commonly necessary to increase the initial dose of analgesia but a plateau is usually reached where further increments are not required unless the clinical state changes. It is sometimes possible to reduce the dose once the child gains in confidence and loses the fear of his pain. If narcotics are suddenly withdrawn after a period of regular administration, the patient is likely to experience a number of unpleasant symptoms. However, these can usually be avoided or minimized if narcotics are withdrawn slowly, possibly temporarily substituting a less potent narcotic during the withdrawal phase.[24] Addiction may be defined as a 'behavioural pattern of compulsive drug use, characterized by overwhelming involvement with the use of a drug, the securing of its supply, and a high tendency to relapse after withdrawal'.[25] Thus defined, addiction appears to be extremely uncommon in patients receiving opiates for pain relief. Porter and Jick[26] reviewed the records of 11 882 adult patients receiving narcotics during general hospitalization. Only 4 cases of documented addiction were recorded in patients who did not have a prior history of addiction.

The management of some specific pain syndromes

Bone pain
Several childhood malignancies may invade bone in their advanced stages. Leukaemia and neuroblastoma are notable examples. The character of the pain varies with site but is generally constant and progressively increases in severity. Narcotic analgesics alone frequently fail to control the pain completely. Non-steroidal, anti-inflammatory analgesics are frequently effective, possibly as a result of the inhibition of prostaglandin synthesis. This is one situation where aspirin is likely to be useful, possibly given in combination with a narcotic analgesic. An alternative approach is to use palliative radiotherapy which can be dramatically effective in relieving bone pain due to leukaemic infiltration and neuroblastoma.

Nerve and nerve root invasion
Peripheral nerve and nerve root invasion results in a constant burning pain occurring in the area served by the involved nerve. The anti-inflammatory effects of corticosteroids, prednisolone or dexamethasone may be effective by reducing perineural oedema and diminishing the pressure on the nerve. Occasionally, a nerve block may be necessary.

Raised intracranial pressure
Raised intracranial pressure due to an intracranial tumour or malignant meningitis may present with unremitting headache exacerbated by movement, coughing and sneezing. The misery may be compounded by vomiting and drowsiness. Corticosteroids are frequently effective in reducing cerebral oedema surrounding the tumour and therefore reducing intracranial pressure. Unfortunately, Cushing's syndrome and excessive weight gain are a real problem. If the interval between commencing steroid therapy and the child's death is long, increasing obesity exacerbates the difficulties of nursing the child, especially at home. High doses of dexamethasone or betamethasone should be given initially to obtain relief and then the dose should be reduced to the smallest effective. Raised intracranial

pressure due to leukaemic infiltration of the meninges may be relieved by intrathecal methotrexate.

OTHER COMMON SYMPTOMS

Anxiety and sleeplessness

Much can be done by communication without the use of specific anxiolytic drugs. Children and parents may have misconceptions and unwarranted fears about their illness and symptoms. Parents are particularly likely to be frightened of the events surrounding the moment of death itself. If pain is effectively relieved, the child and parents may be able to focus on their other worries and opportunities for discussion should be made available. If discussion does not bring relief of anxiety then anxiolytic drugs may be appropriate. Chlorpromazine is a useful drug in children but excessive dosage may result in drowsiness and extrapyramidal reactions. The benzodiazepines may be helpful. Diazepam may be given by mouth or rectally. Temazepam has a short period of action and may be particularly useful for the relief of insomnia without leaving a hangover effect the following morning. Alternative drugs for insomnia include chloral hydrate, promethazine hydrochloride and trimeprazine.

Depression

Depression in children generally improves with improved well-being, the relief of physical symptoms and the improved morale of parents and caregivers. Attention should be paid to the relief of physical and emotional distress and the facilitation of communication. Diversional activity, such as play, is important. Sometimes tricyclic antidepressant drugs may be helpful. Small doses of amitriptyline or imipramine may be prescribed, the dosage being increased gradually as necessary. These drugs are potentiated by chlorpromazine and, in larger doses, may produce confusion.

Dyspnoea

Dyspnoea should be treated symptomatically according to the perceived cause. Bronchospasm, for example, should be treated with bronchodilators in the usual way. Whether or not to treat pneumonia with antibiotics is always a subject for discussion. Antibiotics may possibly prolong life a little but do not, of course, influence the underlying malignancy. The guiding principle should be the relief of symptoms. If physiotherapy and antibiotics are likely to make the dying child more comfortable then they should not be withheld. On the other hand, if the child is too ill to be discomforted by his infection, then antibiotics are inappropriate. The same principles should apply to the treatment of urinary tract infections. Opiates are useful in relieving the subjective appreciation of breathlessness without causing marked respiratory depression.

Skin ulceration

Prevention of pressure sores depends on meticulous nursing care and the use of aids such as sheepskins and ripple mattresses. Even with very high standards of nursing care, pressure sores may develop in immobile patients. They are likely to heal very slowly, if at all. Skin sepsis can be treated locally with dressings and cleansing agents such as eusol or systemic antibiotics may be prescribed if necessary. Foul-smelling lesions may be infected with anaerobic organisms and may respond to treatment with metronidazole or augmentin (amoxycillin plus clavulanic acid).

Death rattle

In the last few hours, the accumulation of saliva in the mouth and pharynx results in an unpleasant bubbling sound which, although of no consequence to the child who is usually unconscious, is extremely distressing to the parents. Subcutaneous injections of hyoscine are useful in drying up the secretions and reducing the rattle. The injections may be repeated 4–6-hourly if necessary. Atropine may also be used but is less effective.

CONCLUSION

The management of terminal illness in adults has been greatly advanced by the research and teaching of the hospice movement, but terminal care in children has only recently received major attention. Many of the principles of care employed in adults are also applicable to the management of children. Because children rarely die, few doctors or nurses have experience of caring for dying children. There remains a need for greater co-operation between hospital and community teams to ensure that these children receive the best possible care during their final illness. Given the combined support of the oncology team and the primary health care team, it should be possible for the majority of children with advanced cancer to be cared for in their own homes.

All doctors and nurses working with dying children need to be aware of the principles of management of chronic pain. We should not let our prejudices and unwarranted fears of addiction prevent us from using the potent analgesics which are most likely to bring our patients relief.

Caring for dying children and their families is a major source of stress for the professional teams who themselves need support. This may be provided in part by free discussion between members of the team and some departments have established staff support groups often led by a psychologist or psychiatrist whose role is the facilitation of communication.

The death of a child with cancer is always a time for sorrow. However, with skilful treatment, the child can be kept pain-free and capable of enjoying his life during his final illness.

REFERENCES

1. Burne S. R. (1984) A hospice for children in England. *Pediatrics* **73**, 97–8.
2. Baum J. D. (25 March, 1986) Making a case for child hospices. *The Times,* London.
3. Haines A. and Booroff A. (1986) Terminal care at home: perspective from general practice. *Br. Med. J.* **292**, 1051–3.
4. Martinson I. M., Armstrong G. D., Geis D. P. et al. (1978) Home care for children dying of cancer. *Pediatrics* **62**, 106–13.
5. Lauer M. E. and Camitta B. M. (1980) Home care for dying children: a nursing model. *J. Pediatr.* **97**, 1032–5.
6. Kohler J. A. and Radford M. (1985) Terminal care for children dying of cancer: quantity and quality of life. *Br. Med. J.* **291**, 115–16.
7. Lauer M. E., Mulhern R. K., Wallskog J. M. et al. (1983) A comparison study of parental adaptation following a child's death at home or in the hospital. *Pediatrics* **71**, 107–12.
8. Cotton M., Cotton G. and Goodall J. (1981) A brother dies at home. *J. Matern. Child Health* **6**, 288–92.
9. Binger C. M., Abling A. R., Feuerstein R. C. et al. (1969) Childhood leukaemia: emotional impact on patient and family. *N. Engl. J. Med.* **280**, 414–18.
10. Woodbine G. (1982) The care of patients dying from cancer. *J. R. Coll. Gen. Pract.* **32**, 685–9.
11. Eland J. (1985) The child who is hurting. *Sem. Oncol. Nurs.* **1**, 116–22.
12. Savedra M., Gibbons P., Tesler M. et al. (1982) How do children describe pain? A tentative assessment. *Pain* **14**, 95–104.
13. Levine J. D. and Gordon N. C. (1982) Pain in prelingual children and its evaluation by pain-induced vocalization. *Pain* **14**, 85–93.
14. Richards J. S., Nepomuceno C., Riles M. et al. (1982) Assessing pain behaviour: the UAB pain behaviour scale. *Pain* **14**, 393–8.
15. Melzack R. (1975) The McGill Pain Questionnaire: major properties and scoring methods. *Pain* **1**, 227–99.
16. Miser A. W., Davis D. M., Hughes C. S. et al. (1983) Continuous subcutaneous infusion of morphine in children with cancer. *Am. J. Dis. Child.* **137**, 383–5.
17. Miser A. W., Miser J. S. and Clark B. S. (1980) Continuous intravenous infusion of morphine sulfate for control of severe pain in children with terminal malignancy. *J. Pediatr.* **96**, 930–2.

18. Mannheimer J. and Lampe G. (1984) *Clinical Transcutaneous Electrical Nerve Stimulation*. Philadelphia, Davis.
19. Inturrisi C. E., Max M. B., Foley K. M. et al. (1984) The pharmacokinetics of heroin in patients with chronic pain. *N. Engl. J. Med.* **310**, 1213–17.
20. Twycross R. G. (1979) The Brompton Cocktail. In: Bonica J. J. and Ventafridda V. (eds.) *Advances in Pain Research and Therapy*. Vol. 2. New York, Raven Press, pp. 291–300.
21. Schecter N. L., Allen D. A. and Hanson K. (1986) Status of pediatric pain control: a comparison of hospital analgesic usage in children and adults. *Pediatrics* **77**, 11–15.
22. Stimmel B. (1985) Pain, analgesia and addiction: an approach to the pharmacological management of pain. *Clin. J. Pain* **1**, 14–22.
23. Jaffe J. H. and Martin W. R. (1975) Narcotic analgesics and antagonists. In: Goodman L. S. and Gilman A. (eds.) *The Pharmacologic Basis of Therapeutics*, 5th edition. New York, Macmillan, pp. 245–83.
24. Hasday J. D. and Weintraub M. (1983) Propoxyphene in children with iatrogenic morphine dependence. *Am. J. Dis. Child.* **137**, 745–8.
25. Jaffe J. H. (1975) Drug addiction and drug abuse. In: Goodman L. S. and Gilman A. (eds.) *The Pharmacologic Basis of Therapeutics*, 5th edition. New York, Macmillan, pp. 284–324.
26. Porter J. and Jick H. (1978) Addiction rare in patients treated with narcotics. *N. Engl. J. Med.* **302**, 122.

FURTHER READING

Chapman J. and Goodall J. (1980) Symptom control in ill and dying children. *J. Matern. Child Health*, **5**, 144–54.
Newburger P. E. (1981) Chronic pain: principles of management. *J. Pediatr.* **98**, 180–9.
Saunders C. and Baines M. (1983) *Living with Dying: the Management of Terminal Disease*. Oxford, Oxford University Press.

15. The Late Effects of Treatment

A. Oakhill

Patient:	When will you want to stop seeing me? I've been off treatment for 4 years now.
Physician:	We never discharge our patients and will want to see you, albeit infrequently, for the rest of your life.
Patient:	But why?
Physician:	The treatment of cancer in children is itself still in its infancy. We need to see how you grow, how well you perform at school, to make sure your cancer never returns, to see how your children are. We need to make sure that there are no side-effects from your treatment that may show themselves as problems when you are an adult. We have a great deal to learn from you, information that may well help us to treat children like you in the future.

This fictional conversation is a common one for the paediatric oncologist in the follow-up clinic for children who have completed therapy. The reasons for close follow-up include recurrent disease, second tumours and late effects of treatment. Practically, this will involve at least a full physical examination on each visit to the clinic. It is important to be aware of late sequelae so that they can be avoided in the treatment of future patients and pre-empted and minimalized in the individual patient under review.

The simplest approach is, therefore, to look at each organ system.

THE RESPIRATORY SYSTEM

Lung toxicity, secondary to drugs and radiation, is rare in childhood. This is because the 2 drugs, busulphan and bleomycin, most commonly implicated in pneumonitis and pulmonary fibrosis are rarely used for paediatric tumours. Other agents, including the nitrosureas, methotrexate and cyclophosphamide, can also lead to pneumonitis, however.

Problems usually arise when the patient is still receiving treatment, but may be evident later (for example, after using busulphan in bone marrow transplantation) or produce long-term effects.

The differential diagnosis of the pneumonitides is discussed in the chapter on bacterial infections. The child presents with a dry cough and dyspnoea. There may be few signs on auscultation but, unlike infection due to pneumocystis, crepitations are heard. A chest X-ray will reveal alveolar infiltrates. If a biopsy is performed early, there is a proliferation of type II pneumocytes and the alveolar space contains proteinaceous fluid and cellular debris. If lung toxicity is discovered at this stage, it is possible to reverse it with steroids. If, however, fibrosis occurs, then this is a more difficult management problem.

The earliest signs of lung toxicity will be a change in the diffusion of carbon monoxide. For patients at risk, therefore, monitoring CO transfer factor is recommended.

If pulmonary fibrosis does develop, the patient will become progressively debilitated, with decreased diffusion capacity, restrictive lung function, cyanosis and clubbing. There is little that can be done at this stage.

Radiation pneumonitis may also occur with doses of greater than 2000 rad. This has been seen in children with metastatic Wilms' tumour and has led to decreased doses to the whole lung[1] and 'rifle shooting' to the pulmonary metastases. Adriamycin and actinomycin D (2 drugs frequently used in the management of Wilms' tumour) may enhance the effect of pulmonary radiation. Steroids again may be beneficial in the early course of the disease.

THE CARDIOVASCULAR SYSTEM

The most sinister late effects of treatment on the cardiovascular system are cardiomyopathy and pericarditis. These are associated with anthracyclines and radiation as both single and combined modalities.

The incidence of cardiomyopathy in children treated with the 2 commonest anthracyclines, adriamycin and daunorubicin, is reportedly between 5 and 30 per cent.[2] The incidence depends on the total cumulative dose and as it is now unusual for any chemotherapy protocol to prescribe more than 500mg/m^2 (total dose) severe toxicity is a rare event. Precautions taken during administration, such as regular echocardiography and radionucleotide angiocardiography have elicited sub-clinical cardiac muscle malfunction, alerting the oncologist to the dangers of continuing therapy.

Cardiomyopathy leading to congestive failure does, however, still occur. It may be seen in patients who, by necessity, are treated with more than 550mg/m^2 of adriamycin. Younger children may develop sequelae at lower total doses and patients who concomitantly receive radiation, actinomycin and cyclophosphamide are also at greater risk.

Awareness of these dangers and regular echo- and radionucleotide angiocardiography are very important. If cardiac failure should occur, it is often difficult to reverse and the majority of patients will succumb from therapy rather than disease. Anti-failure treatment with digoxin and diuretics, having discontinued the anthracycline, is the only measure available.

It is to be hoped that the newer anthracyclines currently under investigation will have less cardiotoxicity.

Pericardial effusion and pericarditis may occur when radiation is given to the mediastinum. The commonest situation in which this is seen is in the treatment of mediastinal Hodgkin's disease. The prior use of chemotherapy, however, allows lower doses and smaller fields of radiation to be given and, consequently, problems are rare.

When pericardial effusion does occur, it is often self-limiting. Steroids and stripping of the pericardium may be necessary with persisting problems.

THE CENTRAL NERVOUS SYSTEM

The late effects of radiation and chemotherapy on the CNS are dealt with in detail in Chapter 13.

OCULAR PROBLEMS

The late effects on the eye are related to primary ocular disease and its treatment, primary brain tumour, CNS radiation and the use of steroids.

Radiation treatment of primary orbital disease, such as rhabdomyosarcoma, will have an effect on the growth of the orbit and may lead to cataract formation. The latter is also seen when high doses of steroids are used and if the globe is not shielded during radiation to the head.

Scant regard has been shown to the sequelae of posterior fossa tumours. In our own experience, 60 per cent of children who survive medulloblastoma have gaze-evoked nystagmus with a considerable effect on their schooling.

HEARING PROBLEMS

The use of the platinum compounds for treating paediatric malignancies has led to toxic effects on the 8th nerve. This is irreversible and auditory tests are advised throughout treatment.

The aminoglycoside antibiotics frequently used in the management of neutropaenic fever can also damage the 8th nerve.

These drug effects, coupled with the high incidence of ear infections, underline the need for careful, continuing auditory assessment.

THE URINARY SYSTEM

Chemotherapy (including antibiotics) and radiation can cause toxicity to the kidney and bladder. Cisplatin, CCNU, high dose methotrexate, BCNU and 6MP have all been reported to cause damage to the nephron and it is advised that regular investigation of the creatinine clearance is performed during long-term therapy with these compounds.

Cyclophosphamide and ifosfamide damage the bladder epithelium and if no precautions are taken, will lead to haemorrhagic cystitis. This painful condition presents with frequency and haematuria and blood loss on occasion is severe. The symptoms may be recurrent and lead to a telangiectatic, small, fibrosed bladder. This should be prevented by giving adequate hydration during and after administration of cyclophosphamide and ifosfamide, with frequent voiding of urine. When ifosfamide or high dose cyclophosphamide are given, concomitant Mesna should be used to protect the bladder epithelium. The risk of haemorrhagic cystitis is increased with the use of radiation to a field including the bladder.

Radiation nephritis, presenting with proteinuria, hypertension and progressing to chronic renal failure is seen in children who have received more than 3000 rad to the kidneys.[3] If this is not suspected, the problem may occur long after treatment is completed.

Children who have had spinal cord compression, often have residual problems with voiding urine. Specialist assessment and advice regarding manual expressing, and intermittent and long-term catheterization needs to be taken and patients need to be taught these procedures when appropriate. Recurrent urinary tract infection is common and regular culture of urine and prophylactic antibiotics should be considered.

It should be evident that, by continuously assessing the patient during treatment and after successful completion, many problems can be pre-empted. For example, with Wilms' tumour, it is important to check blood pressure and renal function regularly to assess how well the remaining kidney is performing. In addition, urinary tract infections are common in children and mid-stream urine microscopy and culture should be a regular investigation in the follow-up of children who have been treated for Wilms' tumour.

THE GASTROINTESTINAL SYSTEM

Dentition is affected by several processes. There may be an increased intake of sweets and sugar-containing medicines. This is a preventable complication and advice is given to parents. Radiation has an effect on enamel formation and salivary secretion. In addition, there are often changes in oral flora. Poor oral hygiene is, therefore, common but eminently preventable.

The only other common toxicity seen in the gastrointestinal tract is hepatic. Both chemotherapy and radiation cause hepatotoxicity. Methotrexate is the most commonly implicated drug, followed by 6-Mercaptopurine. As the maintenance therapy of acute lymphoblastic leukaemia (ALL) contains both these drugs, children with this disorder are at risk. Regular estimation of bilirubin and hepatic enzymes should be performed on children with ALL and treatment interrupted when an abnormality is detected (although the degree of abnormality at which this should be done is controversial). It is to be hoped that, by employing this precaution, the high incidence of hepatic fibrosis reported in some series[4] will be prevented. It must be emphasized, however, that patients with early hepatic fibrosis may be both asymptomatic and have normal hepatic enzymes. This has led to some investigators performing liver biopsies on patients with ALL.

There may be acute and chronic effects from radiation to the liver. Severe acute effects are seen with large doses of radiation to a large volume of liver. Hepatic failure with hepatomegaly, jaundice, ascites and coma can ensue. Treatment is supportive.

The anthracyclines and actinomycin D are radiomimetic and also excreted by the liver. Their use, during whole abdominal radiation, may therefore lead to complications.

Hepatic fibrosis is the commonest late effect. When radiation is used in the management of right-sided Wilms' tumour, part of the right lobe of the liver will be in the treatment field and acute and chronic effects will be seen.[1]

It is unusual to use large doses of radiation to the whole abdomen in paediatric practice. Chronic malabsorption and direct bowel toxicity leading to stricture formation are now rarely seen. The author has, however, seen oesophageal strictures in 2 children with acute leukaemia who were fed with a nasogastric tube. The combination of a nasogastric tube, chemotherapy damaged mucosa and oral-oesophageal candida was present in both patients. The thinner nasojejunal tubes are, therefore, recommended.

MUSCULO-SKELETAL SYSTEM

This is a complex area when considering late effects of treatment. The great variety of problems that follow surgery, radiation, chemotherapy and primary cerebral disease requires careful assessment by orthopaedic surgeons, physiotherapists and occupational therapists, so that children can be allowed to return to as normal function as possible.

Children with bone tumours treated by amputation, limb salvage or other complicated procedures require highly specialized assessment and advice. In order that the amputee returns to normal schooling, for instance, not only is a good prosthesis necessary, but also a review of the school architecture, to assess the ease of moving from class to class. These practical aspects of life are of great importance.

Radiation causes damage to the epiphysis, metaphysis and diaphysis of a growing bone. Shortening, necrosis and pathological fractures can be problems in limb bones. Little can be done to prevent this when high doses of radiation are deemed necessary.

The inclusion of the spine in the radiation field will affect the growth of the vertebral body. If there is a uniform dose given, the sitting height will be reduced. If there is only part of the spine included, then kyphosis and scoliosis may be detected as the child grows. These can be accentuated by damage to soft tissues, also within the radiation field. Thus, not only should standing height be assessed in the follow-up clinic, but also sitting height.

Bone mineralization can be affected by poor nutrition when the patient is first ill or following intensive chemotherapy. Methotrexate and steroids can cause osteopenia and osteoporosis with long-term administration (for example, in ALL) and, therefore, bone pain and pathological fractures may be seen during the course of treatment or immediately after.

Primary tumours of the nervous system leading to paraplegia and hemiparesis will need assessment by physiotherapists, occupational therapists and educational advisers to allow as full activity and as normal schooling as possible.

THE ENDOCRINE SYSTEM

The endocrine system may be affected by primary disease of an organ or disease secondary to treatment.

THE HYPOTHALAMIC-PITUITARY AXIS

Primary tumours of the pituitary and central nervous system obviously can have permanent effects on this axis, which may range from panhypopituitarism to a single deficiency. In addition, the predilection of the histiocytosis X for invasion of the pituitary fossa will lead to diabetes insipidus, which usually requires long-term therapy with vasopressin.

The most important effect on the axis, however, is that of cranial and craniospinal irradiation. This is most commonly seen after the treatment of CNS tumours, head and neck tumours and rarely after the prophylactic treatment of ALL. The age of the patient and dose of radiation are 2 crucial factors, young children and treatment with more than 3000 rad leading to serious risk of growth hormone deficiency.[5]

The importance of measurement in children considered at risk of growth hormone deficiency cannot be emphasized strongly enough. If weight and height can be obtained from the patient's normal child health records, these should be plotted at the time of diagnosis. Regular measurements should be taken thereafter.

Patients who have the posterior fossa tumours, medulloblastoma and ependymoma, are treated with whole CNS radiation and, therefore, a sitting height to measure spinal growth should be obtained, as well as a standing height. Growth velocity curves should then be constructed.

Head and neck rhabdomyosarcoma may invade the CNS, particularly when there is involvement of a cranial nerve. To prevent this, radiation is now given in a condensed field to the base of the skull. It is likely that this practice will increase the incidence of growth hormone deficiency in long-term survivors.

The contentious issue of whether prophylactic CNS radiation in ALL causes growth hormone deficiency is unresolved and is unlikely to be so now that lower doses (and in some patients no radiation) are given. Poor growth may often be seen in children treated for ALL due to the combined effects of chronic disease prior to diagnosis, steroids and chemotherapy. The majority of patients will have normal or even catch-up growth after completing treatment.

Should poor growth or an abnormal growth velocity be evident, careful investigation of the pituitary axis should be undertaken. Results are often difficult to interpret and an experienced endocrinologist is vital in the decision whether growth hormone replacement therapy is necessary.

THE GONADS

Radiation and chemotherapy can profoundly affect the ovary and testis, leading to infertility and sex hormone dysfunction. The effects are seen in pre- and post-pubertal patients.

Irradiation of the ovary leads to a high incidence of sterility, although this again appears to depend on age, older post-pubertal patients having a higher chance of ovarian failure than younger pre-pubertal patients. It would appear that even small doses of radiation may affect the sensitive ovary.

Ovarian failure in pre-pubertal patients will be manifested by failure of development of secondary sexual characteristics. The elevated gonadotropins accompanied by low ovarian hormones emphasize the failure of the ovary to respond to the pituitary drive. In post-pubertal patients, ovarian failure will be evident from complaints of infertility, amenorrhoea and menopausal symptoms such as hot flushes.

It is difficult to assess the risk of ovarian failure but a careful study by Stillman et al.,[6] looking at pre-pubertal girls, showed that 68 per cent were affected by 3000 rad and 14 per cent were affected when their ovaries were at the edge of the field. Patients and their parents should be made aware, therefore, of the problem of ovarian failure and the clinician alerted to the possibility of its development.

The ovary can be repositioned in the pelvis to remove it from the radiation field. This should be attempted whenever possible.

When the testis is treated with radiation, for example, in the management of leukaemic infiltration, where a dose of 2400 rad may be given, sterility will usually ensue, in spite of the age of the patient. Leydig cells are little affected, even by such large doses and, therefore, testosterone levels will usually be normal leading to normal sexual development. FSH and LH will, however, be raised. It is difficult to assess the effect of lower doses of radiation which may only be a temporary lowering of the sperm count. Perhaps the only valid test is to see if the patient is fertile.

Chemotherapy has a definite toxic effect on the gonads of adults, but children have a more variable response. Similarly to radiation, abnormalities depend on pubertal status, sex and the drugs used.

Alkylating agents and, in particular, cyclophosphamide, have the worst reputation. Unfortunately, most investigations have centred on adult women, where it is well recognized that a high incidence of ovarian failure follows the use of cyclophosphamide. Pre-pubertal girls are much less sensitive, although Shalet et al. have reported biochemical evidence of dysfunction.[7]

The pre-pubertal testis is not sensitive to chemotherapy. The Leydig cells function normally and boys who have received combination chemotherapy would be expected to enter a normal puberty.

The same is not true for post-pubertal teenagers. Cyclophosphamide again causes the most serious problems, with low sperm counts. It may also affect the Leydig cells as has been suggested by Chapman et al. who reviewed the use of mustine in the treatment of Hodgkin's disease.[8]

It should not be forgotten that the underlying disease itself may lead to low sperm counts and lack of libido. This explains the difficulties in obtaining quality semen in patients in whom the use of a sperm bank prior to therapy is considered.

THE THYROID

The thyroid gland commonly falls in the radiation field in the treatment of Hodgkin's disease, head and neck rhabdomyosarcoma, and in craniospinal radiation. This can lead to hypothyroidism, carcinoma and thyroid nodules. Age and dose of radiation are related to the severity of problems, young patients being most at risk.

Whilst clinical hypothyroidism is rare, there is commonly a raised serum thyroid stimulating hormone. There is considerable difference of opinion whether to treat this biochemical abnormality, the argument of the interventionists being that switching off the pituitary drive will make nodular disease and perhaps carcinoma less likely.[9]

SKIN AND HAIR

It is common to see hyperpigmentation after radiation. Unfortunately, this often looks like dirt and parents may complain that they cannot get their child's neck clean! Moisturizing creams and, in girls, cosmetic creams may help. Telangiectasis may also be seen within the radiation field.

Skin rashes due to methotrexate, particularly on the face, may be seen after the completion of therapy. This is often seasonal and responds to moisturizing cream although, in severe cases, steroids are necessary.

Hair loss associated with intensive chemotherapy and low dose cranial irradiation is not permanent. Severe patchy alopecia occurs, however, with higher doses of radiation. It is common, therefore, after treatment of the posterior fossa, to have a bald patch. Advice should be sought from an experienced hairdresser, ideally one who is involved in wig-making for oncology patients.

SECOND TUMOURS AND LEUKAEMIAS

Early reports suggest that 17 per cent of survivors of childhood cancer at 20 years from diagnosis will have developed a second malignancy.[10] There appear to be 2 major reasons for this. Firstly, there may be a genetic predisposition and, secondly, radiation and chemotherapy alone and, even more so in combination, are oncogenic.

Genetic predisposition is best illustrated by retinoblastoma where there is a high incidence of secondary osteogenic sarcoma. The incidence is greatest in the inherited form of the disease, which is often bilateral or has more than one primary tumour. Initially, osteogenic sarcoma in these patients was seen in the radiation field and it was believed that radiation was the cause of the second tumour. With more refined treatment, however, there is still a high incidence, but the sarcoma develops outside the radiation field.

It is likely that, with longer follow-up, other primary malignancies such as Wilms' tumour will also be associated with second malignancies.

Radiation, as a single modality, increases the risk of cancer. Thyroid carcinoma, acute myeloid leukaemia and osteogenic sarcoma are the commonest reported second malignancies. The unfortunate practice of irradiating enlarged thymi in infants during the 1940s led to a 30 per cent incidence of thyroid nodules, a third of which were carcinomas.

Chemotherapy alone may also increase the risk of second malignancies. The alkylating agents are the most commonly associated drugs, the commonest cancer being leukaemia.

Hodgkin's disease treated with radiation and chemotherapy leads to a reported incidence between 2 and 10 per cent of acute leukaemia.[11] The picture is complicated by the fact that acute leukaemia may co-exist with Hodgkin's disease and that, in at least one patient transplanted for acute myeloid leukaemia, Hodgkin's disease has occurred as a second tumour.

CHILDREN OF PAEDIATRIC CANCER SURVIVORS

Apart from the offspring of patients with a known genetic component to their cancer (i.e. retinoblastoma, neurofibromatosis, etc.), there appears to be no increased risk of malignancy or serious malformation in children of long-term survivors of childhood cancer.

SUMMARY

There are many unknowns for the physician and the child cured of cancer. Only with careful history, measurement and examination can the risk of late sequelae be elicited. An awareness of what can happen will help us to shape treatment for future patients and, hence, there is a need for considerable vigilance in the follow-up of our 'successes'.

REFERENCES

1. Tefft M. (1977) Radiation related toxicities in national Wilms' tumour study I. *Int. J. Radiat. Oncol. Biol. Phys.* **2**, 455–63.
2. Von Hoff D. D., Rozencweig M. and Piccart M. (1982) The cardiotoxicity of anti-cancer agents. *Semin. Oncol.* **9**, 23–33.
3. Madrazo A., Schwarz G. and Chung J. (1975) Radiation nephritis. *J. Urol.* **124**, 822–7.
4. Perry M. C. (1982) Hepatotoxicity of chemotherapeutic agents. *Semin. Oncol.* **9**, 65–74.
5. Ramshi C. A., Zipf W. B. and Miser A. (1984) Evaluation of growth hormone release and human growth hormone treatment in children with cranial irradiation associated short stature. *J. Pediatr.* **104**, 177–81.
6. Stillman R. J., Schinfield J. S. and Schiff I. (1981) Ovarian failure in long-term survivors of childhood malignancy. *Am. J. Obstet. Gynecol.* **139**, 62–6.
7. Shalet S. M., Beardwell C. G. and Jones P. H. M. (1976) Ovarian failure following abdominal irradiation in childhood. *Br. J. Cancer* **33**, 655–8.
8. Chapman R. M., Sutcliffe S. B. and Malpas J. S. (1981) Male gonadal dysfunction in Hodgkin's disease. *JAMA* **245**, 1323–8.
9. Constine L. S., Donaldson S. S. and McDougall J. R. (1984) Thyroid dysfunction after radiotherapy in children with Hodgkin's disease. *Cancer* **53**, 878–83.
10. Li F. P., Cassady J. R. and Jaffe N. (1975) Risk of second tumours in survivors of childhood cancer. *Cancer* **35**, 1230–5.
11. Nelson D. F., Cooper S. and Weston M. G. (1981) Second malignant neoplasms in patients treated for Hodgkin's disease with radiotherapy or radiotherapy and chemotherapy. *Cancer* **48**, 2386–93.

Index

Academic achievement, 215
Acute lymphoblastic leukaemia (ALL)
  calcium levels, 81–3 (*Fig.* 5.3)
  chemotherapy complication
    prevention, 86, 264
  CNS disease, 95
  intellectual development, 215–17
  metabolic problems, 76–83
    correction, 84–6
  phosphorus levels, 81–3 (*Fig.* 5.2)
    management, 87
  potassium levels, 79–81 (*Fig.* 5.1)
    treatment, 86
  raised intracranial pressure, 94, 95
  renal failure, 77–9
    management, 87
  thymic mass, 86
  wide mediastinum, 91
Acute medical problems, 90–6
Acyclovir, 18, 36
Addiction, 254, 255
Adolescence, special needs, 226
AIDS
  transfusion risk, 73
  virus infections, 37
Alcohol avoidance, 111
Alloimmunization, transfusion, 73
Allopurinol, purine load, 85
Alopecia and cytotoxic drugs, 100
Aluminium hydroxide, phosphorus
    binding, 85, 86
Aminoglycosides, 8
Amphotericin B, 12
  aspergillosis, 52
  candidosis, 47
  cryptococcosis, 54
  empirical treatment, 58
  mucormycosis, 57

Amphotericin B (*cont.*)
  reactions to, 48
  renal impairment, 48
Amputation, 265
Amsacrine, features and side-effects,
    101
Anaemia prevention, 63
Anaesthesia, catheterization, 164, 165
Analgesics *see also* individual drugs
  addiction, 254
  doses, 251
  routes, 248, 249
  scheduling, 249
  side-effects, 253–5
Anaphylaxis, cytotoxic drugs, 99
Anorexia, chemotherapy, 127
Antibiotics *see also* individual drugs
  antifungal, 11, 18, 19, 47–9
  antiviral, 18
    herpes simplex, 36, 37
    toxicity, 36–9
  course duration, 9
  empiric combinations, 7, 8
  gut sterilization, 3
Antibody testing
  measles, 28, 29
  varicella, 28
  viral infections, 27–9
Antiemesis, 129–39
  distraction, 129
  management, 128, 129
  pharmacological, 129–38
  route, 130
  sedative, 129
Antiemetics *see also* individual drugs and
    drug classes
  classification, 131
  combinations, 138

Antiemetics (*cont.*)
  drugs used, 131–8
  sites of action, 131
Antigen detection
  candidosis, 47
  cytomegalovirus, 34
  fluorescent membrane (FAMA), 35
  vesicular rashes, 31
Anxiety, management terminal care, 256
Apheresis techniques, 74
  risk, 69, 70
  uses, 74, 75
Asparaginase, 101
  liver toxicity, 117
  neurotoxicity, 116
Aspergillus spp.
  allergen, 49
  cerebral, 18
  cranial abscesses, 94
  environmental, 49, 50
  filtration, 3
  spread, 18
A. fumigatus, 49
Aspergillosis, 49–52
  clinical signs, 50, 51
  cutaneous, 51
  diagnosis, 51, 52
  gastrointestinal, 50
  lesion types, 50
  occurrence, 49
  serum tests, 51, 52
  sputum, 51
  treatment, 52
Aspirin, 251
Astrocytomas, 93
Attendance allowance, 195, 196
Azacytidine
  bone marrow depression, 115
  features and precautions, 102

Bacterial infections, 1–20, 261
  catheter-related, 12–15
  CNS infections, 17, 18
  febrile neutropaenia, 7
  management, 9
  prevention, 2–6
  pulmonary complications, 10–12
BACUP, 201
Behavioural problems, 217, 218
  questionnaires, 218
  siblings, 220
Bereavement, 190, 191
  reactions, 234, 235

Biopsy
  lymph node, 91
  open lung, 11, 12
    risk, 12
Bleomycin, 102
Blood, plasma-reduced, 61
Blood product support, 61–71
  age, 61
  irradiation, 74
Blood transfusion *see also* individual
      blood components
  reactions, 62
  uses, 63
Body fluids, virus sampling, 33
Body integrity threat, 215
Body surface area, height–weight ratio,
      99
Bone marrow depression, cytotoxic
      drugs, 99, 114, 115
Bone marrow transplantation (BMT)
  infections, 7
  neutropaenia, 1, 2
  role, 60
  viral pathogenicity, 17
Bone tumours, late effects of treatment,
      265
Borderline Substances, prescribable,
      156–8
Brain *see also* central nervous system
  acute syndromes, 17
  central herniation, 96
  focal disease, 18
  tonsillar herniation, 96
  uncal herniation, 95, 96
Buffy coat, 69
Buprenorphine, 252
Busulphan, 102
Butyrophenones, antiemetic, 132

Cachexia, 142
Calcium levels and treatment, 81–3
  (*Fig.* 5.3)
Cancer Link, 201
Candida albicans, 43–8
  deep form, 44
  defences to, 44
Candidaemia, 45
Candidosis, 43, 44
  antigen detection, 47
  clinical signs, 44
  deep forms, diagnosis, 46, 47
  disseminated, 45, 46
    lesions, 46

Candidosis (*cont.*)
    gastrointestinal, 45
    oesophageal, 45
    oral, 44, 45
    serological tests, 46
    treatment, 47–9
Cannabinoids
    antiemetic activity, 135, 136
    hallucinations, 136
Carboplatin, 103
    renal function, 103
Cardiac function
    cyclophosphamide, 105
    cytotoxic drugs, 99, 115
    mitozantrone, 110
Cardiomyopathy, 261, 262
Cardiovascular system, late treatment
        effects, 261, 262
Catheters, central venous, 163–70
    access sites, 164
    anaesthesia, 164, 165
    asepsis, 169
    blockage, 170
    breaks, 170
    cuffs, 163, 164
    fixing, 169
    implantable devices, 167
    insertion techniques, 165
        open operation, 165, 166
        percutaneous, 167, 168
    parents' role, 170
    position, 168
    problems, 167, 168
    removal, 169
    types, 163, 164
    venous malformations, 167
Catheters and venous lines
    indwelling, 7
        types, 12
    -related infections, 12–15
        antibiotics used, 14
        eradication success, 14, 15
        incidence, 13
        rate, 13, 14
        skin commensals, 13, 15
    use and coagulase-negative infections,
            13, 14
Central nervous system
    disease prevention, 94–6
    infections, 17
    tumours invading, 266
Chemoreceptor trigger zone (CTZ)
    ablation, 124
    brain, 123
    dopamine role, 123, 125

Chemoreceptor trigger zone (*cont.*)
    drugs affecting, 131
    and vomiting, 123
Chemotherapy *see also* cytotoxic drugs
    anxiety, 129
    checklist, 114
    cytoreductive, 92
    malnutrition, 143, 144
    personnel risk, 98, 119, 120
    problems, 98–120
    toxicity, 143
Chlorambucil, 103
Chlorpromazine, antiemetic use, 132
CHOP regimen, 92
Chronic disease
    achievement, 205
    cancer as, 204, 205
    maladjustment, 205
Chronic granulocytic leukaemia (CGL)
    granulocyte count, 68, 69
    granulocyte donations, 69
Cisplatin, 104
    emetic activity, 125, 133, 134
    renal damage, 116
Clostridium difficile
    antibiotic use, 16
    toxin effect, 15
Clotting factors, 63–5 *see also*
            disseminated intravascular
            coagulation
    bleeding, 63
Coagulation screen, 64
Compassionate Friends, 201
Complement fixation, viral antibody
            testing, 27
Constipation
    analgesic, 253
    nutritional management, 154
Coping strategies, 220–3
    child, 221, 232
    maladaptive, 222
Corticosteroids, antiemetic, 137
Cost, antibiotic prophylaxis, 3–5
Counsellor, 224–6
    aims, 225
    roles and timing, 225, 226
Creatinine, normal values, 77
Cryptococcus neoformans, 52–5
    meningitis, 95
    sources, 52
Cryptococcosis, 52–5
    cerebrospinal fluid, 53, 54
    clinical signs, 53, 54
    cutaneous, 53
    diagnosis, 54

Cryptococcosis (*cont.*)
  dissemination, 53
  symptoms, 53
  treatment, 54, 55
Cryptosporidium sp., AIDS, 17
Cyclophosphamide
  bladder mucosa, 116
  bone marrow depression, 115
  dose, 105
  precautions, 105
  vomiting, 125
Cystic fibrosis, behavioural problems, 217, 218
Cystitis, haemorrhagic, 106, 110, 116
Cytosine, 106
Cytotoxic drugs *see also* individual drugs
  chemoreceptor trigger zone, 124
  dose calculation, 99
  emetic activity, 125, 126
    relative, 126
    sites, 124, 125
  extravasation, 117, 118
  handling hazards, 119, 120
    guidelines, 119
  side-effects, 99–117
  types and features, 99–114

Dacarbazine, emetic activity, 126
Dactinomycin, 106
  irradiation, 106
The Damocles Syndrome, 213, 214
Daunorubicin, features and precautions, 107
Death, 190, 191 *see also* bereavement, dying, mourning
  age and attitudes, 190
  age and cancer, 243
  anniversary, 236
  awareness, dying child, 230, 231
  child's concepts, 230
  concepts, 190
  DHSS leaflet, 197
  home, 239, 240
  pathological reactions, 235
  play therapy, 175
  practical aspects, 190
  rattle, 257
Death grant, 190, 196
Depression management, terminal care, 256
Development
  cognitive, 230

Development (*cont.*)
  intellectual and treatment, 215–17
    assessment, 216
DHPG-9 and cytomegalovirus, 37
DHSS, assistance, 185, 195
Diamorphine, 251
  in terminal care, 252, 253
Diarrhoea
  nutritional management, 155
  organisms causing, 15–17
Diet, therapeutic, 152
Dihydrocodeine, 251, 252
Disseminated intravascular coagulation (DIC), 63
  clotting factors, 65
  fresh frozen plasma, 64
  process, 64
Divorce, 219
DNA probes, viral diagnosis, 32
Domperidone
  antiemetic use, 134, 135
    dose, 135
    formulations, 135
  chemoreceptor trigger zone, 134
Dose calculation, 99
Doxorubicin, 107
Drugs
  irritant, administration, 117, 118
  tissue necrosis, 117
Dry mouth, 155
Dying child
  anxiety, 231
  attitudes to death, 233
  awareness, 230, 231
  communicating with, 232, 233
  family, 233, 234
  isolation, 231
  parents' support, 234
  symptom control, 245–56
  withdrawal, 234
Dyspnoea management, terminal care, 256, 257

Eland Color Tool, 247
Electron microscope in virology, 31
  uses, 33
Employers, role, 186
Endotoxin
  fibrinolytic system, 64
  vascular injury, 63, 64
Enzyme-linked immunosorbent assay (ELISA)
  viral antibody testing, 27, 33

Epirubicin, 108
 liver function, 108
Etoposide, 108
Extravasation
 antidotes, 118
 occurrence, 117
 prevention, 118
 treatment plan, 118
Eye, late treatment effects, 262

Family *see also* parents
 anxiety, 210
 bereavement, 234, 235
 coping, 221
 diagnosis, 210, 211
 disturbance, 218
 dying child, 233, 234
 effects of illness, 210
 psychological problems, 204–35
The Family Fund, 199
Feeds
 chemically-defined, 148, 149, 157
  indications, 148
 commercial, 148
 sip, 156
 tube, 157
Fibrin degradation products, 64
Fibrinolytic system, 64
Financial help, 185
Flucytosine, 48
 cryptococcosis, 54
Fluid overload, 83
Follow-up, 260
Food *see also* feeds, nutrition
 advice to parents, 153–5
 aversions, 147
 contamination in immunosuppression,
  147
 preferences, 145, 146, 153–5
 presentation, 146, 153
Foscarnet, cytomegalovirus infection,
  38
FRACON, 3
Funeral expenses, 196, 197
Fungal infections, 43–58 *see also*
  individual diseases
 empirical treatment, 58
 opportunistic, 43
 prevention, 58
 unusual, 57, 58
Fungi
 invasive disease, 9, 19
 overgrowth, 9

Gastroenteritis, viral causes, 32, 33
Gastrointestinal tract
 cytotoxic drug effects, 100, 115, 124,
  125
 flora and antibiotics, 15
 late treatment effects, 264, 265
 selective decontamination, 4, 5
 sterilization, drug combinations, 3
Gastrostomy, feeding, 149
Genetic predisposition to cancer, 269
Glucose polymers, 156
Graft versus host disease (GVHD), 17,
  73, 74
 blood transfusion, 73
 fatal, 73
Granulocytes, 68–71
 collection, 68, 69
  hazards, 69, 70
 cryopreserved, 74
 prophylactic, 71
 therapy, 68
Granulocyte transfusion, 10, 69
 HLA matching, 71
 neonates, 69
 role, 71
 side-effects, 70
Granulocytopenia, 9
Groups
 roles, 228, 229
 staff, 229
 support, 187, 199–201
Growth hormone, 266

Haematological support, 60–75
Hair loss, 268
Hearing, late treatment effects, 263
Helen House, 240
Hepatitis, transfusion-associated, 72
High energy drinks, 156
HLA antibodies, 62
 detection, 67
 platelet destruction, 68
Hodgkin's Disease Association, 201
Hodgkin's disease and leukaemia, 269
Hodgkin's lymphoma, wide
  mediastinum, 91
Home care, 239, 240, 242, 243
 cost, 245
 desirability, 242–5
 organization, 240–3
 parents' role, 244
 practice, 242, 243
Hospices, 240

Hospital
  cost of terminal care, 245
  fear of, 244
  role, 241
Hydrocortisone, extravasation, 118
Hydroxyethyl starch, 69, 70
Hyperkalaemia
  cardiac, fatal effects, 81
  leukaemia, 79, 80 (*Fig.* 5.1)
  levels and treatment, 80 (*Fig.* 5.1)
  lymphoma, 80 (*Fig.* 5.1)
  pseudo-, differentiation, 80
  sudden death, 79
  treatment, 86, 87
Hyperphosphataemia
  levels and treatment, 81, 82 (*Fig.* 5.2)
  management, 87
Hypertensive crisis, 107
Hyperuricaemia
  nephropathy, 77, 78
  renal function, 79
Hypocalcaemia, 77, 78, 83
  levels and treatment, 81–3 (*Fig.* 5.3)
Hypomagnesaemia, 83
Hypoparathyroidism, 83
Hypothalamic-pituitary axis, treatment
      effects, 266

Ifosfamide, 108
  and mesna, 108, 109
Illness, child's concept, 205, 206, 226 *see
      also* parents
  cognitive leaps, 209
  concrete logical, 207
  and coping, 221
  definitions, children, 206
  development in cancer, 208–10
  formal-logical, 207, 208
  leukaemia, 209
  prelogical explanations, 207
Immunofluorescence
  viral antibody testing, 27, 28
  viral identification, 33
Immunoglobulins, prophylactic, 5, 6
Immunosuppression
  food sterility, 147
  gastrointestinal problems, 15–17
  vaccination role, 34–6
Infection *see also* bacterial, fungal and
      viral
  parenteral nutrition, 151
Information, publications for parents,
      192–4

Interferon, prophylaxis, 38
Isle of Wight Survey, 205

Ketoconazole, 49
  prophylaxis, 58

Laminar air flow systems, 3
Latex agglutination, 54
Leucocytes, harvesting, 74
Leucopheresis, 69, 74
Leukaemia *see also* acute, chronic
  publications, 192–4
Leukaemia Care Society, role, 198,
      200
Levonantradol, 137
Liver function
  cytotoxic drugs, 99, 117
  toxic effects, 264
Lorazepam, 137
Low ionic strength saline (LISS), 62
Lung
  function, 116
  infections, 10–12
    immunosuppression, 12
  toxicity, cytotoxic drugs, 115
Lymphocytotoxicity tests, 67

McGill pain questionnaire, 247
Malcolm Sargent Fund
  applications, 198
  role, 197
  social workers, 202
Malnutrition, protein-energy, 142, 143
  risk factors, 142
Marital breakdown, 219
Measles vaccination in
      immunosuppression, 34, 35
Mediastinum
  causes of wide, 90, 91
  regions, 90
Meningitis, 17, 18
  organisms, 18
  viral causes, 33, 34
Mercaptopurine features and
      precautions, 109
Mesna
  bladder effects, 116, 117
  doses, 109
  features and precautions, 109

Metabolic problems, leukaemia and
    lymphoma, 76–87
Methotrexate, 110
    excretion, 116
    folinic acid rescue, 110
    photosensitivity, 110
Metoclopramide
    antiemetic use, 132, 133
    and cisplatin, 133
    dopamine blocker, 125
    side-effects and diphenhydramine, 133
Miconazole, 47
    intravenous, 48, 49, 55
Mitozantrone, 110
Mobility, factors affecting, 172
Monoamine oxidase inhibition, 111
Morphine, terminal care, 252, 253
Mortality, 238
    causes, 60
    cytomegalovirus pneumonitis, 11
    febrile neutropaenia, 6
Mourning, 191
    anticipatory, 233
    tasks, 235
Mucormycosis
    debridement, 57
    diagnosis, 55–7
    disseminated, 56, 57
    microscopy, 56
    pathogens, 55
    pulmonary, 56
    rhinocerebral, 55, 56
    treatment, 57
Mucosa, drugs damaging, 1
Multimodal therapy, 143
Myelography, 93

Nabilone, antiemetic use, 136
Nasogastric feeding, 147
    commercial feeds, 148, 157, 158
    complications, 148
    pump, 147
National Society for Cancer Relief, 198
Nausea
    anticipatory, 126, 127
        treatment, 138, 139
    feeding, 154
NEOCON, 3
Neoplatin, 104
Nephritis, radiation, 263
Neuroblastoma
    metastatic CNS, 95
    spinal cord compression, 93

Neuroblastoma Society, 200, 201
Neurological function
    cisplatin, 104
    cytotoxic drugs, 99, 116
Neutropaenia
    bacterial infections, 1
    counts, 68
    definition, 6
    febrile, 6, 7
Non-Hodgkin's lymphoma (NHL)
    calcium levels, 81–3 (Fig. 5.3)
    chemotherapy complication
        prevention, 86
    metabolic problems, 76–83
        correction, 84–6
    phosphorus levels, 81–3 (Fig. 5.2)
        management, 87
    potassium levels, 79–81 (Fig. 5.1)
    renal failure, 77–9
        management, 87
    thymic mass, 86
    tumour assessment, 84
    wide mediastinum, 91
Nuclear magnetic resonance (NMR),
    93
Nurses
    community oncology, 242
    MacMillan, 242
    terminal care, 239
Nutrition, 142–60
Nutritional status
    assessment, 144
    improved, advantages, 145
    investigations, 144
Nutritional support
    Borderline Substances, 156–8
    chemically defined, 148, 149
    feeding routes, 145 (Fig. 9.1)
    gastrostomy, 149
    liquid supplements, 146, 147
    methods, 144, 145 (Fig. 9.1)
    nasoenteric, 147
    oral, 145, 146
    parenteral, 149–51
    parents' advice, 153–5
    protein, 159, 160
    therapeutic diet, 152
Nystatin
    candidosis, 47
    prophylactic, 58

Ommaya reservoir, 12
    infections, 14, 15

Oncology unit
  groups, 199, 200
  terminal care, 189
Open communication
  hazards, 183
  policy, 182, 183, 211, 215, 232
Ototoxicity
  cisplatin, 104
  cytotoxic drugs, 100
Ovarian failure, treatment effects, 267

Pain *see also* analgesics
  aetiology, 246
  assessment, 246–8
    regular, 249, 250
  control, 233, 245–56
    terminal care, 245, 246
  distraction, 250
  fear, 232, 249
  management, 248–56
    bone, 255
    nerve root, 255
    radiotherapy, 250
    routes, 249
  raised intracranial pressure, 255, 256
  treatment, 246
Paracetamol dose, 251
Parenteral nutrition
  candidosis, 46
  carbohydrate, 151
  complete, 150–2
  complications, 151
  fat, 151
  fluid requirements, 150
  indications, 149, 150
  minerals, 151
  preparation, 152
  protein source, 150
  treatment side-effects, 149
  vitamins, 151
Parents
  anger, 182
  anxiety, 211, 219
  caring role, 212
  communication, 182, 183
  coping
    assessment, 181, 182, 189
    strategies, 220–3
    tasks, 222
  counselling, 223, 224
  death, 190, 191, 222, 232
  diagnosis, 210, 211
  expenses, 185

Parents (*cont.*)
  groups, 187, 199–201, 228
  home or hospital care, 189, 244
  informing child, 211
  labelling of, 183
  marital breakdown, 219
  mental health problems, 218, 219
  prognostic views, 212, 213
  psychosocial intervention, 223
  publications for, 192–4
  shock, 181
  sibling handling, 183, 184
  stress, 186
  therapy cessation, 188, 189
  understanding of illness, 210–13
Penicillin
  prophylactic, 5, 8
  synthetic, 8
Perianal sepsis, 16
Peritoneal dialysis, renal failure, 87
Phenothiazines
  antiemetic actions, 131, 132
  side-effects, 131, 132
Phosphorus
  renal retention, 81
  serum levels and treatment, 81, 82
    (*Fig.* 5.2)
Platelets
  bleeding control, 65, 66
  destruction, 67, 68
  dose, 65, 66
  HLA matching, 67, 68
  preparation, 65, 66
  transfusion count, 67
Platelet concentrates, 65
Platinex, 104
Play
  Expert Group, 173
  pain, 250
  preparation, concept, 176, 177
  role, 172, 226
  stress reduction, 173
  teacher, 226
Play therapy
  death, 175
  drawing, 176
  family unit, 175
  and hospitalization, 173, 174
  injections, 177
  postoperative, 178
  role modelling, 176, 177
  worry expression, 174
Pneumocystis carinii
  diagnosis, 11
  pneumonia, incidence, 10, 11

Pneumonia, organisms causing, 10
Pneumonitis
    cytomegalovirus, 11, 34
        treatment, 37, 38
    radiation, 261
Potassium, serum levels and treatment,
        80 (*Fig.* 5.1)
Procarbazine, features and precautions,
        111
Prognosis
    data weighting, 213
    improving, 220, 221
    parents' and paediatricians' views, 212
        213
Prophylaxis
    bacterial infections, 2–6
    fungal infections, 58
    nausea and vomiting, 128, 129
Protein supplements, 156
    high protein recipes, 159, 160
Pseudomembranous colitis, 15, 16
Pseudomonas spp.
    ecthyma gangrenosa, 57
    severity, 19
    typhilitis, 16
Psychosocial support, 223
    staff, 229
Pulmonary fibrosis, 261
Pyrexia of unknown origin (PUO), 32

Quality of life, 213

Radiation
    CNS, 266
        and development, 215–17
        prophylactic, 266
    malnutrition, 143, 144
    pigmentation, 268
Raised intracranial pressure, 94
    causes, 94
    CNS disease, 94–6
    pain relief, 255, 256
Recipes, high-protein, 159, 160
Red cells
    flow properties, packed, 61
    haematological support, 60–3
    washed and antibodies, 62
Relapse, responses and social work, 188
Relaxation training, 139, 227
Renal failure
    aetiology, 77, 78

Renal failure (*cont.*)
    management, 87
    post-treatment, 81
    signs, 79
Renal function
    cisplatin, 104
    cytotoxic drugs, 99
    radiotherapy, 85
Respiratory infections, viral, 31, 32
Respiratory system, toxic effects, 260,
        261
Retinoblastoma, 269
Ribavirin, 38
Rubella vaccination in
        immunosuppression, 34, 35
Rutter Behaviour Scale, 218, 220

Safety precautions, cytotoxic drug use,
        119, 120
School, 186, 187
    obstacles, 187
Second tumours, 269
Sibling
    behavioural problems, 220
    distress, 244, 245
    groups, 228
    handling and care, 183, 184, 212
    lifestyle changes, 220
    psychological problems, 219, 220
Side-effects, 214, 215
    actinomycin D, 264
    amphotericin B, 48, 50
    antiemetic combinations, 137
    antifungal therapy, 9
    antivirals, 36, 37
    blood use, 61
    cannabinoids, 136, 137
    cyclophosphamide, 267, 268
    cytotoxic drugs, 99–117, 263
        infertility, 117
        severity, 99, 100
    dexamethasone, 137
    granulocyte transfusion, 70
    lorazepam, 137
    lung damage, 11
    6-mercaptopurine, 264
    methotrexate, 246, 264
    metoclopramide, 133, 137
    nausea and vomiting, 121
    nephrotoxicity, 7, 8
    nutritional, 143
    opiates, 253, 254
    phenothiazines, 131, 132

Side-effects (*cont.*)
  psychological, 214, 215
  trimethoprim-sulphamethoxazole, 4, 11
  urinary system, 263, 264
  vidarabine, 37
  vincristine, 246
Skin, treatment effects, 268
Skin ulceration, management in terminal care, 257
Social work, 180–202
  bereavement, 190, 191
  communication role, 182, 183
  development, 202
  DHSS liaison, 183
  at diagnosis, 181, 182
  family life, 184
  maintenance, 186
  relapse, 188
  voluntary help, 185
Social worker
  advice, 196
  'Malcolm Sargent', 202
  paediatric oncology, 180, 181
  role, 181, 223
Spinal cord compression, 92–4
  causes, 93
  diagnosis, 93
  paralysis, 92
  sites, 93
  therapy, 94
  tissue diagnosis, 94
Splenectomy risks, 2
Staff, needs, 229
Staphylococcal infections, intravenous line use, 13, 14
Staphylococcus epidermidis, catheter-related, 13
Surgery, malnutrition, 143
Survivors, children of, 269

Teachers, information for, 187, 217
Team
  composition, 224
  counsellor, 224–6
  death, 190
  role, 224, 241, 242
Teniposide, 111
Terminal care, 189, 190, 229–35, 238–58
  cost, 245
  domiciliary *see also* home care
  home and hospital, 239, 240, 242, 243
    see also home care

Terminal care (*cont.*)
  inexperienced staff, 241
  nurse, 239
  quality of life, 243
  pain, 245–56
  stress, 258
Terminal illness, 204
Testes
  pre-pubertal immunity, 268
  treatment effects, 267
Tetrahydrocannabinol (THC), antiemetic, 135, 136
Thioguanine, 111
Thrombocytopenia, 63
  platelets, 65, 66
Thyroid, treatment effects, 268
Travelling expenses, 195
Treatment
  cessation, 188, 189, 238 *see also* terminal care
  failure, 241
  late effects, 260–70
  pain, 246
  preparation for, 227, 228
    model, 227
  psychological effects, 227
  stress, 214
Trimethoprim-sulphamethoxazole
  antifolate, 4
  gut selective decontamination, 4, 5
  pneumonia, 10, 11
Tumour breakdown, rapid, 81
Tumour lysis
  complication prevention regimen, 84, 85
  monitoring, 85
  syndrome, 76
Typhilitis, 16

UAB Pain Behaviour Scale, 247
Urinary system, late treatment effects, 263, 264
Urine, red, 107
Urological effects, cytotoxic drugs, 100, 116, 117

Vaccination in immunosuppression, 34–6
  measles, 34, 35
  mumps, 34
  varicella, 35, 36

Vaccine
  anti-*Pseudomonas*, 5
  -boosted immune whole blood
    transfusion, 30
  varicella zoster, 35
Varicella
  vaccination and immunosuppression,
    35, 36
  vaccines, 35
Vena cava
  persistent left superior, 167
  superior, obstruction, 90–2
    cytoreduction chemotherapy, 92
    radiotherapy, 86, 92
    tissue diagnosis, 91, 92
    treatment, 86, 92
    X-ray, 91
Vidarabine, 37
Vinblastine, 112
Vincristine, 112
  neurotoxicity, 116
Viral infections, 26–39
  antibody testing, 27
    patients, 27, 28
  cytomegalovirus, 30
    laboratory diagnosis, 34
    therapy, 37, 38
  herpes simplex, 29, 30
    acyclovir, 36, 37
  immune state, 31
  influenza treatment, 38
  life-threatening, 26, 29
  procedures, 31
    therapy, 37, 38
  respiratory, 31, 32
  respiratory syncytial, 31, 32
    treatment, 38, 39
  varicella-zoster, 30
    acyclovir, 37

Viral infections (*cont.*)
  reactivation, 30
  vesicular rashes, 31
Virus
  cytomegalovirus, 11, 26
    hyperimmune immunoglobulin, 38
    transfusion risk, 72
    transmission, 30
  Epstein-Barr, 29
    transfusion, 72
  herpes group, 26
  herpes simplex, 29, 30
  HTLV and transfusion, 73
  identification methods, 33
  influenza, 36
  measles, 28, 29
  non-A, non-B hepatitis, 72
  polyoma, 26
  transfusion-associated, 71–3
  varicella, 28, 30
Voluntary organizations, 185, 197–9
Vomiting, 121 *see also* antiemesis,
    chemoreceptor trigger zone
  aetiology, 128
  anticipatory, 126, 127
    treatment, 138, 139
  centre, 122
    drugs affecting, 131
  chemotherapy-induced, 128, 129
  epidemic, 129
  initiators, 124
  management, 254
  neurophysiology, 122, 123
  stages, 122

Wilms' tumour, 261, 263, 264